MANUAL of
CHILD NEUROLOGY

MANUAL of CHILD NEUROLOGY

Owen B. Evans, M.D.

Director, Pediatric Neurology
Associate Professor of Pediatrics and Neurology
The University of Mississippi School of Medicine
Jackson, Mississippi

CHURCHILL LIVINGSTONE
New York, Edinburgh, London, Melbourne 1987

Library of Congress Cataloging-in-Publication Data

Evans, Owen B.
  Manual of child neurology.

  Includes bibliographies and index.
  1. Pediatric neurology—Handbooks, manuals, etc.
I. Title. [DNLM: 1. Nervous System Diseases—diagnosis—
handbooks.   2. Nervous System Diseases—in infancy &
childhood—handbooks,   3. Neurologic Examination—in
infancy & childhood—handbooks.   WS 39 E92m]
RJ486.E83   1987   618.92'8   86-21569
ISBN 0-443-08435-1

Distributed in the United Kingdom by Churchill Livingstone,
Robert Stevenson House, 1–3 Baxter's Place, Leith Walk,
Edinburgh EH1 3AF, and by associated companies, branches, and
representatives throughout the world.

Accurate indications, adverse reactions, and dosage schedules for
drugs are provided in this book, but it is possible that they may
change. The reader is urged to review the package information
data of the manufacturers of the medications mentioned.

Acquisitions Editor: *Robert A. Hurley*
Copy Editor: *Ann Ruzycka*
Production Designer: *Michiko Davis*
Production Supervisor: *Sharon D. Tuder*

Printed in the United States of America

First published in 1987

PREFACE

This manual has been written for pediatricians and other physicians involved in the primary medical care of children. Not only are they most likely to be the first to encounter neurologic problems, but they also manage most of them. This work is not a textbook and the reader should refer to the references and the several excellent texts for more detailed information. As a manual, it should be a practical guide and ready reference for the differential diagnosis of neurologic problems and examination findings.

I have tried to stress the clinical approach to neurologic diagnosis, especially history-taking and the interpretation of general physical and neurologic examination findings. Most neurologic disorders do not require that specialized examination techniques or tests be made in order to make a diagnosis and initiate therapy.

The references at the end of each chapter were selected because the articles are good reviews on the subject, were published in widely circulated journals, and are relatively recent. The pediatric literature was cited preferentially.

I would like to thank Drs. Menkes, Ford, Farmer, Swaiman, and Wright for their textbooks on child neurology. I consider them old friends and valuable references. The texts on neonatal neurology by Fenichel and Volpe are invaluable references on that growing subspecialty. Herskowitz and Rosman have produced an excellent work emphasizing the behavioral and developmental aspects of pediatrics and child neurology.

I am indebted to a number of colleagues, residents, and students who have helped review parts of this manual. Drs. Blair Batson, Howard Nichols, Paul Parker, Don Raggio, Phil Rhodes, and Bernard Blumenthal made a number of helpful suggestions. Drs. Les Jones, Bill Perkins, Mike Graeber, and Tree Clemmons, residents in neurology and pediatrics, helped with some of the research, as did students Tony Males and Virginia Payne. Ann Swisher, R.N., not only reviewed parts of the manuscript but also assisted in the clinical management of patients, which is the greater help. Nancy Kerr did much of the early typing. Cindy Morgan made the manuscript possible because of her typing skills and persistence. The illustrations are my own.

Finally, I acknowledge my wife, Lynn, whose patience, criticism, encouragement, and tolerance made this manual possible.

Owen B. Evans, M.D.

CONTENTS

MANUAL of
CHILD NEUROLOGY

SECTION 1

Neurologic Evaluation

Assessing the child with a neurologic illness is similar to approaching any other pediatric problem. One obtains a history and performs a physical examination to establish a presumptive diagnosis, a differential diagnosis, and a plan for laboratory evaluation. In pediatrics, the age of the patient determines much of the differential diagnosis and the development assessment is an equally important part of the evaluation. Almost all neurologic diseases impair normal development. This section reviews those aspects of the history, developmental assessment, physical examination, and laboratory procedures which are important in the approach to a child with a neurologic illness.

1

HISTORY

The most common error in making a neurologic diagnosis is obtaining an inadequate history. Hence the taking of the history requires more effort and time than any other portion of the evaluation (Table 1-1). One should always take a history from the patient if the child is verbal. The interview begins with a "warm-up" conversation about school, family, or other interests. The child can use this opportunity to diffuse anxieties and the physician can obtain an impression of the child's social, intellectual, and verbal skills. If asked why he or she is at the doctor's office, the child will often show surprising insight about the illness. Once a chief complaint has been established the child should be encouraged to describe the symptoms in detail. Because the young child's verbal skills are limited, questions of the multiple-choice type are better received than open-ended questions. At the conclusion of this introduction the physician should explain what will occur during the examination. If one can assure the patient that no painful procedures will be performed, one should do so at this time.

After the child has given his information it can be verified with the parent. In the preverbal or uncooperative child, the history must be obtained solely from the parent. One should avoid asking leading questions and encourage a factual description of the patient's symptoms. Frequently the patient's information will be secondhand from a teacher or a relative, and direct communication with the primary observer is then indicated. If a parent cannot recall specific events, then reviewing old diaries or photographs can be helpful. One should ask the parent for his or her impressions or diagnosis. Frequently the parent's diagnosis is correct.

The onset, duration, and rate of progression of the illness will sort most neurologic illnesses into specific categories: acute, episodic, static, and progressive (Table 1-2). Acute neurologic illnesses are often rapidly progressive emergencies that require immediate therapy. After the patient has been adequately stabilized, a detailed history of the events leading to the present illness can be obtained. The past medical history should be explored for predisposing pediatric diseases. Some examples of relevant associations are stroke and sickle cell disease, cerebral abscess and cyanotic congenital heart disease, and status epilepticus in the patient with epilepsy. Ingestions are especially common in young children and a list of all possible intoxicants should be obtained.

Episodic and relapsing illnesses are the most common neurologic problems in childhood; the majority will be seizures. Other episodic illnesses include

Table 1-1. Medical History for Neurologic Diseases

Chief complaint

Present history
  Symptoms
  Onset
  Duration
  Progression
  Recurrence

Past history
  Perinatal history
    Pregnancy: duration, exposures, complications
    Labor: duration, monitoring, complications
    Delivery: presentation, Apgar scores, complications
    Neonatal course: hospital stay, complications
  Past medical illnesses
    Accidents and injuries
    Hospitalizations
    Acute infectious disorders and exposures
  Review of systems
  Immunizations
  Allergies
  Medications and dosages
  Environmental

Family history
  Neurologic and developmental disorders
  Other medical diseases and general health
  Causes of death
  Pedigree

Development

School performance
  Grades
  Academic and psychological testing
  Conduct

breath-holding spells, vascular headaches, intoxications, and some of the rare metabolic and neuromuscular diseases. An observer's history is often necessary because the patient may be amnesic for the event. Illnesses which have been episodic over many years are unlikely to represent serious underlying disease. Those which have had a more recent onset and particularly those showing a crescendo progression cause more concern. Most children with episodic illnesses are normal between attacks. Those who fail to regain normal function are likely to have a metabolic or degenerative disease.

The static illness presents with a fixed deficit in either neurologic function or intellectual performance. The child's function improves with time but never at the rate of siblings or peers. The static disorder is usually congenital but may be acquired from a specific illness or injury. In this case, neurologic and intellectual function may have been normal before the injury. The diagnosis may be found by careful exploration of the pregnancy and birth history, past medical history, and family history. Frequently it is necessary to obtain records of the birth or other hospitalizations.

Table 1-2. Classification of Neurologic
Disorders by History

Acute neurologic disorders
    Intoxications
    Animal and insect bites
    Head trauma
    Cerebrovascular disease
    Acquired metabolic encephalopathies
    Infections
    Postinfectious neurologic syndromes
    Acute increased intracranial pressure
    First episode of a recurrent neurologic disorder
    Hysteria

Episodic or relapsing neurologic disorders
    Seizures
    Migraine and other causes of headache
    Breath-holding spells
    Syncope
    Vertigo
    Substance abuse
    Inborn errors of metabolism
    Behavioral disorders
    Sleep disorders

Static nonprogressive neurologic disease
    Mental retardation
    Cerebral palsy
    Learning disabilities
    Behavior disorders

Progressive neurologic disease
    Inborn errors of metabolism
    Degenerative diseases
    Neurocutaneous syndromes
    Chronic infections
    Intracranial masses
    Chronic intoxication
    Neuromuscular diseases
    Psychiatric disorders

Progressive disorders are the most worrisome in pediatric neurology. In general, the more slowly progressive the signs and symptoms, the more likely the child has a degenerative disease. The elements of the illness have often been present for years prior to the parents seeking medical attention. Therefore one should examine carefully the child's early development, particularly noting at what age the child stopped performing at the level of his peers. The rapidly progressive neurologic illness is more likely an acquired disease secondary to an infection, neoplasm, intoxication, or other insult.

After the history of the present illness has been obtained, the past medical history is documented. The details of the pregnancy, labor and delivery, and nursery course are valuable clues to many neurologic diseases. Information should be obtained for any serious illness or injury requiring hospitalization. A review of systems will frequently disclose systemic illnesses predisposing to neu-

Table 1-3. Neurologic Manifestations of Systemic Disease

System	Disease	Neurologic Manifestation
Ear, nose, and throat	Chronic infections	Intracranial abscess
	Local infection	Headache, dural sinus thrombosis
Pulmonary	Cystic fibrosis	Vitamin E deficiency (ataxia, other)
	Tuberculosis	Chronic meningitis
Cardiovascular	Valvular heart disease	Embolic stroke, mycotic aneurysm, abscess
	Congenital cyanotic heart disease	Cerebral abscess, paradoxical embolism
	Myxoma	Embolic stroke, aneurysm
Gastrointestinal	Malabsorption	Vitamin E deficiency: ataxia, neuropathy
	Malnutrition	Vitamin A: pseudotumor cerebri Protein: weakness, developmental delay Pyridoxine: seizures Thiamine deficiency: Wernicke's encephalopathy Vitamin B_{12}: spasticity, neuropathy
Genitourinary	Renal disease	Hypertensive encephalopathy
Endocrine	Hypothyroidism	Mental retardation
	Hyperthyroidism	Weakness
	Cushing's disease	Myopathy, opportunistic infections
	Diabetes mellitus	*Nocardia* infections, polyneuropathy, hypoglycemia
Hematopoetic/neoplasms	Hemoglobinopathies	Strokes
	Thrombocytopenia	Intracranial hemorrhage
	Neuroblastoma	Ataxia, myoclonus, opsoclonia
	Cancer chemotherapy	Polyneuropathy, dementia, strokes, opportunistic infections
Musculoskeletal	Down's syndrome	Atlanto-occipital subluxation
	Neuromuscular diseases which cause scoliosis	Myelopathy
Immune	Immunosupression	Opportunistic infections, chronic viral encephalitis

Table 1-4. Systemic Manifestation of Neurologic Disease

System	Neurologic Disease	Systemic Manifestations
Ear, nose, and throat	Ataxia telangiectasia	Chronic sinusitis, otitis
	Dermoid sinus	Recurrent meningitis
Pulmonary	Ataxia telangiectasia	Chronic bronchitis, bronchiectasis
Cardiovascular	Friedreich's ataxia	Cardiomyopathy
	Mitochondrial myopathies	Cardiomyopathy
	Glycogen storage disease	Cardiomyopathy
	Progressive myopathies	Cardiomyopathy
	Tuberous sclerosis	Cardiac tumors
Gastrointestinal	Wilson's disease	Acute hepatic disease, cirrhosis
	Glycogen/lipid storage disease	Hepatosplenomegaly, hypoglycemia
	Abetalipoproteinemia	Malabsorption
Genitourinary	Hypothalamic, pituitary tumors	Syndrome of inappropriate secretion of antidiuretic hormone (SIADH), diabetes insipidus, precocious or delayed sexual development
	Cerebral aneurysms	Polycystic kidneys
	Fabry's disease	Hypertension
	Tuberous sclerosis	Renal and heart tumors
	Myelopathies	Incontinence
Endocrine	Hypothalamic, pituitary tumors	Failure to thrive, delayed maturation, hypothalamic syndrome, diabetes insipidus
	Metabolic encephalopathies	Acidosis, hypoglycemia
Hematopoetic	Metabolic encephalopathies	Thrombocytopenia, anemia
Musculoskeletal	Neuromuscular diseases	Joint contractures, scoliosis
	Mucopolysaccharidosis	Dwarfism, kyphosis
	Friedreich's ataxia	Pes cavus, scoliosis
	Neurofibromatosis	Scoliosis

rologic disease (Table 1-3) or systemic manifestations of neurologic disease (Table 1-4). The physician should record immunizations and dates, any infectious diseases, any known allergies, and present medications and their dosages. The environmental history may disclose chronic exposure to toxins or infections. The patient's school performance in both academic and social areas must be recorded and compared to previous years' performance. Finally, the history should conclude with a detailed family history (Table 1-5) and ethnic background. One should not accept an established diagnosis in a family member without verifying the symptoms and signs for that disease. On the other hand, a parent may be unaware or deny the presence of disease which can be determined by examining the parent.

If one is unsure of the differential diagnosis after taking a history, then it is unlikely the diagnosis will be found on examination or by performing laboratory tests. In this case one should seek to obtain further information from

Table 1-5. Inheritance of Common Neurologic Disease[a]

Inheritance	Category	Disease
Dominant	Neurocutaneous disorders	Tuberous sclerosis
		Neurofibromatosis
		Von Hippel-Lindau disease
	Neuromuscular disease	Myotonic dystrophy
		Facioscapulohumoral dystrophy
		Familial distal myopathies
		Charcot-Marie-Tooth disease
	Degenerative diseases	Huntington's disease
		Familial spastic paraparesis
	Other	Mental retardation
		Epilepsy
		Migraine
X-Linked recessive	Muscular dystrophies	Duchenne dystrophy
		Becker dystrophy
		Emery-Dreifuss dystrophy
	Inborn errors of metabolism	Hunter's mucopolysaccharidosis
		Fabry's disease
		Adrenoleukodystrophy
		Lesch-Nyhan disease
		Menkes' kinky hair syndrome
	Other	Leber's optic atrophy
		Pelizaeus-Merzbacher disease
		X-Linked mental retardation
		X-Linked hydrocephalus
X-Linked dominant, male lethality		Incontinentia pigmenti
		Aicardi syndrome
		Ornithine transcarbamylase
		Rett syndrome
Sporadic		Sturge-Weber syndrome
		Dermatomyositis
		Multiple sclerosis

[a] Recessively inherited diseases are too numerous to list and have been omitted.

the parent or child or other hospital records. Unless it is an emergency, an evaluation should be deferred until a working diagnosis has been established.

SELECTED READINGS

Dodge PR: Neurologic history and examination. p. 1. In Farmer TW (ed): Pediatric Neurology. Harper & Row, New York, 1964

Gamstorp I: History—general outline. p. 1. In Pediatric Neurology. 2nd Ed. Butterworth, New York, 1985

Swaiman KF: Neurologic history in childhood. p. 1. In Swaiman KF, Wright FS (eds): The Practice of Pediatric Neurology. 2nd Ed. CV Mosby, St. Louis, 1982

2

CHILD DEVELOPMENTAL ASSESSMENT

The nervous system is the least developed of all the organ systems at birth. Maturation continues throughout childhood and possibly beyond. As a result the child's repertoire of behavior not only increases but also becomes more sophisticated as the child matures. This change in behavior is termed *development* and reflects the functional abilities of the nervous system. In order for a child to develop completely there must be both physical development of the nervous system and interaction with the environment for training and learning. An incompletely formed or injured nervous system or an impoverished environment will inhibit the child's development. This chapter reviews developmental maturation and developmental assessment.

DEVELOPMENT OF THE NERVOUS SYSTEM

Neurulation, prosencephalization, and histogenesis are the major embryologic processes which determine the gross morphology of the brain prior to birth. The embryology is discussed in more detail in Chapter 13. Further maturity of the nervous system occurs following birth because the nervous system is not completely myelinated. Myelin is an insulating fatty material around the nerve processes. In the peripheral nervous system it is formed by Schwann cells, whereas in the CNS it is formed by oligodendroglia. Myelin prevents the dispersion of an electrical impulse and thus speeds the conduction velocity of an action potential down an axon. A neuron is not functional until myelinization is completed. Most of the growth of the brain following birth is due to myelinization. Thus a newborn brain of 400 reaches an adult weight of 1200 to 1400 g mainly as a result of myelinization (Fig. 2-1).

Myelinization is a major determinant of development. Myelinization continues, perhaps through adulthood, and results in the normal time delays in achieving developmental goals (Fig. 2-2). At birth, the structures which are predominately myelinated are the bulbar structures, optic pathways, and peripheral nervous system. For these reasons, sucking and crying, visual fixation, and primitive reflexes are present in the newborn. In the ensuing months after birth the acoustic system, cerebellar system, and cerebrospinal tracts are myelinated. This coincides with the increasing sophistication and coordination of motor movements. The cerebrospinal tracts myelinate in a cephalocaudal di-

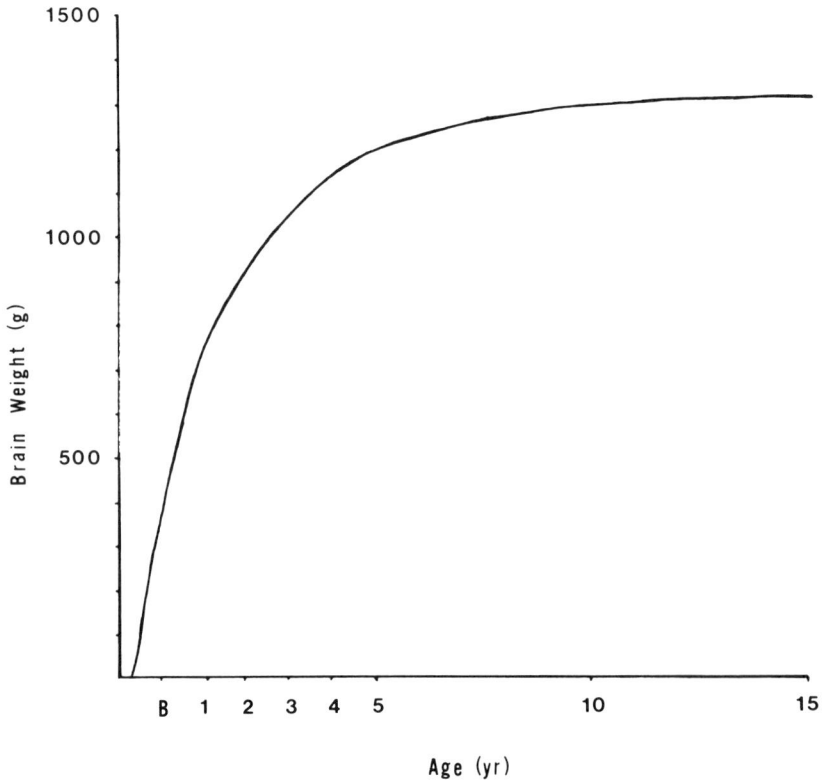

Fig. 2-1. Brain growth. (Adapted from Lemire RJ, Loeser JD, Leech RW, Alvord EC: Normal and Abnormal Development of the Human Nervous Center. Harper & Row, New York, 1975.)

rection, which is reflected in the earlier skills obtained by the hands prior to the ability to walk and later by the ability to control urinary and bowel functions.

The last areas to be myelinated are the corpus callosum and commissures and the association tracts of the cerebral cortex. This latter may myelinate well into adulthood. These structures are important for higher cortical function and correspond to the development of cerebral dominance and cognitive abilities. Delays in myelinization of certain tracts may contribute to disparity in the normal attainment of milestones. Variations in the times of walking and of the ability to learn to read are examples.

ENVIRONMENTAL INFLUENCES

The other major determinant of normal development is interaction with the environment. Children reared in an impoverished environment do less well than those reared in an enriched environment. This is true not only in the general sense but also for specific areas, such as deafness causing language delay. Interaction with the physical environment and social interaction contribute to the

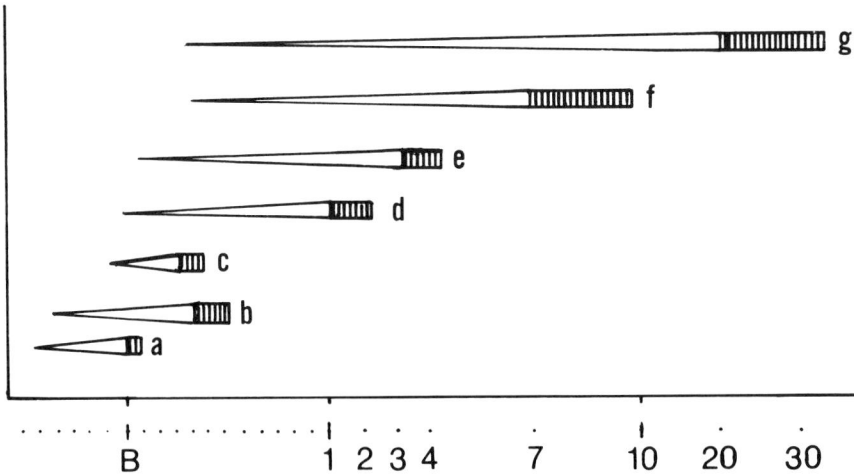

Fig. 2-2. Development of selected myelinated pathways: (*a*) motor roots, (*b*) sensory roots, (*c*) optic nerve and tract, (*d*) pyramidal tracts, (*e*) acoustic radiations, (*f*) cerebral commissure, (*g*) intracortical association tracts. (Modified from Yakolev PI, Lecours AR: The myelogenetic cycles of regional maturation of the brain. In Minkowski A (ed): Regional Development of the Brain in Early Life. Davis, Philadelphia, 1967, pp. 1–70.)

development of higher cortical function. The physical substrate of this interaction may be the development and elaboration of dendritic processes of the neurons. In animal models, learning or training is associated with an increase in dendritic processes.

Through interaction with the environment, certain cognitive concepts are developed. These concepts contribute much to the developing behavior of the child and include problem solving, causality, object permanence, locomotion, and communication. These concepts are either encouraged or repressed through the child's interaction with the environment. With normal morphologic development, myelinization, and environmental interaction, the child goes through a complex pattern of behavioral development which is surprisingly similar from culture to culture.

DEVELOPMENTAL RECRUITMENT AND PLASTICITY

Developmental abnormalities will be discussed in other sections of this text, but two important concepts are mentioned briefly here. Many lesions of the nervous system will be silent until those parts of the nervous system are developmentally recruited. Thus a child may "grow into" a disorder. For example, abnormal development of the language areas of the brain is not apparent in the newborn. A language disorder is recognized only at the time language abilities normally develop.

The second concept is plasticity. Plasticity is the mechanism by which the developing brain functionally recovers from brain injury. Thus the child with an early injury to the dominant hemisphere may develop speech at the normal time. It is thought that plasticity occurs either through regeneration of destroyed neural tissue or, more likely, through the brain developing alternative methods for problem solving and learning. It may be that either hemisphere has a full capacity for developing higher cortical function during early development. As one hemisphere becomes more specialized, the versatility of the other is suppressed. In early stages of development, alternative parts of the brain may be utilized to perform a function of an injured part of the brain.

NORMAL DEVELOPMENT

Normal child development is as reassuring as the daily sunrise. Parents and pediatricians await developmental milestones with eager anticipation. Failed milestones are a source of anxiety for parents and frequently lead to neurologic consultation. Normal growth and development should be the core of pediatric knowledge. Experienced pediatricians recognize the relatively broad range and variability of normal achievement. A knowledge of development allows for both early recognition of significant developmental delays and appropriate reassurance for minor variations.

Motor milestones are the most obvious developmental landmarks in the first year. An infant progresses from minimal head control to walking within 12 to 15 months. Sitting is the first major motor milestone and depends upon acquisition of head control and extinction of some of the primitive reflexes (e.g., Moro and tonic neck). Learning to sit progresses through a typical schedule (Fig. 2-3). Creeping or crawling is the next major milestone, although the method is highly variable (Fig. 2-4). Walking is the best-remembered motor milestone. The ability to walk is determined by both the maturity of the nervous system and the concept of locomotion. Without the latter, there is no perceived need for moving from one place to another. The child progresses from weight bearing to cruising to walking (Fig. 2-5). The mature gait with synchronous arm–leg motion is not fully developed until about 30 to 36 months. Subsequent motor activity is one of increasing coordination, particularly in fine motor development. The most significant fine motor achievement in the first year is the pincer grasp (Fig. 2-6). Motor development is outlined in Table 2-1.

Language development is not as obvious during the first year as it is in subsequent years. Failure to talk by the second year is a serious problem. In order for a child to talk there must be an accurate speech mechanism, intact nervous system, adequate environmental stimulation and reinforcement, and the concept of communication. The concept can be present without the other prerequisites and the child will communicate by gesture instead of words. Table 2-2 outlines the development of speech and language.

Social development is obvious throughout development. One of the earliest skills a child learns is the responsive smile. Indeed, there would probably be fewer children born if this skill were not mastered early. Civilization of the toddler is one of the more important tasks a parent must accomplish and by age 6 the child has mastered many of the social skills of his culture. Table 2-3 summarizes social development. *(Text continues on p. 16).*

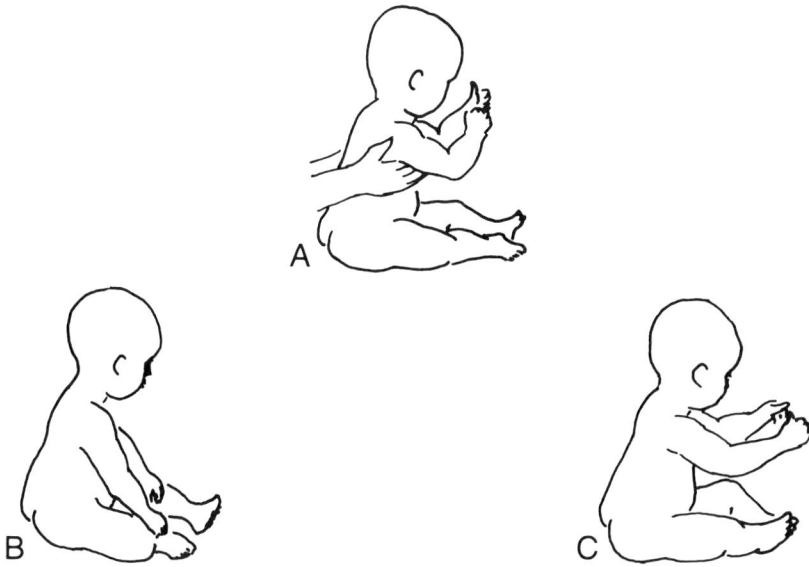

Fig. 2-3. Development of sitting: (A) 3 months, sitting with support and with head control; (B) 4 to 6 months, tripod position; (C) 6 to 8 months, sitting without support.

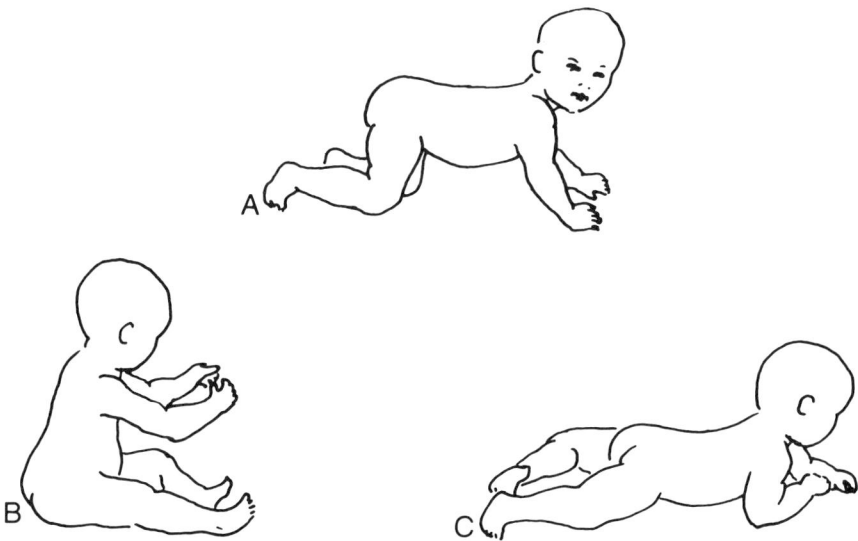

Fig. 2-4. Creeping and crawling: (A) traditional four-extremity reciprocal crawl, (B) "bottom scoot," (C) "army crawl."

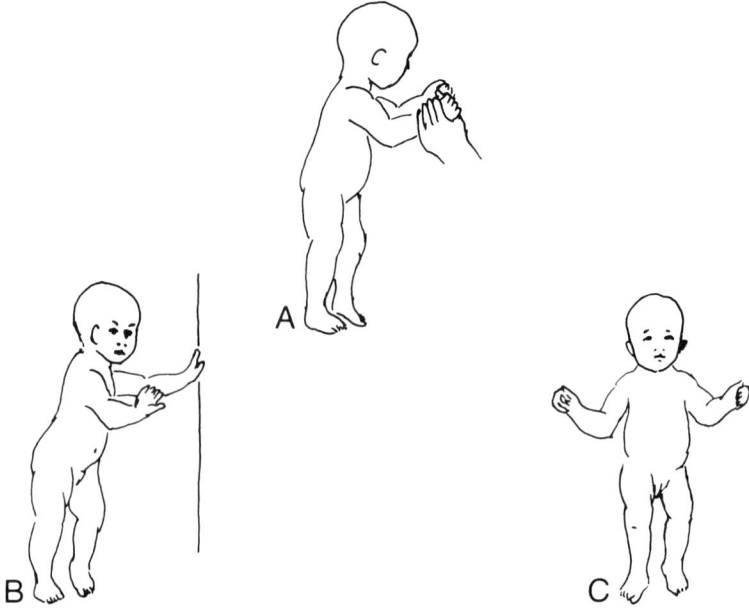

Fig. 2-5. Development of walking: (A) 4 to 6 months, weight bearing; (B) 6 to 10 months, cruising; (C) 10 to 15 months, walking.

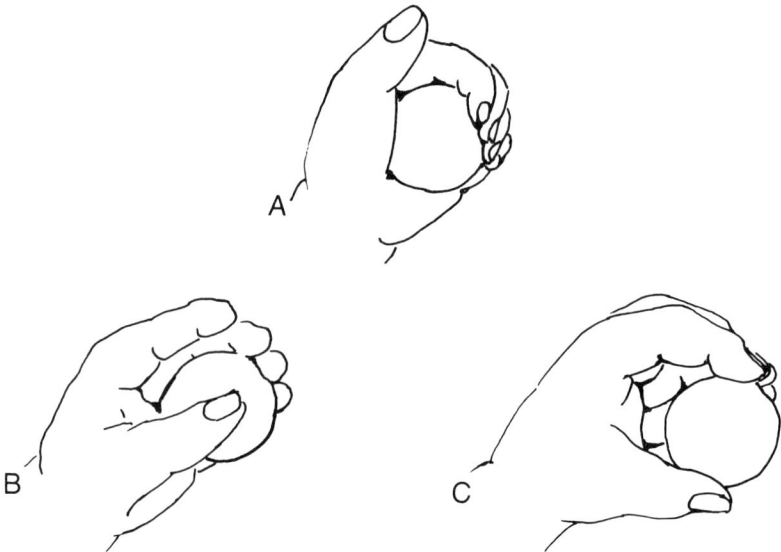

Fig. 2-6. Development of grasp: (A) 2 to 6 months, palmer grasp; (B) 6 to 8 months, apposition grasp; (C) 8 to 12 months, pincer grasp.

Table 2-1. Motor Development[a]

Age	Fine Motor Development	Gross Motor Development
1 month		Raises head slightly when prone
3 months		Head control
4–5 months	Voluntary grasp	Sits with support, bears weight
6–8 months	Transfers objects	Sits alone
7–9 months	Claps hands	Creeps and/or crawls
8–11 months	Opposes thumbs and finger	Stands holding on
9–15 months		Walks independently
12–15 months	Tower of two blocks	
18–24 months	Imitates vertical line	Throws ball, jumps, and "runs"
25–30 months	Imitates horizontal line Tower of six blocks	Climbs well
30–36 months	Draws circle	Goes up and down stairs independently
3–4 years	Draws square	Stands on one foot, rides tricycle, throws ball overhanded
4–5 years	Uses scissors Draws person with several parts	Throws ball with fair accuracy
5–6 years	Draws triangle Prints letters	
6–7 years	Draws diamond	Runs and jumps well

[a] The mean age for some milestones may vary from one authority to another.

Table 2-2. Language Development

Age	Development
1 month	Reflexive vowel vocalizations
2–4 months	Coos, laughs
6–8 months	Mimics sounds
8–10 months	Associates word and action (*no, bye-bye, patty cake*)
10–15 months	First words
12–18 months	3–50 words
16–24 months	Jargon, knows body parts, obeys simple commands
24 months	Combines words, intelligible to strangers 25% of time
2–3 years	50–300 words, intelligible to strangers 75% of time, three- to four-word sentences
3–4 years	Prepositions, plurals, pronouns, normal dysfluencies
4–5 years	Conjunctions, past tense, clear articulation, knows some colors, counts

Table 2-3. Personal–Social Development

Age	Development
1 month	Regards face
2–3 months	Smiles responsively
4–6 months	Recognizes nipple, poises for feeding
8–10 months	Finger feeds, plays simple games (*peekaboo, patty cake*), recognizes parent, stranger anxiety
12–15 months	Uses cup, attempts spoon
18–24 months	Communicates wants, imitates parental activity
2–3 years	Verbalizes toilet needs, independent and parallel play, removes and puts on clothing
3–4 years	Toilet trained, washes and dries face, cooperative play, turn taking
5–6 years	Dresses self, performs errands, group activities

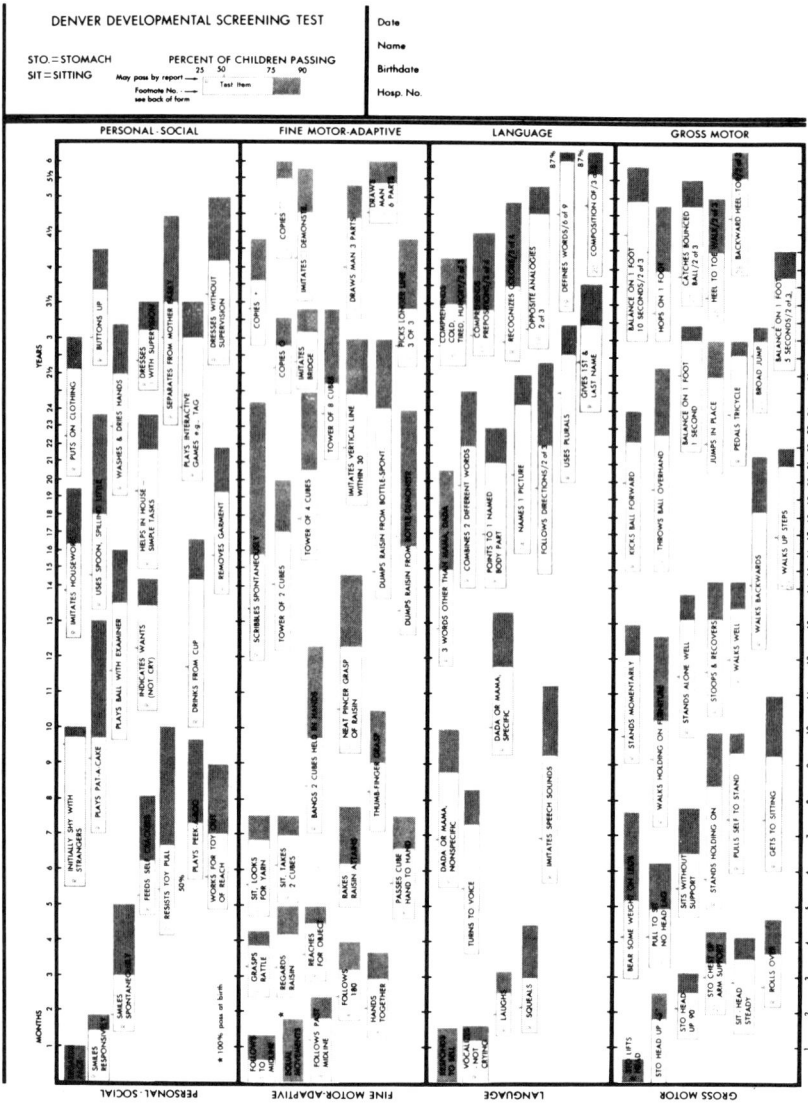

Fig. 2-7. (A,B) Denver Developmental Screening Test. (From Frankenberg WK, Dodds JP: Denver Developmental Screening Test. © 1969 University of Colorado Medical Center, Denver with permission.)

DEVELOPMENTAL ASSESSMENT

A knowledge of development is essential to the practice of pediatrics and pediatric neurology. Motor, language, and social development contribute to the overall pattern of development. Because development is a function of the nervous system, delays in development alert the physician to underlying neurologic

DIRECTIONS

DATE
NAME
BIRTHDATE
HOSP. NO.

1. Try to get child to smile by smiling, talking or waving to him. Do not touch him.
2. When child is playing with toy, pull it away from him. Pass if he resists.
3. Child does not have to be able to tie shoes or button in the back.
4. Move yarn slowly in an arc from one side to the other, about 6" above child's face. Pass if eyes follow 90° to midline. (Past midline; 180°)
5. Pass if child grasps rattle when it is touched to the backs or tips of fingers.
6. Pass if child continues to look where yarn disappeared or tries to see where it went. Yarn should be dropped quickly from sight from tester's hand without arm movement.
7. Pass if child picks up raisin with any part of thumb and a finger.
8. Pass if child picks up raisin with the ends of thumb and index finger using an over hand approach.

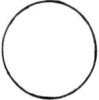

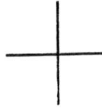

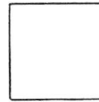

9. Pass any enclosed form. Fail continuous round motions.
10. Which line is longer? (Not bigger.) Turn paper upside down and repeat. (3/3 or 5/6)
11. Pass any crossing lines.
12. Have child copy first. If failed, demonstrate

When giving items 9, 11 and 12, do not name the forms. Do not demonstrate 9 and 11.

13. When scoring, each pair (2 arms, 2 legs, etc.) counts as one part.
14. Point to picture and have child name it. (No credit is given for sounds only.)

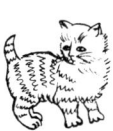

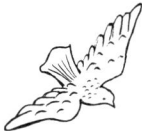

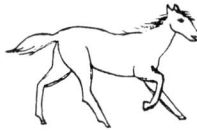

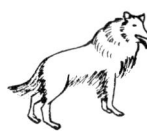

15. Tell child to: Give block to Mommie; put block on table; put block on floor. Pass 2 of 3. (Do not help child by pointing, moving head or eyes.)
16. Ask child: What do you do when you are cold? ..hungry? ..tired? Pass 2 of 3.
17. Tell child to: Put block on table; under table; in front of chair, behind chair. Pass 3 of 4. (Do not help child by pointing, moving head or eyes.)
18. Ask child: If fire is hot, ice is ?; Mother is a woman, Dad is a ?; a horse is big, a mouse is ?. Pass 2 of 3.
19. Ask child: What is a ball? ..lake? ..desk? ..house? ..banana? ..curtain? ..ceiling? ..hedge? ..pavement? Pass if defined in terms of use, shape, what it is made of or general category (such as banana is fruit, not just yellow). Pass 6 of 9.
20. Ask child: What is a spoon made of? ..a shoe made of? ..a door made of? (No other objects may be substituted.) Pass 3 of 3.
21. When placed on stomach, child lifts chest off table with support of forearms and/or hands.
22. When child is on back, grasp his hands and pull him to sitting. Pass if head does not hang back.
23. Child may use wall or rail only, may not person. May not crawl.
24. Child must throw ball overhand 3 feet to within arm's reach of tester.
25. Child must perform standing broad jump over width of test sheet. (8-1/2 inches)
26. Tell child to walk forward, ⚬⚬⚬⚬→ heel within 1 inch of toe. Tester may demonstrate. Child must walk 4 consecutive steps, 2 out of 3 trials.
27. Bounce ball to child who should stand 3 feet away from tester. Child must catch ball with hands, not arms, 2 out of 3 trials.
28. Tell child to walk backward, ←⚬⚬⚬⚬ toe within 1 inch of heel. Tester may demonstrate. Child must walk 4 consecutive steps, 2 out of 3 trials.

DATE AND BEHAVIORAL OBSERVATIONS (how child feels at time of test, relation to tester, attention
B span, verbal behavior, self-confidence, etc,):

Fig. 2-7. (*continued*).

dysfunction. Developmental assessment is a necessary part of the neurologic exam.

There are a number of developmental assessments available for clinical application. Perhaps the most widely used and easiest to perform in an office setting is the Denver Developmental Screening Test (Fig. 2-7). Through a number of questions asked of the parent and simple procedures performed in the office, an indication can be obtained as to whether the child is developmentally normal or at risk of having a developmental disorder. Because it is easy to miss or ignore a developmental problem, it is recommended that all children have developmental screening during their well-baby examinations. All children suspected of having a neurologic disorder must be tested. The division of the Denver Developmental Screening Test into gross motor, fine motor, personal–social, and language functions is useful. Assessing each area not only measures the major behavioral functions of a child but also gives an indication as to whether there is a global disorder or isolated disorders in one or more functions. Longitudinal assessments can determine if there is a delayed but progressive improvement or if there is an increasing lag between expected and actual performance. Persistent abnormalities can thus be referred for more detailed testing.

Certain patterns of development are diagnostically useful. If one could plot development by measuring the maturation of a neurologic behavior as a function of age, one would see a pattern similar to body growth. There is rapid initial development followed by a deceleration phase and finally a plateau at maturity. Static neurologic disorders show a curve that is shifted to the right but which parallels normal development. Degenerative or progressive diseases show a pattern of initial improvement, a plateau of stationary development, and then subsequent regression.

SELECTED READINGS

Donoghue EC, Shakespeare RH: The reliability of pediatric case history milestones. Dev Med Child Neurol 9:64–69, 1967

Frankenburg W, Dodds JB: Denver Developmental Screening Test. J Pediatr 71:181–191, 1967

Horowitz FD: Child development for the pediatrician. Pediatr Clin North Am 29:359–376, 1982

Levine MD, Carey WB, Crocker AC, Gross RT (eds): Developmental–Behavioral Pediatrics. WB Saunders, Philadelphia, 1983

3

GENERAL PHYSICAL
EXAMINATION

The diagnosis of many neurologic diseases can be determined from a careful general physical examination. This chapter highlights those areas of the general examination which are relevant to neurologic disease.

A careful examination of the head is important and should begin with a measurement of the head circumference (Fig. 3-1). The greatest measurement around the fronto-occipital diameter is used. This is a vital piece of information, in that head size reflects brain growth. Abnormalities in the size or shape of the head may suggest an underlying neurologic disease. The causes for megalocephaly, microcephaly, and frontal bossing are listed in Tables 3-1 through 3-3. One should then assess the anterior fontanelle (Fig. 3-2) and head shape (Fig. 3-3) and any dysmorphic features which may be present in the face or scalp. The causes for an enlarged fontanelle are listed in Table 3-4. Transillumination is a helpful screen for hydrocephalus, hydranencephaly, and porencephalia, although ultrasonography is a more sensitive screen for these abnormalities. Percussion of the head produces a "cracked pot" sound in children with increased intracranial pressure (Macewen's sign). A bruit on auscultation is usually normal in the young child but may signify an arteriovenous malformation in the older child.

The funduscopic examination is sufficiently important that dilatation of the pupils is indicated if the fundus cannot be adequately visualized (Table 3-5). Because this may be traumatic in the young child it is often deferred to the end of the examination. A slit-lamp exam by an ophthalmologist is indicated for suspected cataracts or Wilson's disease. Figure 3-4 illustrates some of the important funduscopic abnormalities.

An examination of the ears and percussion of the sinuses may reveal evidence of chronic infection. Neurologic disorders associated with these infections include ataxia telangiectasia and intracranial abscess. Ethmoidal tenderness, proptosis, and orbital injection with edema are particularly ominous and suggest cavernous sinus thrombosis.

The neck should be mobile in the relaxed patient. A stiff neck may reflect meningism, cervical spine disease, soft tissue inflammation of the neck, tonsilitis, or even upper lobe pneumonia. Meningism is caused by inflammation of the meninges (meningitis) or stretch of this structure (posterior fossa tumor). A short neck is seen in the Klippel-Feil anomaly, platybasia, and basilar impression. The differential diagnosis for a head tilt is listed in Table 3-6. *(Text continues on p. 29).*

19

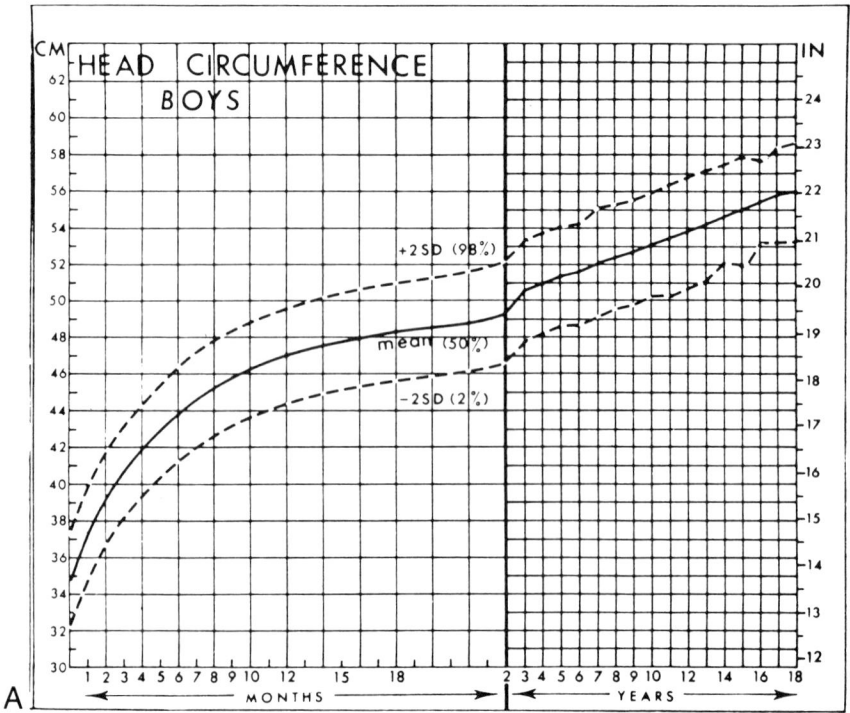

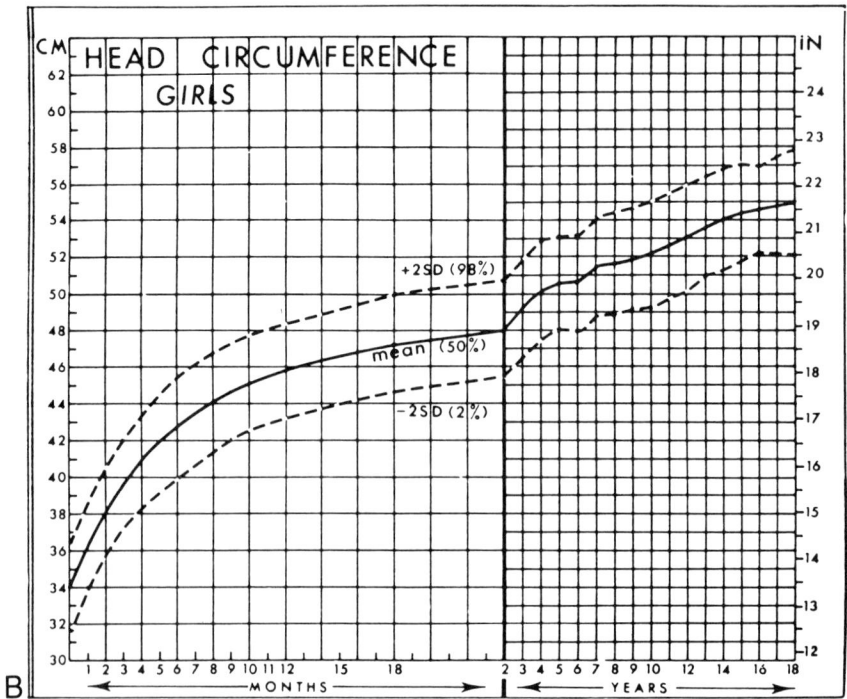

Fig. 3-1. (A,B) Head circumference measurement. (Nelhaus G: Head circumference from birth to eighteen years. Pediatrics 41:106–114, 1968. Reproduced by permission of Pediatrics.)

Table 3-1. Megalocephaly in Children

Hydrocephalus (see Table 30-2)
  Noncommunicating
  Communicating

Cerebral edema (see Table 30-1)

Subdural fluid
  Hematoma
  Hygroma or effusion
  Empyema

Intracranial mass
  Tumor
  Abscess
  Cyst

Megalencephaly
  Anatomic
    Normal
    With gigantism
      Cerebral
      Pituitary
      Arachnodactyly
      Adiposogigantism
    With dwarfism
      Achondroplasia
    With ganglioneuroma
    With neurocutaneous syndromes
      Neurofibromatosis
      Tuberous sclerosis
      Multiple hemangiomatosis
      Ito's syndrome
    Familial
      Dominant
      Recessive
    With miscellaneous malformations
    Idiopathic
  Metabolic
    Aminoaciduria in maple syrup urine disease
    Leukodystrophy
      Canavan's spongy degeneration
      Alexander's disease
    Lysosomal storage diseases
      Tay-Sachs disease
      Generalized gangliosidosis
      Mucopolysaccharidoses
      Metachromatic leukodystrophy

Macrocrania: skull thickening (see Table 6-2)

(Data from DeMyer W: Megalencephaly in children. Neurology 22:634–643, 1972.)

Table 3-2. Microcephaly

Genetic
    Recessive (Penrose syndrome)
    Familial lissencephaly
    Familial micrencephaly with calcifications
    Sex linked micrencephaly with aminoaciduria
    Alper's disease with chorioretinopathy
    Phenylketonuria
    Fanconi's syndrome
    Seckel's syndrome
    Rubinstein-Taybi syndrome
Chromosomal abnormalities
    Down's syndrome (trisomy 21)
    Cornelia de Lange syndrome
    Cri-du-chat syndrome
    Trisomy 13-15 syndrome
    Trisomy 18 syndrome
Intrauterine injuries
    Radiation
    Congenital infections
    Maternal diabetes
Perinatal disorders
    Hypoxic–ischemic injuries
    Acquired infections
    Metabolic, traumatic injuries

(From Harwood-Nash DC, Fitz CR: Neuroradiology in Infants and Children. CV Mosby, St. Louis, 1976.)

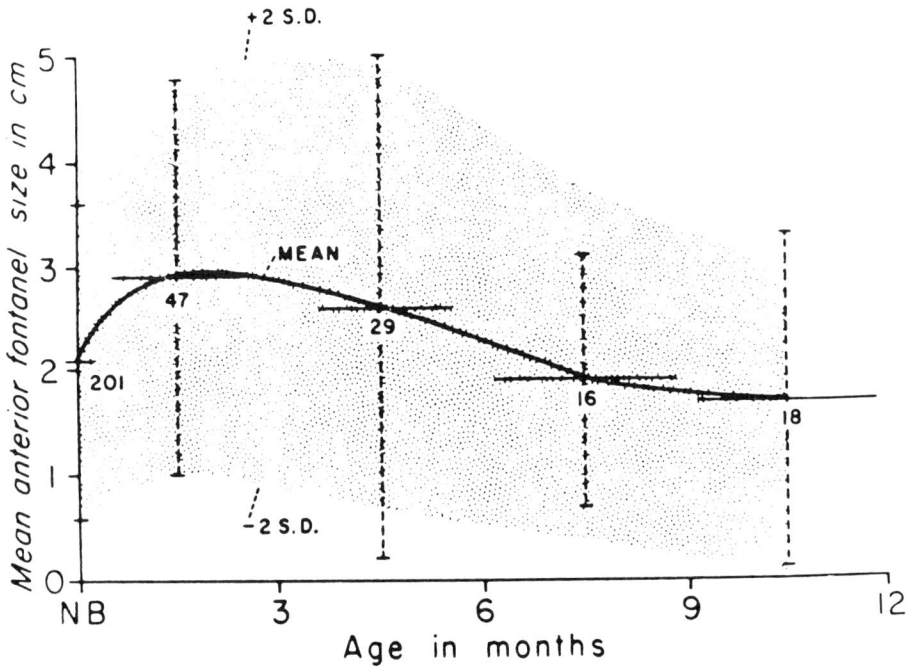

Fig. 3-2. Fontanelle measurement (length plus width divided by 2) during the first year. (From Popich G, Smith DW: Fontanels: range of normal size. J Pediatr 80:749–752, 1972.)

Table 3-3. Frontal Bossing, Hypertelorism, and
Depressed Nasal Bridge

Frontal bossing
  Metabolic: gangliosidoses
  Cranioskeletal dysplasias
  Dysmorphic syndromes
    Rubinstein-Taybi
    Otopalatodigital
    Hallermann-Streiff
    Progeria
  Chronic hydrocephalus
  Calcified subgaleal hematoma
  Familial
Low nasal bridge
  Achondroplasia
  Cleidocranial dysostosis
  Down's syndrome
  Generalized gangliosidosis
  Mucopolysaccharidoses
  Familial
Hypertelorism
  Median cleft face
  Cerebral malformations
    Frontonasal encephaloceles
    Agenesis of corpus callosum
  Cranioskeletal dysplasias
    Cleidocranial dysostosis
    Osteogenesis imperfecta
Metabolic: mucopolysaccharidoses
Fibrous dysplasias of ethmoidal sinuses
Dysmorphic syndromes
  Larsen's
  Crouzon's
  Apert's
  Conradi's
  Cri-du-chat
  Waardenburg's
Familial

(From Harwood-Nash DC, Fitz CR: Neuroradiology of
Children. CV Mosby, St. Louis, 1976.)

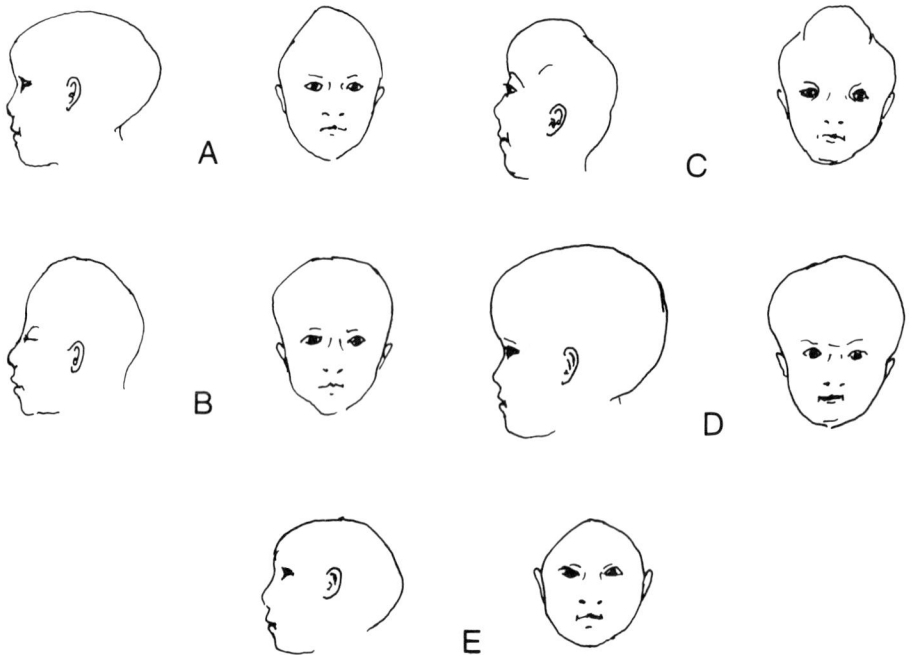

Fig. 3-3. Abnormalities of head shape. (A) Sagittal synostosis with scaphacephaly. (B) coronal synostosis with brachycephaly. (C) "Clover leaf" deformity from coronal and sagittal synostosis. (D) Hydrocephalus with frontal bossing. (E) Microcephaly.

Table 3-4. Causes for Enlarged Fontanelle

Skeletal disorders
  Achondroplasia
  Aminopterin-induced syndrome
  Apert's syndrome
  Cleidocranial dysostosis
  Hypophosphatasia
  Kenny's syndrome
  Osteogenesis imperfecta
  Pyknodysostosis
  Vitamin D deficiency rickets
Chromosomal abnormalities
  Down's syndrome
  Trisomy 13 syndrome
  Trisomy 18 syndrome
Other conditions
  Athyrotic hypothyroidism
  Hallermann-Streiff syndrome
  Malnutrition
  Progeria
  Rubella syndrome
  Russell-Silver syndrome

(Reproduced by permission of Pediatrics from Popich G, Smith DW: Fontanels: range of normal size. J Pediatr 80:749–752, 1972.)

Table 3-5. Eye Abnormalities in Neurologic Disease

Exam	Sign	Neurologic Disorder
Optic disk	Papilledema	Increased intracranial pressure (any cause)
		Acute optic neuritis (papillitis)
		Pseudopapilledema (often hereditary)
		Retro-orbital mass
	Optic atrophy	Demyelinating diseases (many)
		Chronic papilledema
		Leber's optic atrophy
		Neuronal ceroid lipofuscinosis
		Congenital infections
		Vasculitis
		Glaucoma
		Leukodystrophies
Retina	Pigmentation	Congenital infection
		Refsum's disease
		Abetalipoproteinemia
		Neuronal ceroid lipofuscinosis
		Sjögren-Larssen syndrome
		Cockayne's syndrome
		Laurence-Moon-Biedl syndrome
		Chédiak-Higashi syndrome
	Colobomas	Aicardi syndrome
	Hemangiomas	Von Hippel-Lindau
	Cherry-red spot	Tay-Sachs disease
		Gangliosidoses
		Sialidoses, mucolipidoses
		Niemann-Pick disease
		Cherry-red spot, myoclonus syndrome
		Metachromatic leukodystrophy
		Farber's lipogranulomatosis
		Central retinal artery occlusion
		Trauma
	Phakomas	Tuberous sclerosis
Lens	Cataracts	Conradi's syndrome
		Cockayne's syndrome
		Lowe's syndrome
		Marinesco-Sjögren syndrome
		Hallerman-Streiff syndrome
		Pierre Robin syndrome
		Treacher Collins syndrome
		Goldenhar syndrome
		Alport syndrome
		Cerebrotendinous xanthomatosis
		Trisomy 13,18,21
		Incontientia pigmenti
		Congenital infections
		Familial
		Galactosemia
		Myotonic dystrophy
		Congenital hypothyroidism
		Idiopathic
	Subluxation	Homocystinuria
		Marfan's syndrome
		Sulfite oxidase deficiency
Cornea	Clouding	Mucopolysaccharidoses
		Fabry's syndrome
		Congenital rubella
Sclera	Telangiectasia	Ataxia telangiectasia
Iris	Pigmentation	Kayser-Fleischer rings (Wilson's disease)
		Brushfield spots (Down's syndrome)
	Aniridia	Cerebellar aplasia (Gillespie syndrome)

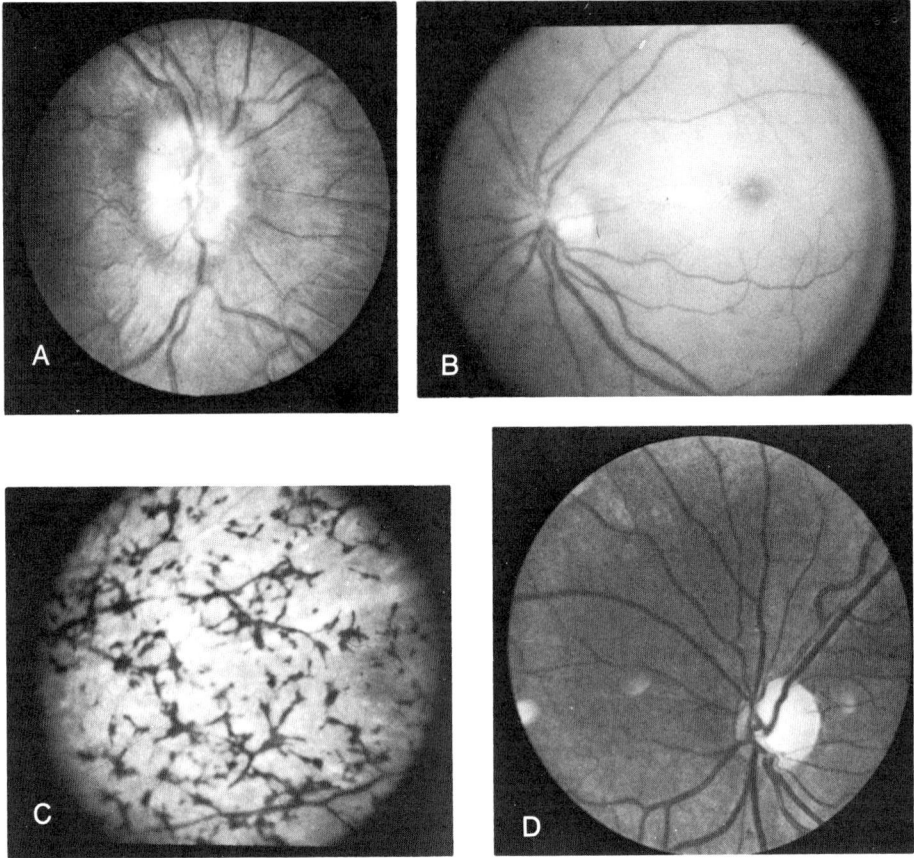

Fig. 3-4. Important funduscopic abnormalities. (A) Papilledema. (B) Cherry-red spot. (C) Retinitis. (D) Optic atrophy.

Table 3-6. Causes for Head Tilt

Neurologic disorders
  Posterior fossa tumor
  Arnold-Chiari malformation
  Syringomyelia
  Skew deviation of the eyes
  Dystonia
  Continuous muscle activity, Isaac's syndrome
  Spasmus nutans
  Spinal tumors
Skeletal disorders
  Klippel-Feil anomaly
  Hemivertebrae
  Rheumatoid arthritis
  Calcification of the intervertebral disks
  Vertebral osteomyelitis
  Subluxation of cervical spine
Other
  Gastroesophageal reflux
  Soft tissue infection of the neck (adenitis, retropharyngeal abscess)
  Congenital torticollis (muscular contraction)
  Muscle spasm/strain ("wry neck")

Table 3-7. Abnormalities of the Chest, Abdomen, and Genitalia Associated with Neurologic Disease

Exam	Sign	Neurologic Disorder
Chest	Chronic infections	Ataxia telangiectasia Cystic fibrosis with vitamin E deficiency
Heart	Heart failure	Pompe's disease Carnitine deficiency Mitochrondrial myopathies Friedreich's ataxia
Abdomen	Hepatosplenomegaly	Gaucher's disease Glycogen storage diseases GM_1 gangliosidoses Mucopolysaccharidoses Niemann-Pick disease Arginosuccinic aciduria
Genitalia	Micropenis Delayed or precocious puberty	Prader-Willi syndrome Pituitary, diencephalic tumors

Table 3-8. Abnormalities of the Back and Extremities in Neurologic Disease

Exam	Sign	Neurologic Disease
Back	Scoliosis	Friedreich's ataxia Neuromuscular diseases (many) Spinal cord tumors Neurofibromatosis Syringomyelia Congenital spinal anomalies
	Kyphosis	Mucopolysaccharidoses
	Mass	Spinal dysraphia with lipoma, myelocele, meningomyelocele
Extremities	Pes cavus	Friedreich's ataxia Charcot-Marie-Tooth disease Other neuropathies
	Joint contractures	Muscular dystrophies Congenital myopathies Arthrogryposis multiplex congenita Dermatomyositis
	Joint laxity	Ehlers-Danlos syndrome
	Limb asymmetry	Hemiatrophy (parietal lobe injury) Leg length (tethered cord, Klippel-Trenaunay syndrome) Beckwith-Wiedemann syndrome

Table 3-9. Neurologic Disorders with Cutaneous Abnormalities

Disorder	Abnormality
Neurofibromatosis	Café au lait patches Axillary freckling Subcutaneous nodules (neurofibromata)
Tuberous sclerosis	Amelanotic nevi Subungual phakomas Shagreen patch Adenoma sebaceum
Sturge-Weber	Port wine angioma of the face
Incontinentia pigmenti	Early: macules, bullae Late: brown, irregular macules Resolution
Klippel-Trenaunay	Angiomas and limb hypertrophy
Linear sebaceous nevus	Midline nevus of face and scalp with yellow nodules
Sjögren-Larsen	Icthyosis
Fabry's disease	Periumbilical and groin angiokeratomas
Dermatomyositis	Maculopapular rash on extensor surfaces, heliotrope around eyes, "butterfly" rash on face
Ataxia telangiectasia	Conjunctival telangiectasia
Spina bifida	Midline hair patch, lipoma, dimple, or skin mark on back
Phenylketonuria	Eczema
Hartnup disease	Photosensitivity, pellagra rash
Biotinidase deficiency	Rash
Trichorrhexis nodosa (hair)	Arginosuccinicaciduria Menkes' syndrome

Significant signs associated with neurologic disease that are found on examination of the chest, heart, abdomen, and genitalia are listed in Table 3-7. One should examine the spine and joints for deformities (Table 3-8), followed by a careful skin examination for stigmas of neurocutaneous and other disorders (Table 3-9). All new patients should be undressed completely, although it may be best to do this in layers as one proceeds through the examination. All children with infantile spasms, unexplained seizures, or mental retardation need a Wood's lamp exam of the skin to identify the amelanotic lesions of tuberous sclerosis.

SELECTED READINGS

DeMyer W: Megalencephaly in children. Neurology 22:634–643, 1972

Kivlin JD, Sanborn GE, Myers GG: The cherry-red spot in Tay-Sachs and other storage diseases. Ann Neurol 17:356–360, 1985

Kohn BA: The differential diagnosis of cataracts in infancy and childhood. Am J Dis Child 130:184–192, 1976

Nelson LB: The visually handicapped child. Pediatr Rev 6:173–182, 1984

Popich G, Smith DW: Fontanels: range of normal size. J Pediatr 80:749–752, 1972

4

NEUROLOGIC EXAMINATION

The purpose of this chapter is to present a method for performing a neurologic examination in children. A neurologic screening examination is relatively straightforward and, if a routine is established, one is unlikely to omit important parts of the examination. The traditional approach is satisfactory at all ages and includes examination of the cranial nerves, motor systems, reflexes, sensation, coordination, and mental status. In pediatrics, one is accustomed to the uncooperative child. Much information can be obtained by careful observation. In many cases this will suffice in lieu of more formal testing. In the child without neurologic complaints, a screening exam consisting of an assessment of motor strength, deep tendon reflexes, eye motility, and gait, a fundus exam, and observation is probably adequate.

CRANIAL NERVES

Table 4-1 summarizes the important function of the cranial nerves and their testing. It is seldom necessary to screen the function of the olfactory nerve. If it is to be tested, it is better to use a familiar odor, such as that of chocolate or of a banana, than a foreign odor. A harsh odor may irritate the nasal mucosa and not test olfaction.

Visual acuity is the most important function of the optic nerve. In the infant, the ability to fixate on a face is the most sensitive test. The ability to follow a face improves with age, so that by 2 to 3 months the child should follow 180°. By the end of 1 year the child can discriminate objects 1 mm in diameter, such as a small candy bead. In older children there are a variety of modified Snellen charts that can be used. Visual loss can be caused by a number of diseases (Table 4-2). Monocular visual loss can only be caused by optic nerve or retinal disease; there will be a diminished direct and consensual pupillary reflex. If the ophthalmoscopic exam and the pupillary light reflex are normal in a child with binocular visual loss, then one should test for optokinetic nystagmus by moving alternating black and white stripes across the visual field. The normal response is nystagmus, with the slow component in the direction of the movement; its absence indicates a disturbance in the visual cortex.

Another important test of cranial nerve II is to examine the visual fields (Fig. 4-1). In small children this can be assessed by moving a bright object into the visual field and observing the child's reaction. Infants 3 months of age or older will turn their heads toward the object. In older children simultaneous finger confrontation is the best method to examine visual fields. The child

Table 4-1. Cranial Nerve Examination

Cranial Nerve	Examination
I, olfactory	Smell
II, optic	Visual acuity and fields, pupillary light reflex
III, oculomotor	Ocular motility (up, medially, down, and in), pupillary light reflex
IV, trochlear	Ocular motility (down and out)
V, trigeminal	Facial sensation, corneal reflex, mastication
VI, abducens	Ocular motility (lateral)
VII, facial	Facial expression
VIII, vestibulocochlear	Hearing, balance
IX, glossopharyngeal	Gag reflex, swallowing, phonation
X, vagus	Palatal motility, phonation
XI, accessory	Head turning, shoulder shrug
XII, hypoglossal	Tongue protrusion

watches the examiner's nose and points to movement of the examiner's finger in the peripheral visual fields.

The pupillary light reflex tests both cranial nerve II and the parasympathetic component of cranial nerve III (Fig. 4-2). A lesion of the afferent limb in one eye causes no difference in the sizes of the two pupils in ambient light. Light shown to the affected eye causes neither pupil to constrict. Light shown to the contralateral eye causes a normal pupillary reaction in that eye (direct response) and in the affected eye (consensual response). The swinging-flashlight test will show paradoxical dilation of the pupil contralateral to the illuminated eye with the afferent defect (Marcus Gunn pupil). Lesions of the efferent limb cause anisocoria, with ipsilateral pupillary dilatation and no direct light reflex but normal consensual pupillary constriction of the contralateral pupil. Lack of sympathetic innervation causes pupillary constriction, ptosis, and decreased sweating on the

Table 4-2. Causes of Loss of Vision in Children

Area of Loss	Cause
Monocular	
Cornea	Keratoconus
	Scarring secondary to herpes
Lens	Cataract (see Table 3-5)
Vitreous	Hemorrhage, glaucoma (Sturge-Weber)
Retina	Detachment, tumor, parasitic infection, ischemia (stroke, migraine)
Optic nerve	Tumor
Amblyopia	Squint
Binocular	
Cornea	Corneal clouding (see Table 3-5)
Lens	Subluxation, cataracts (see Table 3-5)
Vitreous	Retrolental fibroplasia, hemorrhage
Retina	Retinitis, hemorrhages, metabolic storage diseases (see Table 3-5)
Optic nerve	Leber's optic atrophy, leukodystrophies, demyelinating diseases, chronic papilledema
Occipital cortex	Tumor, ischemia (stroke, migraine)

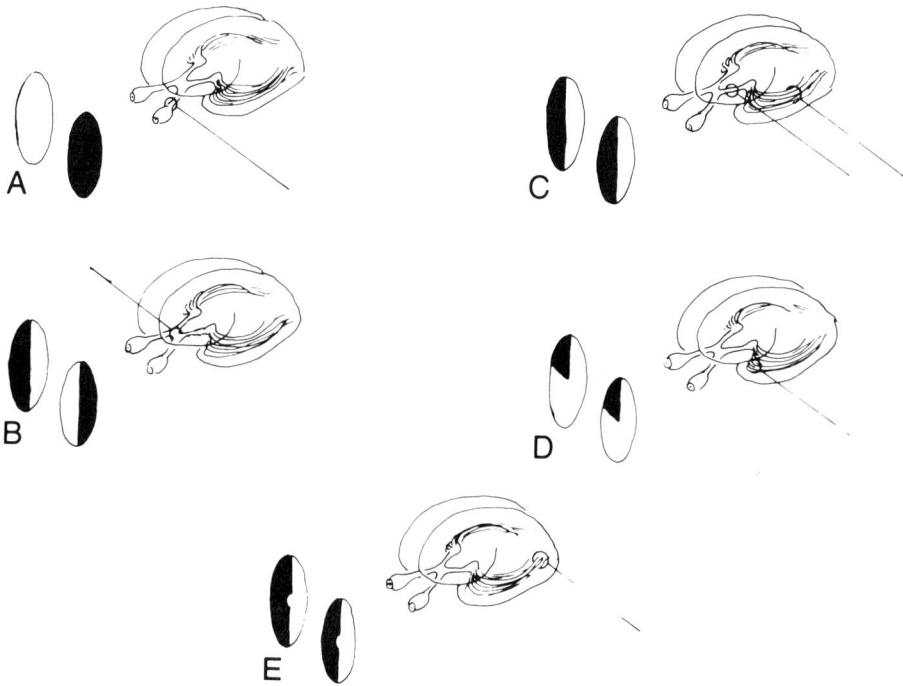

Fig. 4-1. Visual field defects: (A) left optic nerve, left monocular blindness; (B) optic chiasm, bitemporal hemianopia; (C) left optic tract or optic radiations, right homonymous hemianopia; (D) left Meyer's loop, right superior quadrantanopia; (E) left occipital cortex, right homonymous hemianopia with macular sparing.

ipsilateral face (Horner's syndrome). Other pupillary signs are listed in Table 4-3.

The motor function of cranial nerves III, IV, and VI is normally tested simultaneously by having the child look in the six directions of gaze (Fig. 4-3). If there is inconjugate gaze one must determine if there is a paralytic or non-paralytic squint. The latter is due to muscle imbalance rather than a paralysis, and testing each eye separately will differentiate this from a paralytic squint. In the small child ocular motility can be observed by testing the oculovestibular reflex (see below). Disorders of ocular motility are summarized in Table 4-4, and causes of involuntary eye movements in Table 4-5. One should remember that the direction of nystagmus is determined by the fast component.

The trigeminal nerve is examined by testing the corneal reflex in all children and in the older child by subjectively assessing facial sensation (Fig. 4-4) and the muscles of mastication. The facial nerve can be evaluated by observation, particularly in the young infant. Crying, smiling, and grimacing should be symmetric. Peripheral seventh cranial nerve lesions cause ipsilateral weakness of both the upper and lower portions of the face and of eye closure. Facial weakness from upper motor nerve lesions causes maximal weakness in the lower portion

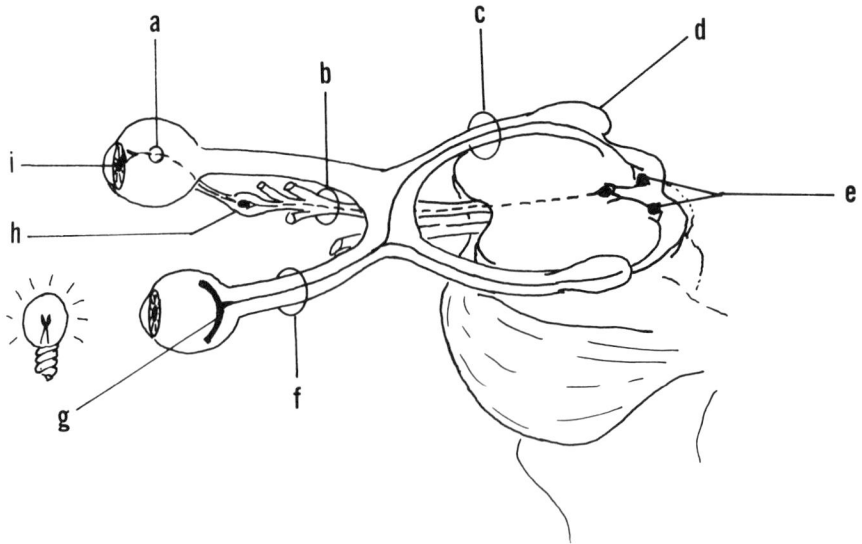

Fig. 4-2. Pupillary light reflex. The diagram illustrates the afferent limb originating from the left eye and the efferent limb causing a consensual pupil constriction in the right eye: (*a*) ciliary nerve, (*b*) oculomotor nerve, (*c*) optic tract, (*d*) lateral geniculate body, (*e*) Edinger-Westphal nucleus, (*f*) optic nerve, (*g*) retina, (*h*) ciliary ganglion, (*i*) pupil.

of the face and frequently spares the forehead. Congenital hypoplasia of the depressor anguli oris is another cause for the asymmetric crying face in the infant.

The auditory nerve is tested in infants by observing a startle reaction to a loud noise. By 3 to 4 months the child will turn toward a sound. The older child can be tested by rubbing the fingertips near the ear. This is performed similarly to the way in which one tests visual field with confrontation. If hearing loss is suspected, an audiogram should be obtained. The vestibular portion of the eighth cranial nerve is easily tested in the young child by holding the infant face-to-face the examiner and spinning him about. The child will develop nystagmus with the slow component in the direction of the spin. If the child can maintain standing or sitting balance without vertigo or nystagmus, then the nerve is intact. In the comatose patient, vestibular function can be assessed by performing caloric testing. Cold water introduced into the ear canal causes the eyes to deviate to that side. In the awake patient, nystagmus will develop toward the opposite side.

Cranial nerves IX and X are examined by observing palatal movement and phonation and by testing the gag reflex. This should be performed on both sides of the pharynx. Weakness of the muscles supplied by these nerves causes drooling, a nasal or weak voice, difficulty swallowing, and a weak suck. The accessory nerve is tested by two simple maneuvers. The strength of the upper trapezius muscle is measured by having the child shrug his shoulders and the strength of the sternocleidomastoid muscle is assessed by having the child turn his head to the ipsilateral side of the muscle being tested. Cranial nerve XII innervates the muscles of the tongue. Lack of innervation causes ipsilateral atrophy as well as

Table 4-3. Pupillary Signs

Abnormality	Description	Etiology
Anisocoria	Less than 1-mm difference	Benign
	Dilation, iridoplegia	Parasympathetic denervation
	Pupillary constriction, reactive	Sympathetic denervation
Abnormal shape	Irregular	Syphilis (Argyll Robertson pupil)
	Oval	Brain stem lesions
Abnormal size (bilateral)	Mydriasis	Decreased parasympathetic innervation, anticholinergic drugs, bilateral retinal or optic nerve disease, congenital aniridia and ataxia (Gillespie syndrome)
	Constriction	Decreased sympathetic innervation, parasympathomimetic drugs, narcotics, pontine lesions
Decreased light reflex	Direct absent but consensual present	Unilateral afferent defect (retina or optic nerve), Marcus–Gunn pupil
	Direct and consensual absent	Efferent defect (cranial nerve III), bilateral afferent defect, anticholinergic drugs
	Direct and consensual absent but near reaction present	Argyll Robertson pupil
Oscillations	Hippus	Brain stem lesion

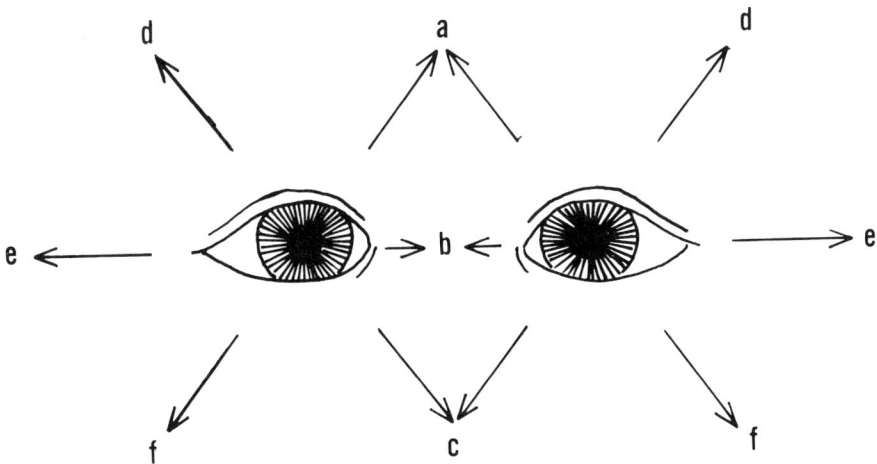

Fig. 4-3. Innervation of ocular motility: (*a*) inferior oblique, cranial nerve III; (*b*) medial rectus, cranial nerve III; (*c*) superior oblique, cranial nerve IV; (*d*) superior rectus, cranial nerve III; (*e*) lateral rectus, cranial nerve VI; (*f*) interior rectus, cranial nerve III.

Table 4-4. Disorders of Voluntary Ocular Motility

Abnormality	Description	Etiology
Forced conjugate gaze	Involuntary, persistent conjugate gaze	Partial seizure, oculogyric crisis (phenothiazines), convergence spasm
Conjugate gaze paralysis	Loss of conjugate gaze	
	Lateral	Contralateral cerebral cortex lesion, ipsilateral pons
	Vertical	Pretectal lesions
	Convergence	Midbrain lesions
Intranuclear ophthalmoplegia	Paralysis of adducting eye with lateral gaze, nystagmus of adducting eye, convergence spared	Medial longitudinal fasciculus
Monocular ophthalmoplegia	Paralysis of movement	Any third, fourth, or sixth cranial nerve lesion, Duane's syndrome, myasthenia gravis
Bilateral monocular ophthalmoplegia	Bilateral mirror ocular palsies	Increased intracranial pressure Möbius syndrome, myasthenia
Ophthalmoplegia	Paresis in all directions of gaze	Neuromuscular diseases, diffuse brain stem dysfunction, Leigh's disease, Wernicke's encephalopathy, myasthenia
Oculomotor apraxia	Inability to break fixation and redirect voluntary gaze without blinking eyes or moving head	Ataxia telangiectasia, Cogan's syndrome, Huntington's disease
Ocular dysmetria	Brief oscillation of eyes after redirecting gaze	Cerebellar lesions

Table 4-5. Involuntary Eye Movements

Movement	Description	Common Etiologies
Nystagmus	Rhythmic jerking	Brain stem, vestibular disease, drug induced, many causes
Congenital	Multidirectional, irregular	Visual loss, albinism
Dissociative	Asymmetric, varying amplitude	Spasmus nutans
Gaze evoked	Present with gaze	Cerebellar degenerative disease
Down beat	spontaneous, down directed	Cervicomedullary disease
Opsoclonia	Brief, shocklike conjugate deviations	Encephalitis, post infectious encephalopathy, occult neuroblastoma
Ocular bobbing	Sudden downward deviation, slow return to neutral	Coma, diffuse encephalopathy
Square-wave jerks	Momentary deviation from gaze	Degenerative diseases
Ocular flutter	Shimmering movements of the eyes	Brain stem and cerebellar lesions

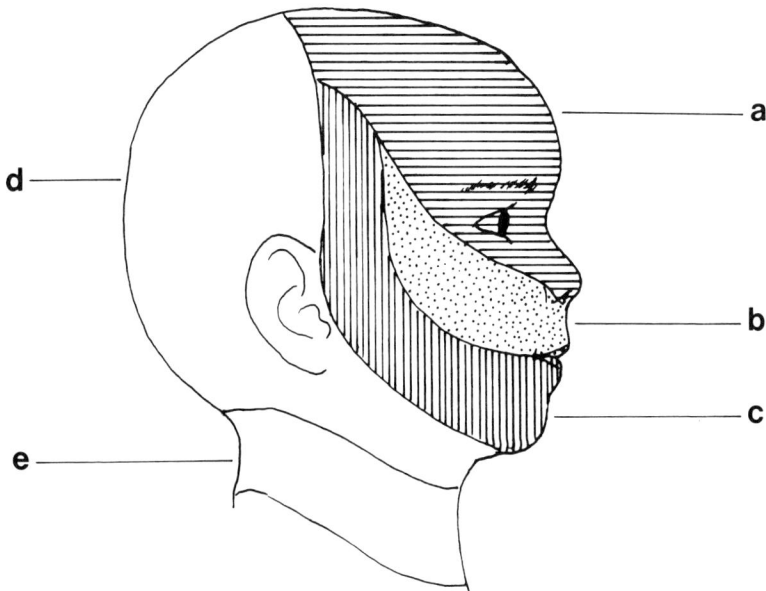

Fig. 4-4. Cutaneous innervation of the head: (*a*) cranial nerve V, ophthalmic division; (*b*) cranial nerve V, maxillary division; (*c*) cranial nerve V, mandibular division; (*d*) C-2 segmental nerve; (*e*) C-3 segmental nerve.

ipsilateral deviation upon protusion of the tongue. Furrowing of the tongue is a sign of denervation.

MOTOR SYSTEM

The motor exam begins with inspection of the muscles for involuntary movements, atrophy, and hypertrophy. The involuntary movements are summarized in Table 4-6. Tics, or habit spasms, can be partially controlled by vol-

Table 4-6. Involuntary Movements of Muscles

Fasciculations	Random contractions of groups of muscle fibers
Myokymia	Rhythmic, undulating contractions of groups of muscle fibers
Myoclonus	Random, single, shocklike contractions of muscles
Chorea	Random brief, repetitive contractions of muscles
Athetosis	Contractions of muscles that cause writhing movements
Tremor	Rhythmic contractions of muscles
Dystonia	Continuous contraction of opposing groups of muscles
Partial seizures	Coarse, semirhythmic contractions of groups of muscles
Tics	Stereotyped repetitive movements

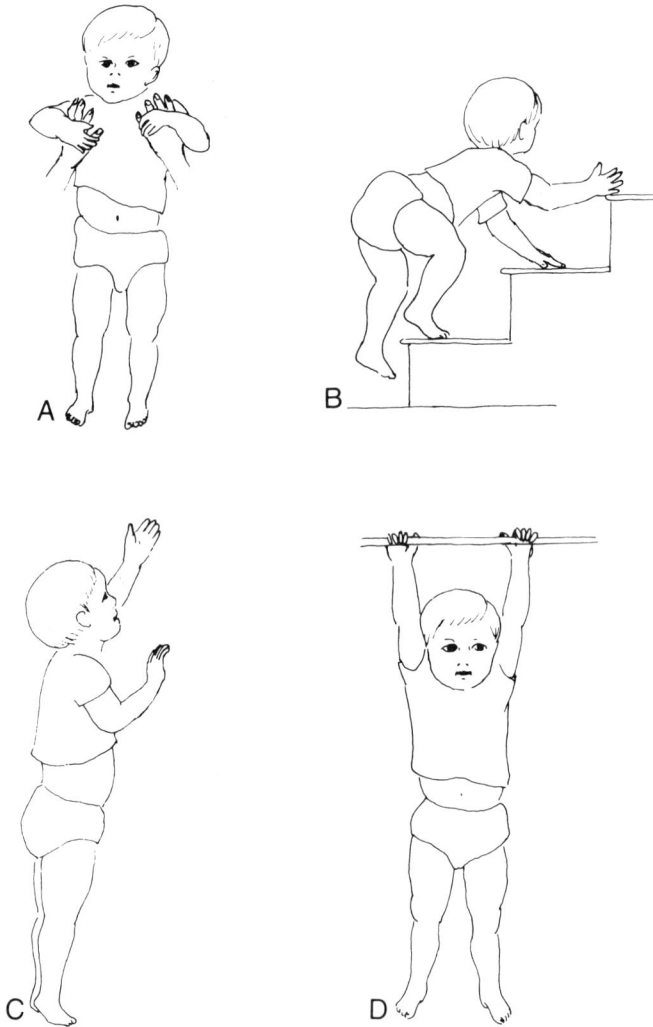

Fig. 4-5. Screening tests for muscle strength. (A) Proximal muscle of upper extremities. (B) Proximal muscles of lower extremities. (C) Distal muscles of lower extremities. (D) Distal muscles of upper extremities.

Table 4-7. Grading of Muscle Weakness

Grade	Level of Weakness
0	No movement
1	Trace movement
2	Movement with gravity only
3	Movement against gravity
4	Mild weakness
5	Normal

Table 4-8. Upper Extremity Muscle Innervation

Nerve	Anatomic Part	Muscle	Spinal Segment
Suprascapular	Shoulder girdle	Supraspinatus	C4–C6
		Infraspinatus	C4–C6
Long thoracic	Shoulder girdle	Serratus anterior	C5–C7
Axillary	Shoulder girdle	Teres minor	C4–C5
		Deltoideus	C5–C6
Musculocutaneous	Arm	Biceps brachii	C5–C6
		Coracobrachialis	C5–C7
		Brachialis	C5–C6
Median	Forearm	Pronator teres	C6–C7
		Palmaris longus	C7–T1
		Flexor digitorum sublimis	C7–T1
		Flexor digitorum profundus	C7–T1
		Flexor pollicis longus	C6–T1
		Pronator quadratus	C7–T1
	Hand	Abductor pollicis brevis	C7–T1
		Opponens pollicis	C8–T1
		Flexor pollicis brevis	C7–T1
		Lumbricales I and II	C8–T1
Radial	Arm	Trioeps (head)	C6–C8
		Anconeus	C7–C8
		Brachioradialis	C5–C6
		Extensor carpi radialis	C6–C8
	Forearm	Extensor carpi radialis Brevis	C6–C8
		Supinator	C5–C6
		Extensor digitorium communis	C6–C8
		Extensor digiti quinti	C6–C8
		Extensor carpi ulnaris	C6–C8
		Abductor pollicis longus	C7–C8
		Extensor pollicis longus	C6–C8
		Extensor pollicis brevis	C7–C8
		Extensor indicis proprius	C6–C8
Ulnar	Forearm	Flexor carpi ulnaris	C7–T1
		Flexor digitorum profundus (medial half)	C7–T1
	Hand	Flexor digiti quinti brevis	C7–T1
		Abductor digiti quinti	C8–T1
		Opponens digitis quinti	C7–T1
		Interossei	C8–T1
		Lumbricales III and IV	C8–T1
		Abductor pollicis	C8–T1
		Flexor pollicis brevis (deep part)	C7–T1

untary effort, whereas the remainder cannot. The only two involuntary movements which persist during sleep are seizures, certain types of myoclonus, and fasciculations. Inspection can also reveal focal atrophy of denervated or disused muscle, and hypertrophy of muscles in patients with certain muscular dystrophies or myotonia congenita. The consistency of a muscle on palpation often suggests an underlying disease. Chronically disused, denervated, or diseased

Table 4-9. Lower Extremity Muscle Innervation

Nerve	Anatomic Part	Muscle	Spinal Segment
Superior gluteal	Buttock	Gluteus medius	L4–S1
		Gluteus minimus	L4–S1
		Tensor fasciae latae	L4–S
Inferior gluteal	Buttock	Gluteus maximus	L4–S2
Femoral	Thigh	Iliopsoas	L1–L3
		Sartorius	L2–L3
		Quadriceps femoris	L2–L4
Obturator	Thigh	Pectineus	L2–L3
		Adductor longus	L2–L3
		Gracilis	L2–L4
		Adductor brevis	L2–L4
		Obturator externus	L3–L4
		Adductor magnus	L3–L4
Sciatic, tibial division	Thigh	Semitendinosus	L4–L5
		Biceps (long head)	S1–S2
		Semimembranosus	L4–S1
	Popliteal space (tibial nerve)	Gastrocnemius	L5–S2
		Plantaris	L4–S1
		Popliteus	L4–S1
		Soleus	L5–S2
	Leg	Tibialis posterior	L5–S1
		Flexor digitorum longus	L4–S1
		Flexor hallucis longus	L4–S1
	Foot	Abductor hallucis	S1–S2
		Abductor digiti minimi	S1–S2
		Interossei dorsales	S1–S2
Sciatic, peroneal division	Thigh	Biceps (short head)	L4–S1
	Leg (deep peroneal nerve)	Tibialis anterior	L4–L5
		Extensor hallucis longus	L4–S1
		Extensor digitorum longus Peroneus tertius	L4–S1
	Foot	Extensor digitorum brevis	L4–S1
	Leg (superficial peroneus nerve)	Peroneus longus	L5–S1
		Peroneus brevis	L5–S1

Table 4-10. Patterns of Muscle Weakness and Neurologic Localization

Pattern	Neurologic Localization
Proximal, symmetric	Myopathies, spinal muscular atrophies
Distal, symmetric	Polyneuropathy
Unilateral (hemiparesis)	Contralateral cerebral cortex, internal capsule, brain stem, ipsilateral spinal cord
Unilateral bulbar, contralateral extremities	Brain stem
Paraparesis	Myelopathy, bilateral cortical or internal capsule
Monoparesis	Plexus, nerve root, peripheral nerve

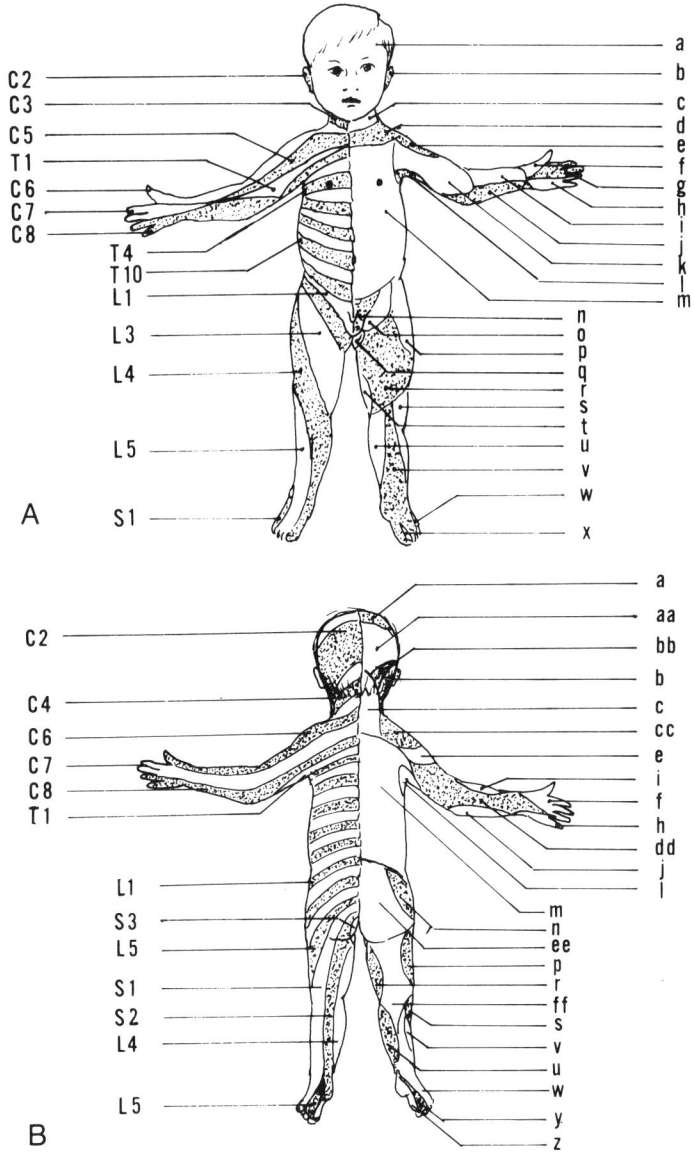

Fig. 4-6. Cutaneous sensory innervation. (A) Anterior; (B) posterior: (*a*) trigeminal n., (*b*) great auricular n., (*c*) cervical cutaneous n., (*d*) supraclavicular n., (*e*) axillary n., (*f*) radial n., (*g*) medical n., (*h*) ulnar n., (*i*) musculocutaneous n., (*j*) medial antebrachial n., (*k*) medial brachial cutaneous n., (*l*) intercostal brachial n., (*m*) thoracic cutaneous nn., (*n*) iliohypogastric n., (*o*) genitofemoral n., (*p*) lateral femoral cutaneous n., (*q*) ilioinguinal n., (*r*) anterior femoral cutaneous n., (*s*) common peroneal n., (*t*) obturator n., (*u*) saphenous n., (*v*) superficial peroneal n., (*w*) sural n., (*x*) deep peroneal n., (*y*) lateral plantar n., (*z*) medial plantar n., (*aa*) greater occipital n., (*bb*) lesser occipital n., (*cc*) posterior supraclavicular n., (*dd*) posterior brachial n., (*ee*) lumbar and sacral cutaneous nn., (*ff*) posterior femoral cutaneous n.

Table 4-11. Patterns of Sensory Loss and Neurologic Localization

Pattern	Neurologic Localization
Unilateral sensation	Contralateral thalamus, sensory cortex
Unilateral pain and touch, contralateral position and vibration	Contralateral hemicord (Brown-Séquard)
Unilateral facial, contralateral extremities	Unilateral brain stem
Bilateral segmental (pain)	Central cord (syrinx)
Unilateral segmental	Spinal root
Bilateral position and vibratory	Demyelinating neuropathy, posterior columns
Distal sensory loss	Polyneuropathy
Spinal level	Myelopathy

muscle feels flabby. Dystrophic muscle with connective tissue infiltration a has a doughy consistency. Muscles which are unusually firm are found in patients with Schwartz-Jampel syndrome, dystonias, and Isaac's syndrome.

Muscle strength is screened using a few simple maneuvers (Fig. 4-5). Distal strength is assessed by having the patient stand on his heels and toes and by having him suspend himself by his hands. Proximal strength in the lower extremities can be tested by having the older child do a deep knee bend or the younger child arise from a sitting position on the floor. In either case the child should accomplish this without using his hands for assistance. Proximal strength in the upper extremities can be determined by performing vertical suspension; all children should be able to support their weight by their proximal arms. If weakness is discovered, it is often helpful to grade the strength (Table 4-7). If there is focal weakness, a lesion in a peripheral nerve root should be suspected (Tables 4-8 and 4-9). Patterns of muscle weakness are often helpful to neurologic localization (Table 4-10).

The last part of the motor exam is determination of muscle tone. Hypotonia in the infant is discussed in Chapter 11. Hypotonia in the older child is manifested by joint laxity (floppiness). Hypertonia is resistance to stretch. Spasticity is greatest in the antigravity muscles. It is characterized by the muscles giving way after an initial resistance ("jackknife" response). Hypertonia secondary to the dystonias and other causes of muscle rigidity gives the muscle a "lead pipe" consistency in which the tone is increased throughout the full movement of a joint.

SENSORY EXAMINATION

Sensory testing is the most difficult part of the neurologic exam at any age. It is purely subjective and fraught with error. A detailed exam is not indicated unless there are complaints of sensory loss or a specific disturbance is suspected. A useful screen is the determination of the presence of pain, touch, and position (or vibratory) sensation in the hands and feet. One has to observe the young child's reaction to the stimulus. Withdrawal from a painful stimulus ensures that the peripheral nerve, but not necessarily the spinothalamic tract, is intact. A grimace or cry to pain is a better test for spinothalamic function. When performing the sensory exam it is useful to have a segmental sensory innervation diagram as well as a peripheral nerve sensory innervation diagram on hand (Fig. 4-6). The pattern of sensory loss is very important for localization (Table 4-11). These primary sensory modalities test the integrity of the peripheral nerve and spinal cord pathways to the level of the thalamus.

Sensory discrimination tests parietal lobe function and can be used if primary sensation is intact. Simultaneous touching of each side of the body will frequently disclose a unilateral sensory neglect which indicates a contralateral parietal lobe injury. It is not uncommon for young children to identify a more proximal stimulation and neglect a distal one. Frequently they will perseverate and indicate bilateral proximal stimulation even though one was distal. It is usually better, when performing simultaneous touch, to have the patient point to the area touched rather than try to name the part. Testing for graphesthesia is another useful assessment of sensory cortex function.

REFLEXES

The simplest reflex is the monosynaptic deep tendon reflex, which depends upon a sensory organ sensitive to stretch, an afferent limb through the peripheral nerve to the spinal cord, a single synapse on the anterior horn cell, and an efferent limb from the anterior horn cell to the muscle which causes reflex muscle contraction. Table 4-12 lists the usual tendon reflexes that are tested with their peripheral nerve and spinal segmental innervation. Grading of reflexes is outlined in Table 4-13 Abdominal and cremasteric reflexes are normally present but are suppressed by recent upper or lower motor neuron lesions. Some reflexes, such as the Babinski sign, are normally absent in the older child but are present with upper motor neuron lesions. Other reflexes, such as the parachute reflex, are an integral part of development and are useful for testing symmetry of the motor system.

Table 4-12. Innervation of Deep Tendon Reflexes

Tendon	Peripheral Nerve	Spinal Segment
Achilles	Sural	S1–S2
Patellar	Femoral	L3–L4
Biceps	Musculocutaneous	C5–C6
Brachioradialis	Radial	C5–C6
Triceps	Axillary	C6–C8

Table 4-13. Grading of Reflexes

Grade	Reflex
0	Absent
1	Trace
2	Normal
3	Brisk
4	Clonus

Table 4-14. Mental Status Testing
Level of consciousness
Orientation
Affect and behavior
Memory
Language
General knowledge and social skills
School performance and/or developmental assessment

COORDINATION

Except for higher cortical function, coordination changes more with age than does any other neurologic function. The newborn infant is highly un-coordinated, to the extent that there are very few skilled movements aside from sucking. As the child matures, coordination improves. Until 3 years of age a child's gait remains unsteady, which makes diagnosing incoordination in the young child difficult. In the older child traditional methods of testing for gait, heel-to-toe walking, finger-to-nose, heel-to-shin, and rapid alternating movements are sufficient to screen for disorders of coordination. In the younger child, the history of developmental achievement and observation of movements are more useful than actual testing. Observing the child reaching for an object such as his bottle or pacifier or watching him as he sits or walks alone will reveal much information. Ataxia in the preambulatory child can be seen as titubation, which is a dysrhythmic truncal and head tremor when the child tries to sit.

Part of the coordination exam includes the Romberg test. This procedure tests many functions. If the child is cooperative, having him stand with his hands outstretched and eyes closed will reveal involuntary movements, posterior column signs (falling), and muscle weakness. This latter is seen by slow drifts of the arm, usually in a down and out position. It must be remembered that few children below the age of 6 can maintain their arms outstretched with no chorealike movements.

MENTAL STATUS

The neurologic exam is not complete without a comment on the mental status (Table 4-14). One should especially note the level of consciousness and, in the older child, orientation to person, place, and time. Alterations in these functions suggest an organic brain disorder. Higher cortical function is tested by the quality of the child's language (both verbal and receptive), testing memory, and obtaining a rough idea of intelligence as determined by simple problem-solving questions. Finally, the child's social skills can be determined by how cooperative he is for his age and whether his behavior is appropriate for the setting. Much of this information can be obtained during the introductory conversation and through reviewing school performance. A developmental assessment is an integral part of the neurologic examination in a patient suspected of having a neurologic disease.

SELECTED READINGS

Brett EM: Normal development and neurological examination beyond the newborn period. p. 24. In Brett EM (ed): Pediatric Neurology. Churchill Livingstone, Edinburgh, 1985

Brown SB, Sher PK, Wright FS: Neurologic examination in children. p. 9. In Swaiman KF, Wright FS (eds): The Practice of Pediatric Neurology. 2nd Ed. CV Mosby, St. Louis, 1982

Dodge PR: Neurologic history and examination. p. 1. In Farmer TW (ed): Pediatric Neurology. Harper & Row, New York, 1964

Paine RS: Neurologic examination in infants and children. Pediatr Clin North Am 7:41–59, 1960

SECTION 2

Neurodiagnostic Procedures

Neurodiagnostic tests and procedures are an extension of the history and physical examination. The selective use of these tests is essential in the practice of neurology. The tests are not inexpensive and can be associated with some risk; therefore they should be used judiciously. As for the neurologic exam, these tests must take into account the patient's age and maturation. This is particularly so for newborn.

The three basic categories of neurodiagnostic tests and procedures are electrophysiologic tests, neuroimaging, and examination of body tissue and fluids.

5

ELECTROPHYSIOLOGIC PROCEDURES

Table 5-1 summarizes the electrophysiologic tests which are available at most facilities. The indications listed for the tests are those which are generally accepted; however, other additional indications are used by some clinicians.

ELECTROENCEPHALOGRAPHY

The EEG measures, amplifies, and records the electrical activity from the surface of the brain, using scalp electrodes. Figure 5-1 demonstrates the general principle of EEG. The cerebral cortex is oriented in a columnar manner, with the cell bodies toward the interior and the arborization of the dendrites toward the exterior. Excitation of the dendrites causes a surface negativity, thus establishing a potential difference or voltages from more positive areas. Inhibitory influences cause the reverse. An EEG electrode placed over the brain surface measures the surface voltage charge and compares it to a reference electrode. If the active electrode is relatively more negative than the reference electrode, then a negative wave is recorded by an upward deflection of the EEG pen. A positive charge is detected as a downward deflection. The farther away the recording electrode is from the voltage source, the more attenuated the signal. The reference electrode can be inert or constant, in which case the input is termed *monopolar*. If the reference is also an active electrode, then a bipolar recording is obtained.

The EEG electrodes are placed about the head in a standardized pattern (Fig. 5-2). Most EEG devices are capable of recording 8 to 16 simultaneous inputs. The pattern of electrodes (montage) varies from laboratory to laboratory, but normally 6 to 12 montages are recorded using both monopolar and bipolar derivations. Over a 20- to 60-minute period the entire available surface of the brain can be sampled.

Recognizing a normal recording is the most important part of interpreting the child's EEG. It is beyond the scope of this book to discuss the interpretation in detail. Figure 5-3 illustrates the normal sleep EEG at different ages. The most significant change in the sleep EEG from infancy to maturity is the development of continuous organization of the record. The development of a posterior dominant rhythm (alpha activity) is the most important change during the awake state (Fig. 5-4).

Table 5-1. Major Indications for Commonly Used Electrodiagnostic Tests

Electrophysiologic Test	Abbreviation	Major Indications
Electroencephalography	EEG	Seizures, sleep disorders, brain death
Brain stem auditory evoked response	BAER	Demyelinating diseases, audiometry, brain stem pathology, brain death
Visual evoked response	VER	Demyelinating diseases, vision loss
Somatosensory evoked response	SER	Demyelinating diseases, myelopathy
Electroretinography	ERG	Retinal degeneration
Electromyography	EMG	Neuromuscular diseases
Nerve conduction velocities	NCV	Neuropathies, myasthenias

Abnormalities in the EEG are basically of two types. The first is paroxysmal discharges, which are helpful in the diagnosis of seizure disorders. The second is abnormalities in the organization of the background activity. Generalized slowing or disorganization of the EEG is frequently seen in diffuse encephalopathies. Focal slowing may indicate an underlying structural lesion of the brain. The different montages are used to locate the source of paroxysmal discharges or focal slowing. Figure 5-5 shows some examples of abnormal EEGs.

EVOKED RESPONSES

The microcomputer has made it possible to determine the brain's response to sensory stimuli. A stimulus is given and the evoked neural response is measured at specific times. Hundreds of evoked potentials are obtained and averaged.

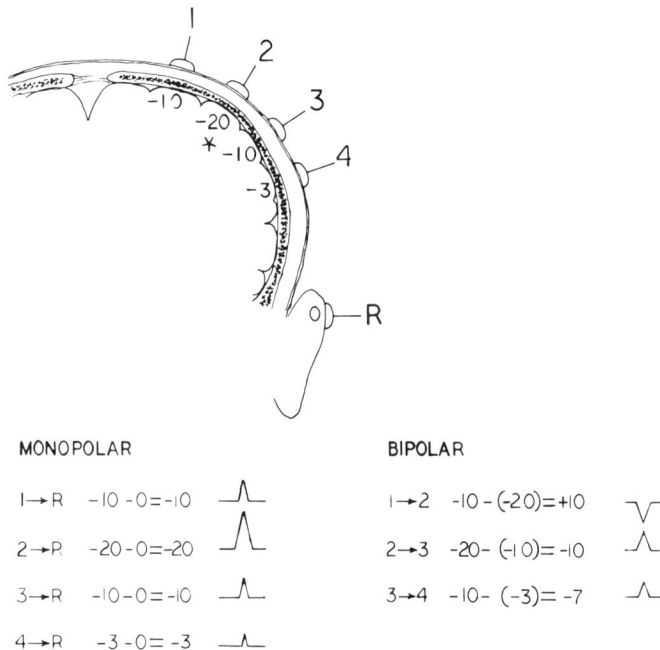

MONOPOLAR

$1 \rightarrow R$ $-10 - 0 = -10$

$2 \rightarrow R$ $-20 - 0 = -20$

$3 \rightarrow R$ $-10 - 0 = -10$

$4 \rightarrow R$ $-3 - 0 = -3$

BIPOLAR

$1 \rightarrow 2$ $-10 - (-20) = +10$

$2 \rightarrow 3$ $-20 - (-10) = -10$

$3 \rightarrow 4$ $-10 - (-3) = -7$

Fig. 5-1. General principle of EEG. Electrodes 1 through 4 record the surface negativity (in millivolts), which varies inversely with the square of the distance from the source. (The asterisk represents a discharge in the cortex.) Monopolar and bipolar EEG recordings are illustrated.

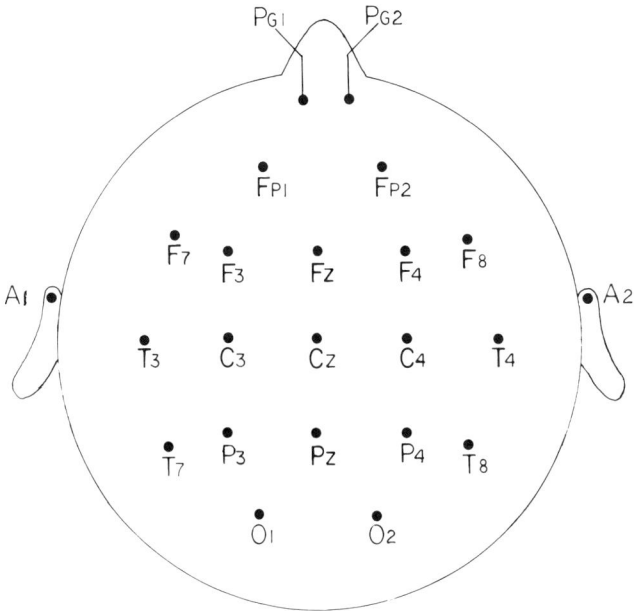

Fig. 5-2. Standard electrode placement for EEG.

A time-locked response will show a consistent relationship to the stimulus, whereas random background activity will be averaged to baseline. The amplitude of the response as well as the latency from the stimulus can be measured. The evoked response therefore gives a relatively sensitive and quantitative examination of those sensory pathways that can be studied. Evoked responses are relatively delayed at birth but with myelinization during maturation, adult values are reached by 1 year of age.

The most sensitive method for measuring the visual evoked response (VER) is using pattern reversals. Usually a checkerboard of black and white squares is flashed with reversal of the pattern 8 to 10 times per second. Simultaneous EEG electrodes record the evoked response. A typical tracing is shown in Figure 5-6. The P100 latency is the most important measurement and probably represents the evoked potential generated in the occipital striate and association cortices. Each eye is stimulated separately. Because of the projection of each optic nerve to both occipital lobes, differences between the P100 values of each eye must reflect disease anterior to the optic chiasm. If the P100 is slowed in both eyes, then defects can exist anywhere in the visual pathway. In general, demyelinating disorders prolong the latency. Cortical diseases or axonal disorders cause a reduction in the amplitude of the evoked response. If a child is unable to fixate on the pattern reversal screen, then the data will not be reliable. Flash evoked responses measured by using a strobe light are not as accurate and should be interpreted with caution. In infants and children with an inability to fixate (e.g., nystagmus and cataracts) the results are also unreliable.

The brain stem auditory evoked response (BAER) is obtained using the same

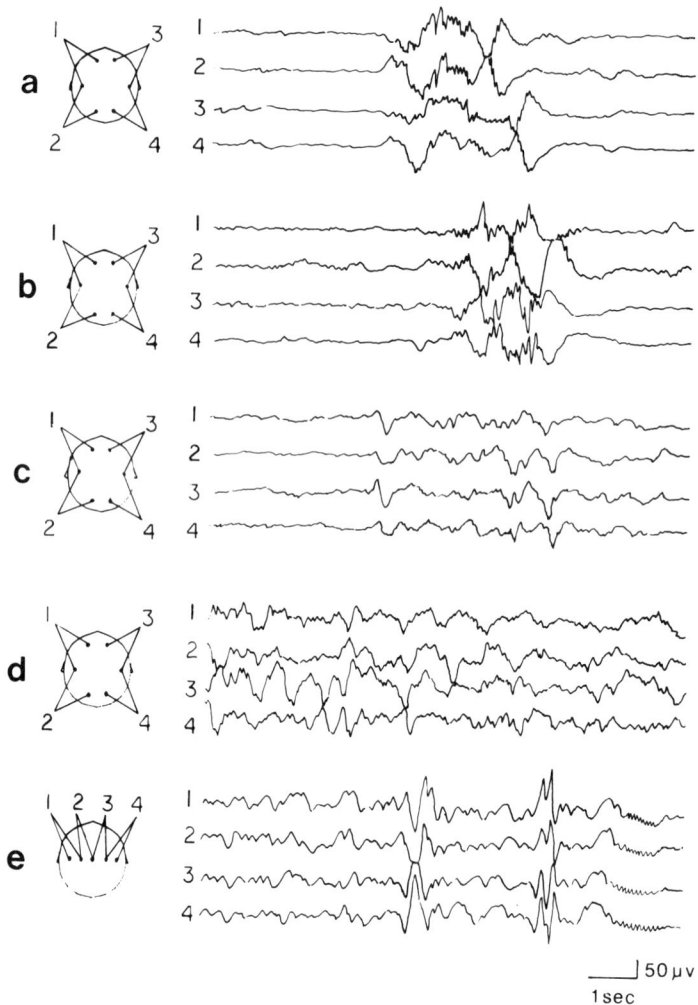

Fig. 5-3. Maturation of the sleep EEG with age: (*a*) 30-week premature infant with bursts of slow waves and low-amplitude fast activity ("delta brushes") on a background of relative electrical silence, (*b*) 34-week premature infant with a discontinuous record and periodic discharge of a variety of wave forms, (*c*) term infant with a continuous record and bursts of slow activity (trace alternant), (*d*) 3-month infant with continuous slow waves, (*e*) 3-year infant with vertex waves and sleep spindles.

principle as the VER. The patient is fitted with earphones, a series of clicks is presented to one ear, and the neural response is recorded over the vertex. A masking noise is presented to the opposite ear. A total of 1,000 or more such clicks are necessary in order to get an averaged response. The wave forms are generated from the peripheral and central auditory pathways. Seven vertex positive waves can be obtained; however, the sixth and seventh waves are usually

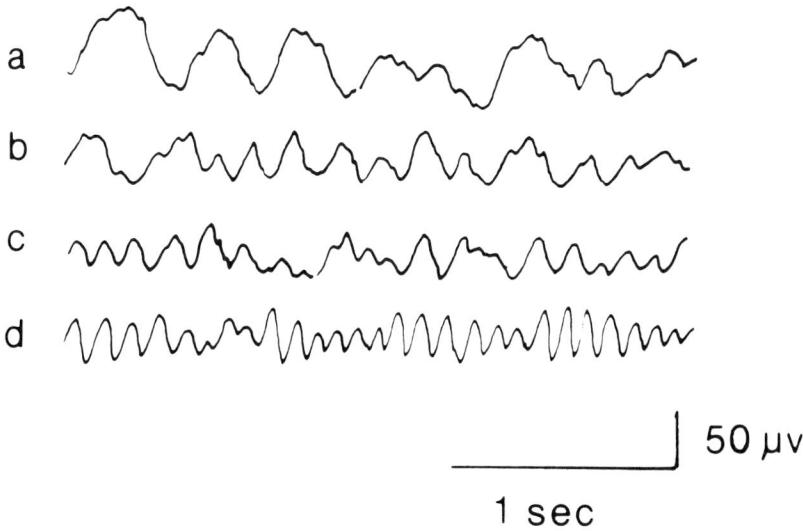

Fig. 5-4. Development of the posterior dominant rhythm: (*a*) newborn, (*b*) 6 months, (*c*) 4 years, (*d*) 10 years.

not clinically significant. Figure 5-7 shows a typical BAER and structures which generate the positive waves.

There are three clinical applications of the BAER in childhood. The first is to investigate the peripheral hearing apparatus by increasing the intensity of the clicks to find the threshold for evoked response. It is a very sensitive method of determining hearing in the young child and does not require active participation. A prolonged latency between waves I and III or I and IV is a sensitive test for disease of the acoustic nerve. The second application is the study of the brain stem structures. For this the clicks are given at an intensity of 65 to 70 above threshold. This technique is a sensitive indicator of the integrity of the auditory pathways and, because of their relationships to other structures, gives some information about the brain stem in general. Patients with intrinsic disease of the brain stem, such as demyelinating, degenerative, or structural abnormalities, have increased latencies between waves and reduced amplitudes of these waves. Another application of the BAER is the determination of brain death. If wave I is present, implying an intact hearing apparatus, then the absence of waves II through V indicates brain death. These waves will be present even with barbiturate coma.

Somatosensory evoked responses (SERs) operate on the same principle as the BAER. In usual practice a peripheral nerve is electrically stimulated and electrodes are placed near the generator sources along the sensory pathway. In the upper extremities Erb's point is used and in the lower extremities electrodes near the conus medullaris are used. The latencies of these peaks from the stimulus can vary, depending on the temperature of the limb and the presence of peripheral nerve disease. However, latencies from these points to other points

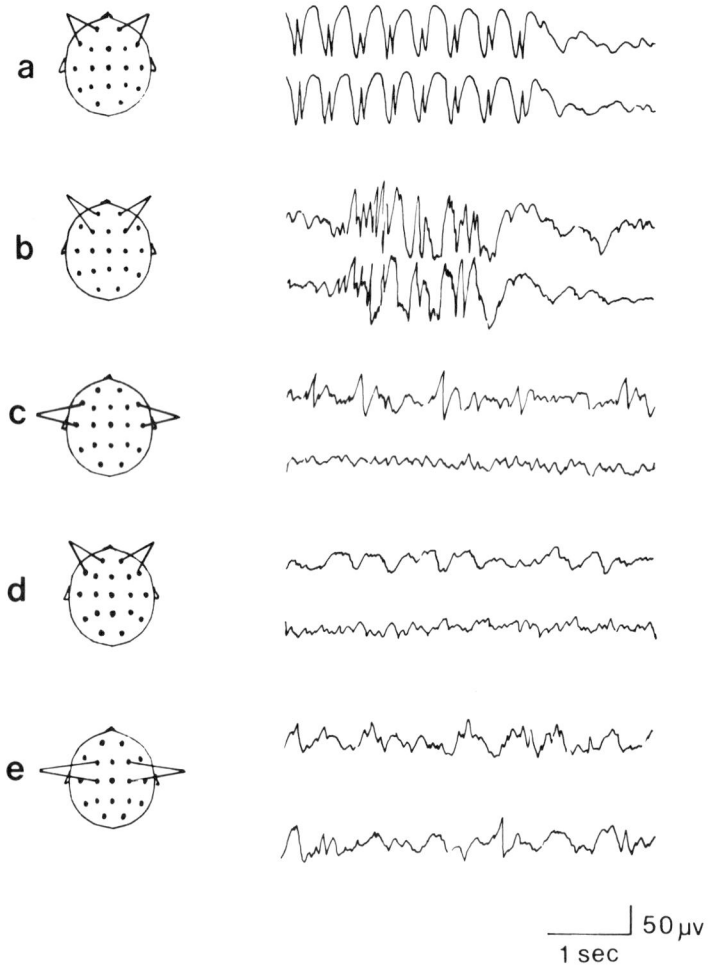

Fig. 5-5. Common EEG abnormalities in children. The bipolar leads are demonstrated on the left and the left-sided EEG recording is represented by the top tracing in each example. (*a*) Petit mal seizure (absence). (*b*) Generalized motor seizures (grand mal). (*c*) Partial seizure (left temporal lobe). (*d*) Focal slowing (left frontal tumor). (*e*) hypsarrhythmia.

along the somatosensory pathway remain relatively constant. Measuring the interpeak latencies provides the physiologic information concerning the integrity of the somatosensory pathway. As in the BAER, the SER is relatively resistant to alterations, with the exceptions of demyelinating or structural diseases. The application of SERs in children is a developing field. At present it has adjunctive value in the diagnosis of demyelinating diseases of the nervous system and structural abnormalities of the cord. Its application to operative procedures is particularly promising in that it gives a continuous physiologic indication of cord function during surgery on the spinal cord.

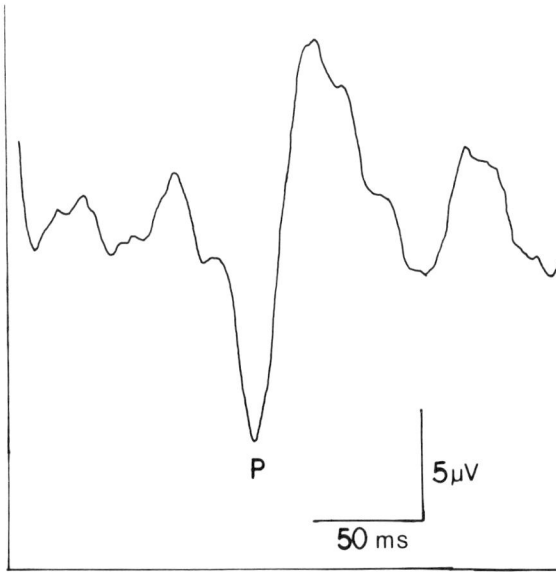

Fig. 5-6. Visual evoked response. P indicates the P100 latency.

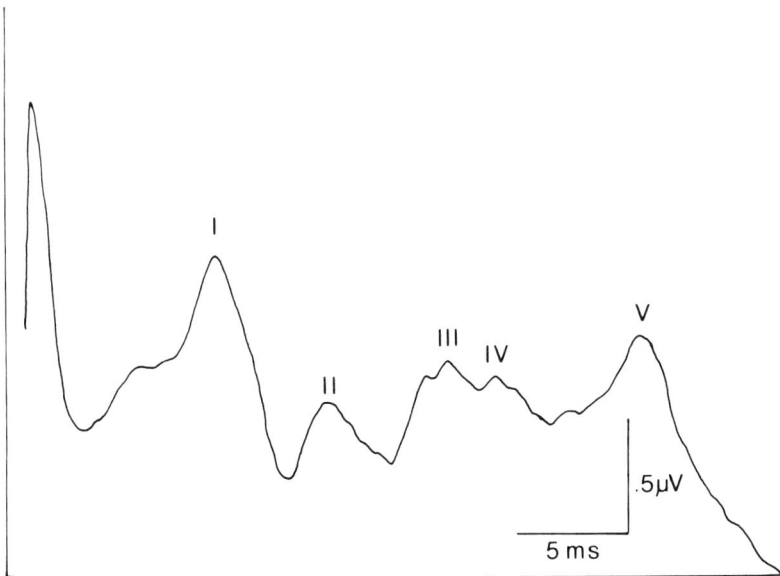

Fig. 5-7. Brain stem auditory evoked response: (I) acoustic nerve, (II) cochlear nuclei, (III) superior olivary complex, (IV) lateral lemniscus, (V) inferior colliculus.

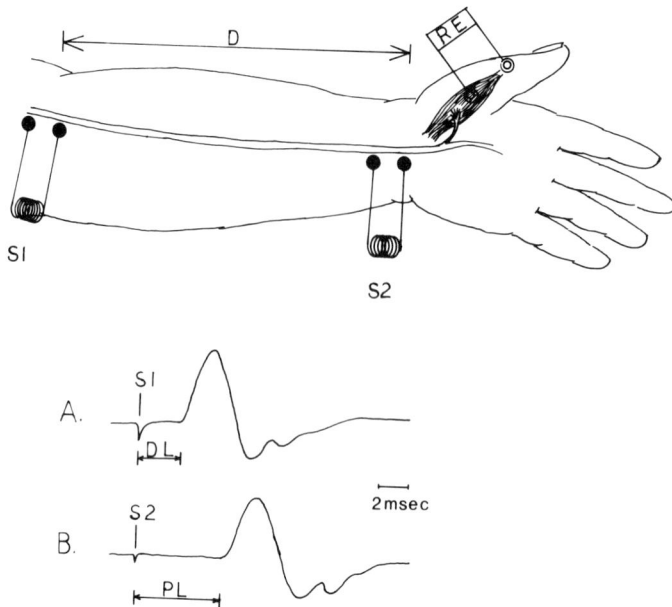

Fig. 5-8. Measurement of motor nerve conduction velocity. The top figure illustrates the method for measuring the median nerve conduction velocity. The recording electrode (RE) is placed over the thenar eminence and the nerve stimulated proximally (S1) and distally (S2). The latencies are displayed on an oscilloscope below. The distal latency (DL) shown in (A), is subtracted from the proximal latency (PL) in (B). The difference (T) is divided over the distance (D) between S1 and S2, and velocity = D/T.

ELECTRORETINOGRAPHY

Electroretinography is the measurement of the electrical activity of the retinal ganglion cells. Electrodes are placed around the eyes and a strobe light is flashed before the eyes. Latencies and amplitudes are recorded as described above. Electroretinography is particularly helpful in the evaluation of retinal degenerations and certain storage diseases which affect the ganglion cells. Abnormalities can be detected before funduscopic abnormalities are seen.

Table 5-2. Motor Nerve Conduction Velocities from Birth to Maturity [a]

Age	Ulnar	Median	Peroneal
1 week	32.3 ± 4.4	29.0 ± 3.7	29.0 ± 4.3
4 months	46.6 ± 8.5	33.9 ± 8.7	36.7 ± 7.3
1 year	49.9 ± 6.8	40.0 ± 5.3	48.2 ± 8.3
3 years	59.8 ± 8.1	49.5 ± 5.9	53.7 ± 8.1
8 years	65.4 ± 8.5	58.3 ± 5.4	57.5 ± 6.9
16 years	67.6 ± 6.0	63.9 ± 5.7	57.6 ± 7.3
Adult	63.2 ± 6.4	63.0 ± 5.6	56.0 ± 5.2

[a] Values in m/sec ± SD.

(Data from Gamstorp I: Normal conduction velocities at the ulnar, median and peroneal nerves in infancy, childhood and adolescence. Acta Pediatr Scand, suppl., 146:68–76, 1963.)

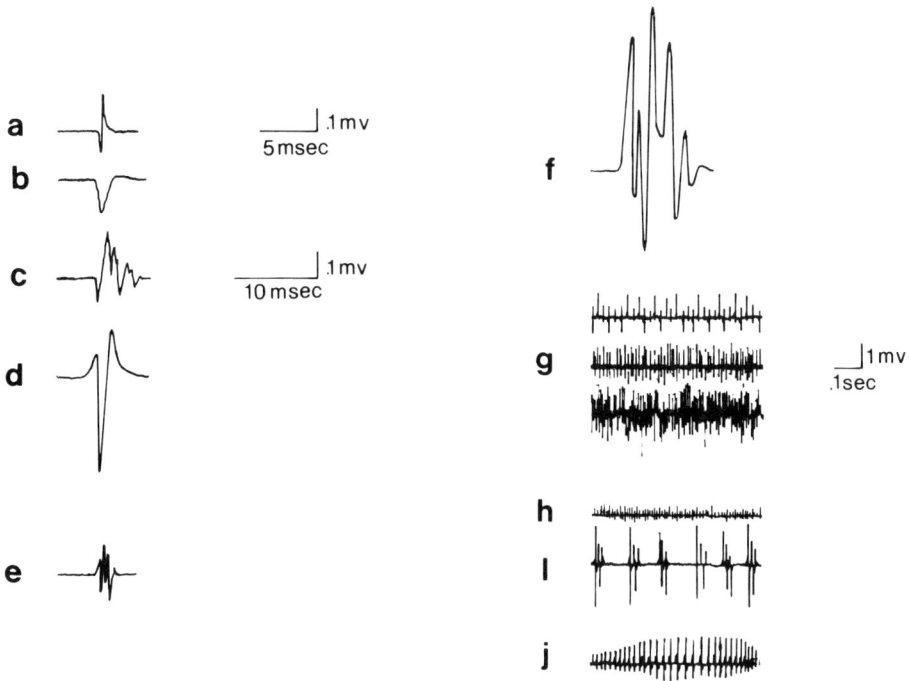

Fig. 5-9. Electromyographic abnormalities. Abnormal spontaneous activities are illustrated in the top three figures. Fibrillations (*a*) and positive sharp waves (*b*) appear in denervating disease after 2 to 3 weeks. Fasciculations (*c*) are usually found in anterior horn cell diseases. A single normal muscle action potential (*d*) is recorded with exertion. Myopathic muscle action potentials are illustrated in *e* and a prolonged polyphasic potential seen in chronic neuropathic disease is illustrated in *f*. Increasing exertion causes increased recruitment of muscle action potentials in the normal patient (*g*). Early recruitment with minimal exertion is illustrated in *h* from a patient with myopathy. Decreased recruitment at full exertion is shown in *i* from a patient with chronic denervation. Myotonia is illustrated in *j* and would cause a "dive bomber" sound on the audio amplication.

ELECTROMYOGRAPHY AND MEASUREMENT OF NERVE CONDUCTION VELOCITY

Electromyography and measurement of nerve conduction velocities are essential parts of the evaluation of neuromuscular diseases. The principle of measuring motor nerve conduction velocities is demonstrated in Figure 5-8. Sensory latencies are obtained by recording directly over the sensory nerve. Conduction velocities are affected primarily by the integrity of the large myelinated fibers. Demyelinating diseases reduce the conduction velocity; therefore measuring conduction velocities and distal latencies is important in the evaluation of neuropathies. Conduction velocities are affected by age and Table 5-2 shows the changes in the conduction velocity of motor nerves from infancy to maturity.

Electromyography consists of inserting a needle electrode into the muscle. The electrode is a coaxial needle with a central active electrode insulated from a surrounding reference electrode. The voltage difference measured between the two is amplified and displayed on an oscilloscope. Recordings are made at rest and with exertion. At rest the muscle is normally electrically silent. On exertion muscle action potentials are recorded. With increasing exertion, more and more motor units are recruited. In normal muscle at full contraction, individual muscle action potentials cannot be observed on the oscilloscope, which causes a complete interference pattern. With chronic denervation there is reinnervation of muscle fibers by surviving axons. Because of the expanded motor unit, many more muscle fibers contract when a single anterior horn cell discharges. This causes the muscle action potential to have multiple phases, prolonged duration, and usually greater amplitude. During contraction fewer motor units are available to be recruited so that a complete interference pattern is not achieved.

In primary muscle disease the number of motor units is intact but the contraction of each muscle fiber is diminished. The muscle action potential is therefore decreased in size, is shorter in duration, and frequently has multiple phases. These brief small-amplitude polyphasic potentials are characteristic of many myopathies. With voluntary contraction more motor units are recruited than normal to give the same amount of work, which causes an increased interference during the early phases of contraction. This early recruitment pattern is also an indication of muscle disease. Figure 5-9 illustrates some electromyographic abnormalities.

Electrophysiology is also used in the diagnosis of myasthenic disorders. The exact mechanism by which this is determined is beyond the scope of this book. In general, a recording electrode is placed over the muscle and the motor nerve supplying that muscle is repetitively stimulated. A patient with myasthenia will show a decrement in the muscle action potential amplitude with repetitive stimulation. A number of maneuvers, such as ischemic exercise, can be performed to enhance this abnormality.

SELECTED READINGS

Davis SL, Aminoff MJ, Berg BO: Brainstem auditory evoked potentials in children with brainstem or cerebellar dysfunction. Arch Neurol 42:156–160, 1985

Lary S, Briassoulis G, de Vries L et al: Hearing threshold in preterm and term infants by auditory brainstem response. J Pediatr 107:593–599, 1985

Lee SI: Electroencephalography in infantile and childhood epilepsy. In Dreifuss FE (ed): Pediatric Epileptology: Classification and Management of Seizures in the Child. John Wright, Boston, 1985

Wagner AL, Buchthal F: Motor and sensory conduction in infancy and childhood: reappraisal. Dev Med Child Neurol 14:189–216, 1972

Weiss IP, Barnet AB: Auditory, visual, and somatosensory evoked potentials in pediatric diagnosis. Clin Proc Child Hosp Nat Med Cent 35:71–84, 1979

6

NEUROIMAGING

Neuroimaging is a rapidly expanding field. Computer application to traditional radiology and the development of new techniques for brain imaging has greatly expanded diagnostic capabilities.

RADIOGRAPHY

The radiograph of the skull is the oldest neuroimaging technique. Although it has been largely replaced by computered tomography (CT) and other techniques in the diagnosis of diseases of the brain, skull radiographs are still helpful in the evaluation of primary diseases and conditions which affect the bone, particularly trauma and malformations, which will be discussed elsewhere in this book.

Because a skull radiograph is more likely to be interpreted by pediatricians than other neuroimaging techniques, this technique will be covered in more detail. The infant's skull is illustrated in Figure 6-1. There is much variation in the closure of sutures and fontanelles (Table 6-1). By 2 years of age the skull has radiographic findings of inner and outer tables, diploic spaces and veins, and vascular and dural markings. A number of abnormalities seen on skull radiographs can be associated with neurologic disease (Table 6-2). Intracranial calcifications in the infant are almost always pathologic. Ultrasound and CT are more sensitive tests for intracranial calcifications. Although the pineal gland is rarely calcified in children, a lateral shift of this structure on radiographs suggests a mass lesion. Table 6-3 lists the occurrence of physiologic intracranial calcifications that do not usually represent disease. Table 6-4 classifies pathologic calcifications and their incidence. Causes for lytic skull lesions are listed in Table 6-5 and abnormalities of the pituitary sella are listed in Table 6-6.

Radiographs of the spine are indicated in the evaluation of spinal trauma, infections and neoplasms involving vertebral bodies, malformations of the spine, and certain metabolic diseases (Table 6-7). Widening of the intrapendicular distance can be associated with intraspinal masses and malformations. Table 6-8 shows maximum intrapendicular distances in children.

ANGIOGRAPHY

Since the widespread use of CT, arteriography has played a lesser role in the diagnosis of intracranial disease. At the present time, the primary indication for arteriography is in the evaluation of vascular disease and both the arterial

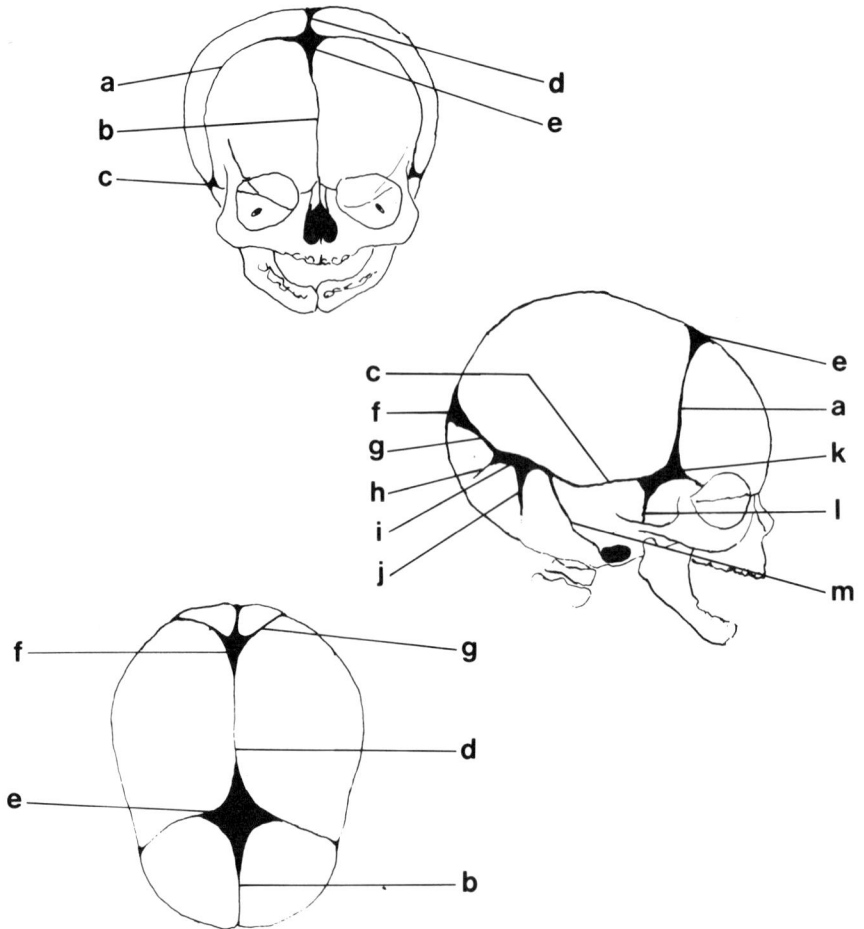

Fig. 6-1. Sutures and fontanelles of the infant skull: (a) coronal suture, (b) metopic suture, (c) squamosal suture, (d) sagittal suture, (e)anterior fontanelle, (f) posterior fontanelle, (g) lambdoidal suture, (h) mendosal suture, (i) posterolateral suture, (j) exoccipto-occipital synchondrosis, (k) anterolateral fontanel, (l) occipitosphenoidal synchondrosis, (m) petrosquamous suture. (Adapted from Harwood-Nash DC, Fitz CZ: Neuroradiology in Infants and Children. CV Mosby, St. Louis, 1976.)

Table 6-1. Closure of Sutures and Fontanelles

Suture	Time of Closure
Mendosal	0–4 weeks
Metopic	18–36 months
Occipital	24–36 months
Occipitosphenoidal	Puberty
Coronal	Adulthood
Lambdoidal	Adulthood
Sagittal	Adulthood

Table 6-2. Radiographic Abnormalities of the Skull

Abnormal size
  Macrocephaly (Table 3-1)
  Microcephaly (Table 3-2)
Suture synostosis
  Sagittal: scaphocephaly (dolichocephaly)
  Coronal: brachycephaly
  Bilateral sagittal and coronal: oxycephaly
  Unilateral sagittal and coronal: plagiocephaly
  Pansynostosis: microcrania
Split sutures: increased intracranial pressure
Calcifications
  Physiologic (Table 6-3)
  Pathologic (Table 6-4)
Lytic lesions (Table 6-5)
Sclerotic lesions
  Meningioma
  Healing infection
  Focal thickening over focal cerebral atrophy (Davidoff–Dyke syndrome)
  Healing histiocytosis X
Abnormalities of pituitary sella (Table 6-6)
Wormian bones
  Chronic hydrocephalus
  Cleidocranial dysostosis
  Osteogenesis imperfecta
  Healing rickets
  Hypothyroidism
  Hypophosphatasia
  Pyknodysostosis
  Normal
Skull thickening
  Arrested hydrocephalus
  Cerebral atrophy
  Myotonic dystrophy
  Hypervitaminosis D
  Renal osteodystrophy
  Chronic anemias
  Mucopolysaccharidoses
  Osteopetrosis
  Treated rickets
  Hyperphosphatasia
  Cranioskeletal dysplasias
Basilar impression and platybasia
  Primary: fusion of atlas to occiput
  Secondary
    Rickets
    Osteomalacia
    Osteogenesis imperfecta
    Achondroplasia

and venous phases should be studied for optimal visualization. Arteriography is indicated for suspected arteriovenous malformations, aneurysms, and other vascular malformations, and children with unexplained cerebrovascular accidents should undergo arteriography. In some instances, arteriography is indicated to visualize the blood supply prior to the excision of tumors or other masses. Figure 6-2 illustrates the major cerebral arteries.

Table 6-3. Occurrence of Physiologic Calcifications

Location	Incidence	Age of Occurrence
Dura		
Falx	Occasional	3 yr onward
Tentorium	Rare	6 yr onward
Interclinoid ligament	Common	Infancy onward
Petroclinoid ligament	Occasional	5 yr onward
Arachnoid granulations	Rare	6 yr onward
Dural plaques	Rare	6 yr onward
Pineal and habenula	Occasional	10 yr onward
Choroid		
Glomera	Occasional	3 yr onward
Plexus	Rare	12 yr onward
Pituitary	Rare	Infancy onward

(From Harwood-Nash DC, Fitz CR: Neuroradiology in Infants and Children. CV Mosby, St. Louis, 1976.)

Digital subtraction angiography is a newer method for the evaluation of large vessel disease. Plain radiographs are made of the head and neck and the image is digitalized and fed into a computer. Contrast material is then injected intravenously and the radiograph repeated. The new radiographic data is fed into the computer and the plain image data are subtracted, leaving an enhanced contrast image of the vasculature. Because small quantities of contrast material and smaller catheters are used, there is much less risk to the patient than with traditional angiography. All but the smallest vessels can be visualized, especially in the small infant who has a thinner skull.

Table 6-4. Pathologic Intracranial Calcifications in Children

	Incidence	
Entity	Among all calcifications	Within entity
Neoplastic		
Craniopharyngioma	Common	70%
Astrocytoma	Occasional	7%
Ependymoma	Occasional	6%
Teratodermoid	Occasional	Common
Other neoplasms		
Meningioma	Rare	Common
Oligodendroglioma	Rare	Common
Choroid plexus neoplasm	Rare	Occasional
Medulloblastoma	Rare	Common
Corpus callosum lipoma	Rare	Common
Secondary retinoblastoma	Rare	Occasional
Pituitary adenoma	Rare	Rare
Chordoma	Rare	Rare
Meningeal leukemia	Rare	Rare
Meningeal neuroblastoma	Rare	Rare
Undifferentiated neuroectodermal neoplasm	Rare	Occasional
Postradiation calcification	Occasional	Occasional

(Continued)

Table 6-4. (*Continued*)

Entity	Incidence	
	Among all calcifications	Within entity
Vascular		
Subdural hematoma	Common	10%
Extradural hematoma	Rare	Rare
Intracranial hematoma	Rare	Rare
Arteriovenous malformation	Occasional	20%
Vein of Galen anomaly	Rare	Rare
Aneurysm	Rare	Rare
Vascular hamartoma	Rare	Rare
Therapeutic radiation	Rare	Rare
Unknown	Rare	Rare
Endocrine		
Hyperparathyroidism	Rare	Occasional
Hypoparathyroidism	Rare	53%
Pseudohypoparathyroidism	Rare	45%
Pseudo-pseudohypoparathyroidism	Rare	Rare
Toxic		
Carbon monoxide	Rare	Occasional
Lead poisoning	Rare	Occasional
Vitamin D intoxication	Rare	Rare
Hypercalcemia	Rare	Occasional
Methotrexate (intrathecal)	Rare	Unknown
Developmental		
Tuberous sclerosis	Common	47%
Sturge-Weber syndrome	Common	50%
Neurofibromatosis	Rare	Less than 1%
Cockayne's syndrome	Rare	Common
Fahr's syndrome	Rare	100%
Lipoid proteinosis	Rare	Common
Miscellaneous familial types	Rare	Common
Basal cell nevus syndrome	Rare	Common
Lissencephaly	Rare	Rare
Wilson's disease	Rare	Rare
Inflammatory		
Cytomegalic inclusion disease	Common	40%
Other viral diseases		
Herpes simplex	Rare	Occasional
Congenital rubella	Rare	Rare
Polioencephalitis	Rare	Rare
Congenital toxoplasmosis	Common	60%
Bacterial infections		
Pyogenic meningitis	Rare	Rare
Tuberculous meningitis	Rare	50%
Tuberculoma	Rare	1% to 8%
Other parasitic infections		
Cysticercosis	Rare	Occasional
Paragonimiasis	Rare	40%
Echinococcosis	Rare	Rare
Trichinosis	Rare	Rare
Coccidioidomycosis	Rare	Rare

(Modified from Harwood-Nash DC, Fitz CR: Neuroradiology in Infants and Children. CV Mosby, St. Louis, 1976.)

Table 6-5. Lytic Lesions of the Skull

Developmental
  Parietal foramina
  Parietal thinning
  Venous lakes
  Pacchionian granulations
  Persistent fontanelles
  Large sinus grooves
  Large emissary foramina
Congenital
  Encephalocele
  Craniolacunia
  Epidermoids and dermoids
  Frontal cranium bifidum
  Hemangiomas of the diploic space
  Neurofibromatosis
Traumatic
  Burr holes and small craniotomy sites
  Local depressed fractures
  Growing fractures
  Radiation necrosis
  Cephalohematomas
  Coronal suture subdural tap sites
Inflammatory
  Osteomyelitis
  Sinus mucocele
Hematologic
  Leukemia, local involvement
  Histiocytosis X
Neoplastic
  Neuroblastomas
  Contiguous cerebral neoplasms
  Sarcomas of the dura and vault
  Aneurysmal bone cysts
  Rhabdomyosarcoma
  Lymphosarcoma
  Meningiomas
Miscellaneous
  Reticuloses (Gaucher's disease)
  Metabolic: hyperparathyroidism and "brown"
    tumors
  Fibrous dysplasia

(Adapted from Harwood-Nash DC, Fitz CR: Neuroradiology in Infants and Children. CV Mosby, St. Louis, 1976.)

Table 6-6. Radiographic Abnormalities of the Pituitary Sella

Decreased sella volumn
  Hypopituitarism
  Growth hormone deficiency
  Primary sellar dysplasia
Increased sella volumn
  Arrested hydrocephalus
  Treated sellar mass
  Increased intracranial pressure
  Parasellar mass lesions
  Intrasellar mass lesions
  Congenital syndromes
Primary bony sellar changes
  Sphenoid bone neoplasms
  Postinflammatory sphenoidal mucoceles
  Fibrous dysplasia

Table 6-7. Radiographic Abnormalities of the Spine Associated with Neurologic Disorders

Disorder	Radiographic Abnormality	Neurologic Syndrome
Congenital anomalies		
Klippel-Feil	Fusion of cervical vertebra	Cord compression
Down's syndrome	Atlanto-occipital subluxation	Cord compression
	Squaring of vertebral bodies	None
Scoliosis, kyphosis	Hemivertebrae	Cord compression
Diastematomyelia	Midline septum, widened canal	Tethered cord syndrome
Spina bifida	Failure of neural arch fusion	Tethered cord, myelodysplasia
Caudal regression	Sacral agenesis	Dysplastic cord
Caudal stenosis	Narrowing of lumbar canal	Cauda equina syndrome
Cervical rib	Cervical rib	Thoracic outlet syndrome
Metabolic and degenerative		
Mucopolysaccharidoses and sialidoses	Dysostosis multiplex, kyphosis	Cervical cord compression
Friedreich's ataxia	Kyphoscoliosis	Cord compression, radiculopathy
Acquired		
Epidural abscess	Osteomyelitis	Cord compression
Syringomyelia	Widened canal, scoliosis	Cord compression
Diskitis	Collapsed disk space	Back pain
Tumor	Bony erosion	Cord, root compression

Table 6-8. Maximum Interpeduncular Distances in Normal Children

	Age					
Vertebra	1 Week	6 Months	2 Years	5 Years	12 Years	20 Years
C2						31.0
C3						32.0
C4	17.0	21.5	25	28.5	32.0	34.0
C5	16.5	21.0	25	28.0	31.5	33.0
C6	15.5	20.5	24	27.5	31.0	34.0
C7	15.0	19.0	23	27.0	30.5	33.0
T1	14.0	18.0	22	25.0	28.0	30.0
T2	12.5	15.5	18.5	21.0	23.5	25.0
T3	11.0	15.0	17.0	19.0	21.0	22.0
T4	11.0	15.0	17.0	18.5	19.5	20.0
T5	11.0	14.0	16.5	18.5	20.0	21.0
T6	11.0	14.0	16.5	18.5	20.0	21.0
T7	11.5	13.5	17.0	18.5	20.5	21.0
T8	11.0	14.0	17.5	19.5	21.5	22.0
T9	11.0	14.0	17.5	19.5	21.0	22.0
T10	12.0	15.0	18.0	20.0	22.0	23.0
T11	12.0	16.0	19.0	22.0	25.0	27.0
T12	13.0	17.5	21.0	24.0	22.5	30.0
L1	13.0	17.5	22.0	26.0	30.0	33.0
L2	14.0	19.5	23.5	27.0	31.0	33.0
L3	14.0	20.5	25.0	28.5	32.5	35.0
L4	15.0	22.5	27.0	30.0	33.5	35.0
L5	17.0	24.0	29.0	33.0	37.0	39.0
S1	18.5	26.0	33.0	37.5	41.0	43.0
S2	16.0	22.0	27.0	30.5	34.5	37.0
S3	15.5	19.5	22.5	25.0	27.0	30.0
S4	15.0	19.0	21.0	23.0	25.0	27.0
S5	13.0	16.5	19.5	21.5	24.5	25.0

(Data from Schwartz GS: The width of the spinal canal in the growing vertebra with special reference to the sacrum. Am J Roentgenol 76:476, 1956.)

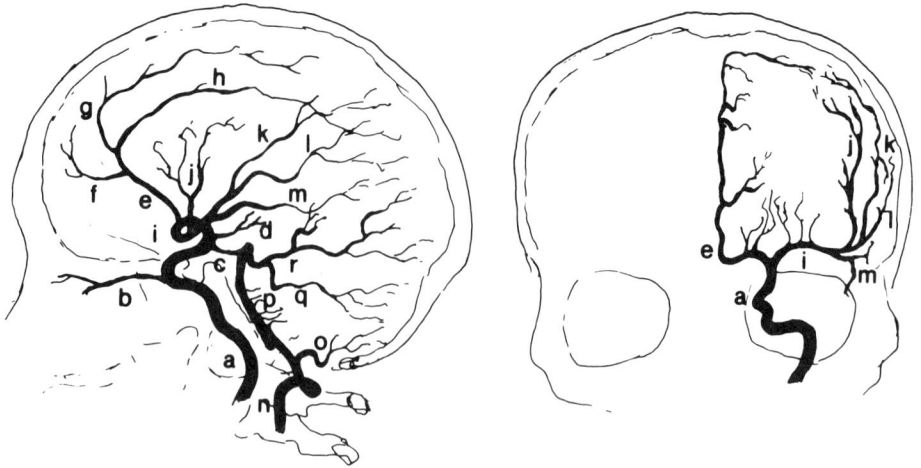

Fig. 6-2. Illustration of the cerebral arteries as seen on arteriography: (*a*) internal carotid a., (*b*) ophthalmic a., (*c*) posterior communicating a., (*d*) anterior choroidal a., (*e*) anterior cerebral a., (*f*) frontopolar a., (*g*) callosomarginal a., (*h*) pericallosal a., (*i*) middle cerebral a., (*j*) frontoparietal a., (*k*) posteroparietal a., (*l*) angular a., (*m*) posteriotemporal a., (*n*) vertebral a., (*o*) posteroinferior cerebellar a., (*p*) basilar a., (*q*) superior cerebellar a., (*r*) posterior cerebral a.

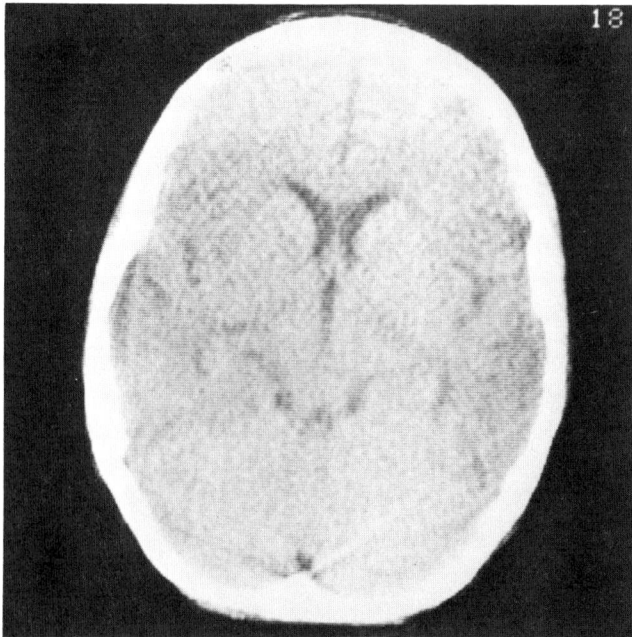

Fig. 6-3. A CT scan image at the level of the frontal horns of the lateral ventricles.

COMPUTED TOMOGRAPHY

Computed tomography (CT) scanning is a major adjunct in the evaluation of patients with neurologic disease. X-rays are projected from one side of the patient in a fixed relationship to an array of detectors on the opposite side. The detectors determine the energy level of the transmitted x-rays, which is a function of tissue absorption. The apparatus is rotated around the patient's head, making exposures at each of hundreds of positions. A computer analyzes the data and calculates a density for small cross-sectional areas of the x-ray path. This produces an image that resembles an anatomic section of the brain (Fig. 6-3). The x-ray exposure is similar to that of skull radiographs.

The CT scan is most useful in the detection of mass lesions such as tumors, hematomas, and abcesses, as well as abnormal anatomy of the brain such as cerebral atrophy, ventricular dilation, and cerebral malformation. Because fresh blood is radiodense, hemorrhages and hematomas are easily detected. It is also helpful in determining infarcts and occasionally demyelinization. The CT scan is much more sensitive than plain radiographs for detecting intracranial calcifications. Many lesions can be enhanced by using a contrast medium which shows areas of altered blood–brain barrier, particularly in abscesses and tumors. Infarcts often enhance 4 to 5 days after the stroke. The CT scan in conjunction with subarachnoid metrizamide contrast media can also be used to evaluate diseases of the spinal cord and abnormalities of the basilar cisterns and ventricular spaces.

MYELOGRAPHY

Myelography is the preferred procedure for the evaluation of diseases of the spinal cord (Fig. 6-4). In most instances metrizamide is used as the contrast medium and it has fewer complications than Pantopaque. It has the advantage of not having to be removed and there is a lower incidence of secondary arachnoiditis. In some patients, however, metrizamide can cause seizures, particularly if the contrast medium passes into the intracranial space. Enhanced resolution can be obtained in conjunction with CT scanning. In acute spinal syndromes myelography should be performed as an emergency procedure. Early detection and possible corrective therapy can often prevent irreversible spinal cord injury. Elective myelography is indicated for male patients with unexplained scoliosis, neurologic deficits associated with spina bifida occulta, and other neurologic deficits localized anatomically to the spinal cord. Because the relationship of the conus of the cord to the vertebral column changes with age, it is helpful to know the normal relationship (Fig. 6-5).

RADIONUCLIDE SCANNING

The radionuclide scan has largely been replaced by the CT scan; however, it continues to be a useful test in the diagnosis of certain conditions. It is probably as sensitive or more so in the early stages of herpes encephalitis and

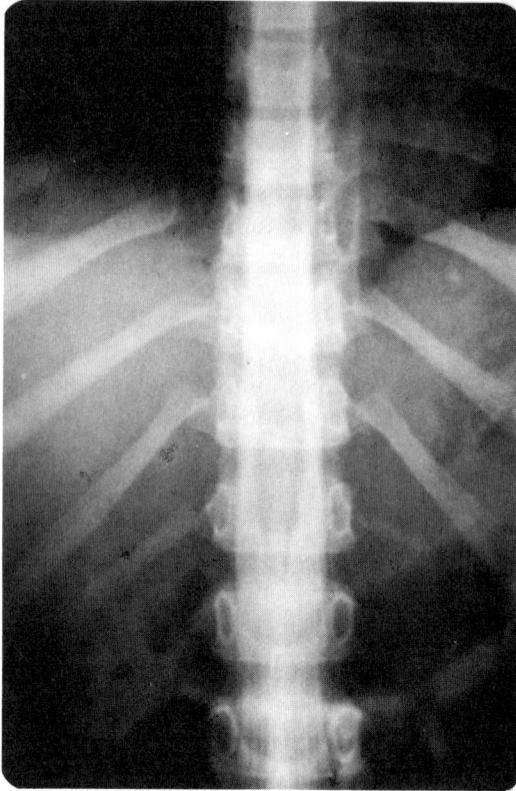

Fig. 6-4. Metrizamide myelography showing the conus of the spinal cord at T12.

is useful in the diagnosis of cerebral abscesses and some tumors. The technique depends upon the alterations of the blood–brain barrier such that radionuclide leaks into the abnormal area. Rapid detection of isotope movement by gamma camera is also available and is used to determine cerebral blood flow. The absence of cerebral blood flow by radionuclide scanning can be used in the diagnosis of cerebral death.

ULTRASONOGRAPHY

Ultrasonography has become a valuable noninvasive, low-risk procedure in the examination of the infant's brain. The technique is based upon echo of ultrasound waves from the tissues in the brain. Echo-dense structures return a higher percentage of the energy delivered and this can be computed into an image. Its greatest use in pediatric neurology is in the assessment of the infant's brain through the portal of the anterior fontanelle. The lack of bone significantly reduces the interference so that adequate images can be obtained (Fig. 6-6). It is particularly helpful in the diagnosis of hematomas and intracranial calcifi-

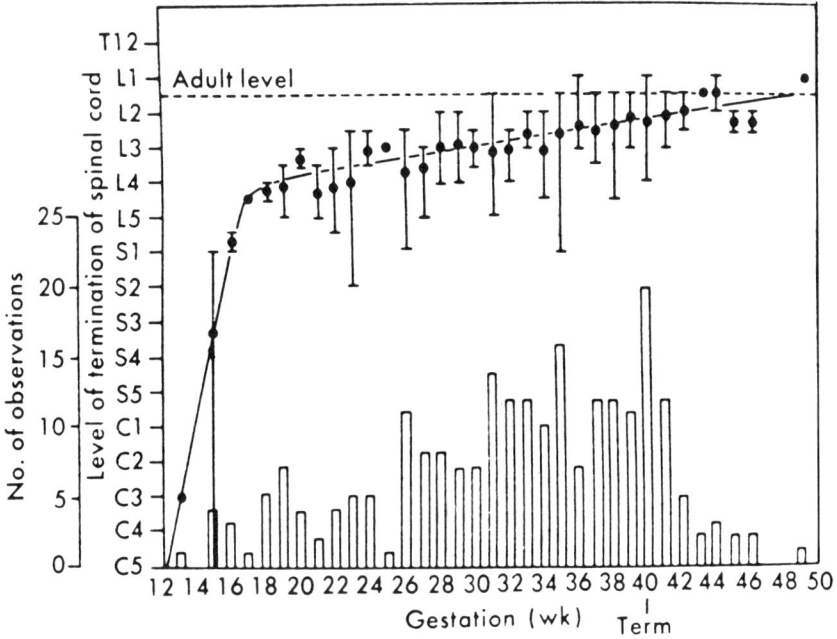

Fig. 6-5. Termination of the spinal cord. (Reproduced with permission from Barson AJ: The vertebral level of termination of the spinal cord during normal and abnormal development. J Anat 106:489–497, copyright 1970, Cambridge University Press.)

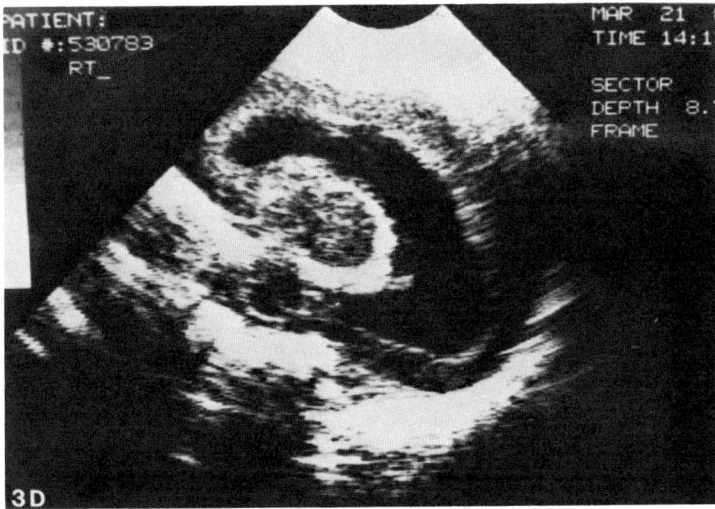

Fig. 6-6. Ultrasonography demonstrating a sagittal image through the lateral ventricle.

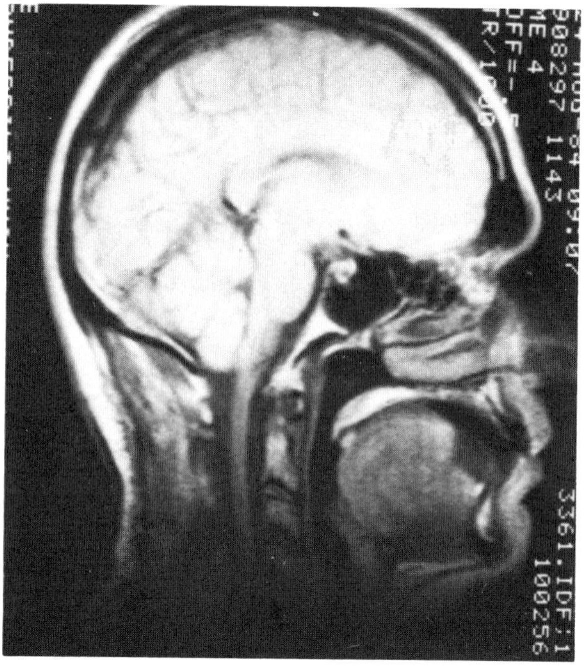

Fig. 6-7. An MRI sagittal scan.

cations and in the evaluation of the ventricular system. It is less useful in the diagnosis of disorders in the posterior fossa and in the evaluation of subdural hematomas and effusions. Many nurseries routinely obtain ultrasound scans of premature infants to screen for intraventricular and periventricular hemorrhages.

MAGNETIC RESONANCE IMAGING

The magnetic resonance imaging (MRI) scan depends upon magnetic characteristics of certain atomic nuclei. In a strong magnetic field, a certain proportion of nuclei align themselves with the field like small magnets (magnetic moment). Within this alignment, nuclei spin or wobble at a given frequency, depending upon the strength of the magnetic field and the nucleus being measured. The frequency of the wobble is the nuclear magnetic resonance. If the tissue is then irradiated by a radio frequency at the same frequency as the nuclear magnetic resonance, there will be displacement of the magnetic moment. After cessation of the radio frequency impulse, the realignment of the magnetic moment generates a radio signal which can be detected. Many parameters can be measured from the characteristics of this radio signal, and with the use of a computer an image is generated.

The MRI scan is particularly useful for the noninvasive examination of the central nervous system. Imaging of the brain can be performed in many different planes so that almost any anatomic part of the brain can be studied in detail (Fig. 6-7). The images separate tissues according to their molecular makeup, which depends largely on whether they are fat or water density. The anatomic representation has more contrast than the CT scan and it is a better test for examining the posterior fossa as well as small tissue changes such as in demyelinization.

OTHER NEUROIMAGING TECHNIQUES

Other methods for neuroimaging includes positron emission tomography and pneumoencephalography. At the present time positron emission tomography is an experimental procedure and only available at certain specialized centers. Pneumoencephalography has been rightfully replaced by the CT scan, ultrasonography, and MRI.

SELECTED READINGS

Bachman DS, Hodges FJ, Freeman JM: Computerized axial tomography in neurologic disorders of children. Pediatrics 59:352–360, 1977

Donn SM, Goldstein GW, Silver TM: Real-time ultrasonography. Am J Dis Child 35:319–324, 1981

Goodnig CA, Brasch RC, Lallemand DP, et al: Nuclear magnetic resonance imaging of the brain in children. J Pediatr 104:509–515, 1984

Harwood-Nash DC, Breckbill DL: Computed tomography in children: a new diagnostic technique. J Pediatr 89:343–357, 1976

Harwood-Nash DC, Fitz CR: Neuroradiology in Infants and Children. CV Mosby, St. Louis, 1976

Schey WL: Intracranial calcifications in childhood: frequency of occurrence and significance. Am J Roentgenol 122:495–499, 1974

Smith FW: NMR imaging in pediatric practice. Pediatrics 71:852–854, 1983

Yalaz K, Treves S: Brain scanning and cerebral radioisotope angiography (CRA) in children. Pediatrics 54:696–701, 1974

7

CEREBROSPINAL FLUID EXAMINATION

Approximately 3 percent of the intracranial volume consists of cerebrospinal fluid (CSF). Figure 7-1 illustrates the circulation of CSF. The fluid is produced primarily by the choroid plexus of the ventricles. The total volume turns over three to four times every 24 hours. The fluid circulates within the lateral and third ventricles, through the aqueduct of Sylvius, and into the fourth ventricle and exits from the foramina of Magendie and Luschka into the posterior fossa subarachnoid space. The fluid communicates with the spinal subarachnoid space and then percolates through the basilar cisterns and subarachnoid spaces to be absorbed by the arachnoid granulations of the major dural sinuses and veins. The maximal rate of absorption is approximately three times the formation rate and increases linearly with increasing CSF pressure. The total volume is 40 to 60 ml in the term infant to 60 to 100 ml in the young child, 80 to 120 ml in older children, and 110 to 160 ml in adults.

The function of the CSF is thought to be support for the brain, which it suspends within the intracranial space. It acts as a cushion, protecting the brain from acute changes in pressure. It also serves an excretory function, since the brain has no lymphatic system. It participates somewhat in the intracerebral transport of metabolites, neurotransmitters, and other substances and it participates in the control of the chemical environment of the CNS.

LUMBAR PUNCTURE

The lumbar puncture is the standard method for obtaining CSF for examination. Figure 7-2 illustrates the method of lumbar puncture. Care should be taken in the selection and preparation of the lumbar puncture site. It is a relatively safe procedure but not without risks. Table 7-1 lists the common indications, contraindications, and complications for performing a lumbar puncture. The absolute indication is evaluation for meningitis. Absolute contraindications are evidence for a focal cerebral mass with increased intracranial pressure and a local skin infection at the site of a lumbar puncture. The most serious complication is the herniation syndrome, which occurs in approximately 1 percent of patients with raised intracranial pressure. It is particularly more likely to occur in patients who have a rapidly expanding focal mass such as a cerebral abcess. In general, a patient presenting with papilledema or a focal

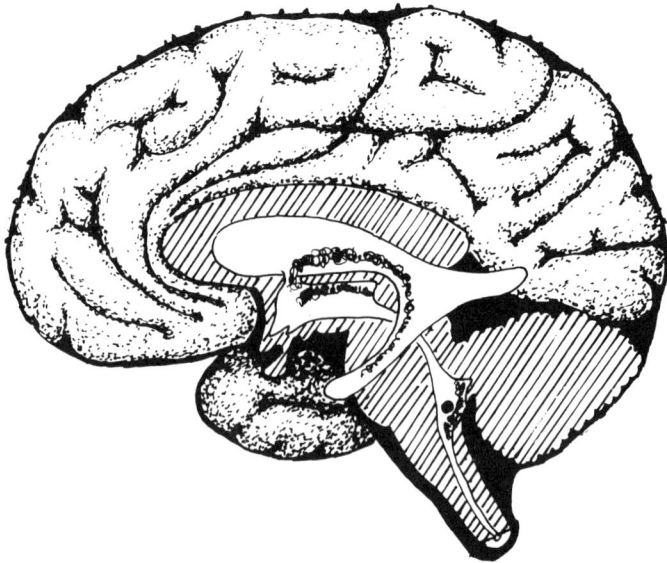

Fig. 7-1. Circulation of CSF. The black area represents the subarachnoid space, and the hatched areas sectioned brain. The clear areas indicate the ventricular space. The CSF is produced by the choroid plexus in the ventricles. It exits to the ventricular system via the foramina of Luschka and Magendie, percolates through the subarachnoid space, and is absorbed in the major venous sinuses through the arachnoid granulations.

neurologic sign should have a computed tomography scan prior to a lumbar puncture. If there is some concern about increased pressure and the performance of the lumbar puncture giving the patient 0.25 g of mannitol per kilogram of body weight approximately 30 minutes prior to performing the tap, using a 22 to 24 gauge needle, and withdrawing immediately if the pressure is greater than 300 mmH$_2$O may reduce the risk somewhat.

CSF PRESSURE

The normal range for CSF pressure is 40 to 200 mmH$_2$O in the horizontal position. Pressure increases considerably if the patient is in the upright position. Normally, there should be a 4- to 5-mmH$_2$O pulsation with respiration and a 2 to 3 mmH$_2$O pulsation with the pulse. Patients with papilledema usually have pressures greater than 200 mmH$_2$O and spontaneous venus pulsations of the retina are lost at pressures greater than 180 mmH$_2$O. Causes of increased CSF pressure are listed in Table 7-2.

CSF APPEARANCE

The CSF becomes cloudy if there are greater than 200 white blood cells per cubic millimeter, becomes pink with 500 to 6,000 red blood cells per cubic millimeter, and is grossly bloody with greater than 6,000 red blood cells per

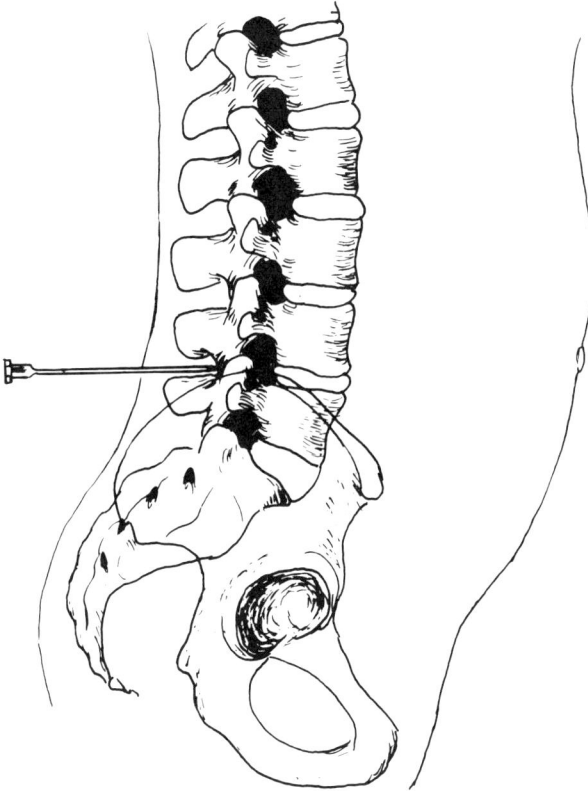

Fig. 7-2. Lumbar puncture. The L4–L5 interspace is palpatated on a plane with the iliac crest. The area is generously cleaned with antiseptic solution and infiltrated with a 1 percent of xylocaine. A 22- to 24-gauge spinal needle is inserted and directed toward the umbilicus with the bevel parallel to the vertebral column.

Table 7-1. Indications, Contraindications, and Complications of Lumbar Puncture

Indications	Contraindications	Complications
Absolute	Absolute	Herniation syndrome
Infections (excluding abscess)	Intracranial mass Local skin, soft tissue, or bone infection	Spinal hematoma
Myelography		Radiculopathy
Spinal anesthesia	Relative	Spinal headaches
Relative	Known spinal arteriovenous malformation	Inoculations
Subarachnoid hemorrhage		Bacteria
Measurement of CSF pressure	Increased intracranial pressure	Tissue (epidermoid tumor)
Measurement of CSF constituents		Cranial nerve palsies
Therapeutic		
Pseudotumor cerebri		

Table 7-2. Causes of Increased CSF Pressure

CSF overproduction (choroid plexus papilloma)
CSF obstruction (hydrocephalus)
    Ventricular (noncommunicating)
    Extraventricular (communicating)
Intracranial mass
    Tumor
    Abscess
    Hematoma
Intoxications
    Estrogens
    Glucocorticoids
    Vitamin A
    Parathormone
    Tetracycline
    Phenothiazines
    Lead
Vascular
    Intracranial hemorrhage
    Venous thrombosis
    Extracranial venous obstruction
    Systemic hypertension
    Heart failure
Infections
    Meningitis, acute and chronic
    Encephalitis
    Abscess
Cerebral edema
    Reye's syndrome
    Cytotoxic (e.g., post anoxia)
    Vasogenic (e.g., abscess, tumor)
Pseudotumor cerebri
High CSF protein (e.g., Guillain-Barré syndrome)

cubic millimeter. The CSF is xanthochromic following a prior bleed of 2 to 12 hours before the spinal tap. A xanthochromic CSF can also be observed in patients who have jaundice, hypercarotinemia, or a CSF protein of greater than 600 mg/dl.

CELL COUNT

Beyond the newborn period the normal cell count is less than $5/mm^3$ monocytes. If there has been blood contamination of the CSF, one can estimate the true CSF white blood cell count by measuring the ratio of white blood cells to red blood cells in the blood. This is normally 1:700 and thus 1 white cell per 700 red cells in the CSF would be expected from the bloody contamination. White blood cells lyse more rapidly than red blood cells, particularly at room temperature. For accuracy, all counts should be obtained as rapidly as possible. A traumatic tap can often be differentiated from subarachnoid hemorrhage if the blood shows clearing from the first to the third tubes and if the spun specimen is not xanthochromic. Pleocytosis is seen in a number of diseases, most of which are infectious. In general, bacterial infections give rise to segmented neutrophil

Table 7-3. Pleocytosis and CSF Glucose Concentrations

Polymorphonuclear pleocytosis, reduced glucose
  Bacterial meningitis
  Parameningeal suppuration (subdural abscess)
  Primary amebic meningoencephalitis
Polymorphonuclear pleocytosis, normal glucose
  Bacterial meningitis
  Viral encephalitis (early stages)
  Eastern equine encephalitis
  Tuberculous or fungal meningitis (early stages)
Acute hemorrhagic leukoencephalitis
Lymphocytic pleocytosis, reduced glucose
  Tuberculous meningitis
  Fungal meningoencephalitis (certain types)
  Partially treated bacterial meningitis
  Viral aseptic meningitis (rare cases of mumps, HVH, LCM, enterovirus)
  Meningeal leukemia, carcinomatosis
  Meningeal sarcoidosis
  Cerebral cysticercosis
  Laboratory error
Lymphocytic pleocytosis, normal glucose
  Viral aseptic meningitis, encephalitis
  Partially treated bacterial meningitis
  Brain abscess
  Parameningeal suppuration
  Rocky Mountain spotted fever
  Lead encephalopathy
  Tuberculous or fungal meningitis (early)
  "Chemical" meningitis
  Leptospiral or mycoplasmal meningitis
  Meningeal leukemia
  Cerebral granulomatous angiitis
  Vogt-Koyanagi-Harada disease
  Behçet's disease
Hemorrhagic fluid
  Spontaneous subarachnoid hemorrhage
  Dural sinus–cortical vein thrombosis
  Herpes simplex encephalitis (infrequent cases)
  Ruptured mycotic aneurysm
  Anthrax meningitis
  "Traumatic" tap

(From Bell WE, McCormick WF: Neurologic Infections in Children. 2nd Ed. p. 47. WB Saunders, Philadelphia, 1981. Reprinted by permission from WB Saunders Co.)

pleocytosis and viral and fungal infections are associated with lymphocytic pleocytosis. Early viral infections and treated bacterial infections can show the opposite characteristics. Table 7-3 lists other causes of pleocytosis.

PROTEIN

The normal CSF protein content is 0.5 to 1.0 percent of the serum protein. A protein gradient exists between the site of CSF formation in the ventricles to the lumbar space. The normal range of lumbar CSF is approximately 15 to 45 mg/dl. The protein can be increased in a number of neurologic disorders, in-

Table 7-4. Neurologic Diseases with
Increased CSF Protein

Metabolic
  Metachromatic leukodystrophy
  Krabbe' leukodystrophy
  Refsum's disease
  Diabetes mellitis
Toxic
  Lead encephalopathy
  Diphtheria polyneuritis
Infectious
  Bacterial meningitis
  Chronic meningitis
  Viral meningitis, encephalitis
  Congenital infections
Postinfectious
  Guillain-Barré syndrome
  Acute cerebellar ataxia
  Leukoencephalitis
Neoplastic
  Brain tumor
  Carcinomatous meningitis
  Spinal block
Other
  Intracranial hemorrhage
  Lupus erythematosis
  Sarcoidosis

cluding infections, certain metabolic diseases, and postinfectious inflammatory disorders. If there has been a bloody contamination, then one can estimate a correction factor by the ratio of the protein in the blood to the red blood cell count. Normally, one can expect a 1 mg/dl increase in protein concentration for every 1,000 blood cells. A protein value greater than 500 is unusual and is most frequently seen in meningitis or spinal block. Causes for increased CSF protein are listed in Table 7-4.

Another test available for the examination of CSF protein is the measurement of immunoglobulins. An increased percentage of γ-globulins may indicate chronic infections and acquired demyelinating diseases of the CNS. Cerebrospinal fluid immunoelectropheresis may also show oligoclonal bands, which suggest an antibody being produced within the CNS. These bands are known to represent specific antibodies such as seen in subacute sclerosing panencephalitis with production of anti-measles antibody. They are seen in a majority of patients with multiple sclerosis and may be found in neurosyphilis, Guillian-Barré syndrome, encephalitis, and certain other disorders. Myelin basic protein is found in a variety of disorders of the CNS but is most frequently associated with conditions which cause CNS demyelinization.

GLUCOSE AND OTHER CSF CONSTITUENTS

The normal CSF glucose is approximately 60 percent that of serum. However, transport of the glucose across the blood–brain barrier can become saturated so that there is proportionately less CSF glucose with hyperglycemia. Levels

Table 7-5. Normal CSF Constituents

Constituent	CSF	Serum
Osmolarity	295 mOsm/L	295 mOsm/L
Sodium	138.0 mEq/L	138 mEq/L
Potassium	2.8 mEq/L	4.1 mEq/L
Calcium	2.4 mEq/L	5.2 mEq/L
Magnesium	2.7 mEq/L	1.9 mEq/L
Chloride	124.0 mEq/L	101.0 mEq/L
Bicarbonate	23.0 mEq/L	23.0 mEq/L
Carbon dioxide tension	48 mmHg	38 mmHg (arterial)
pH	7.31	7.41 (arterial)
Nonprotein nitrogen	19.0 mg/100 ml	27.0 mg/100 ml
Ammonia	30.0 mg/100 ml	70.0 mg/100 ml
Uric acid	0.24 mg/100 ml	4.0 mg/100 ml
Urea	4.7 mmol/L	5.4 mmol/L
Creatinine	1.1 mg/100 ml	1.6 mg/100 ml
Phosphorus	1.6 mg/100 ml	4.0 mg/100 ml
Total lipid	1.25 mg/100 ml	876.0 mg/100 ml
Total cholesterol	0.4 mg/100 ml	180.0 mg/100 ml
Cholesterol esters	0.3 mg/100 ml	126.0 mg/100 ml
Glucose	>45.0 mg/100 ml	90 mg/100 ml
Lactate	1.6 mEq/L	1.0 mEq/L
Protein	10.0–30.0 mg/100 ml	6.0–8.0 g/100 mL
Prealbumin	1–7%	Trace
Albumin	49–73%	56%
α_1-Globulin	3–7%	4%
α_2-Globulin	6–13%	10%
β-globulin ($\beta1$ plus τ)	9–19%	12%
γ-Globulin	3–12%	18%

(Adapted from Fishman RA: Cerebrospinal Fluid Diseases of the Nervous System. WB Saunders, Philadelphia, 1980.)

below 40 mg are almost always abnormal and are most frequently associated with bacterial infections. One can also find depressed glucose in hemorrhage, carcinomatous meningitis, and occasionally viral infections. Normal values for other CSF constituents are listed in Table 7-5. Cerebrospinal fluid lactate can be elevated in bacterial meningitis and certain inborn errors of metabolism. Measurement of other constituents is not routinely performed.

CYTOLOGY

Cytology of the CSF is positive in approximately 60 percent of patients who have carcinomatous meningitis. It is rarely positive in patients who have intracerebral tumors and occasionally false-positive results will be obtained in patients who have chronic inflammatory diseases.

MICROBIOLOGY

The microbiologic examination of the CSF is one of the more critical tests that are performed. There are three basic tests: (1) visual examination for organisms, (2) microbiologic culture, and (3) detection of antigens.

Table 7-6. Normal CSF Values in Premature and Term Infants

Term newborn infant	
Quantity	Approximately 40 ml
Appearance	Clear to xanthochromic
White blood cells	0–32/mm^3 (mean = 8/mm^3)
Red blood cells	0 to several hundred per mm^3
Glucose	70–80% of serum glucose
Protein	60–150 mg/100 ml (mean = 90 mg/100 ml)
Smear and culture	Negative
Premature newborn infant	
Quantity	10–30 ml
Appearance	Clear to xanthochromic
White blood cells	0–15/mm^3 (mean = 7/mm^3
Red blood cells	0 to several hundred per mm^3
Glucose	70–80% of serum glucose
Protein	60–200 mg/100 ml (mean = 115 mg/100 ml)
Smear and culture	Negative

(Adapted from Bell WE, McCormick WF: Neurologic Infections in Children. 2nd Ed. WB Saunders, Philadelphia, 1981. Reprinted by permission from WB Saunders Co.)

Direct visualization uses the Gram stain for bacteria, the India ink preparation for certain fungal infections, and the acid-fast stain for tuberculosis. These tests should be performed as rapidly as possible after the specimen is obtained. Failure to identify an organism does not exclude the diagnosis of an infection. A presumptive identification, however, can direct initial therapy until a specific identification has been obtained from culture material.

In patients with acute meningitis, the CSF should be cultured on blood agar, chocolate agar (place in CO_2 jar), desoxycholate agar, and thioglycolate broth. If a chronic meningitis is suspected, then cultures for tuberculosis and fungi are indicated in addition to bacterial cultures. Viral cultures of the CSF are not helpful for treatment purposes but are helpful in the epidemiology of viral meningoencephalitis. Because of their expense and lack of availability, viral cultures are seldom obtained routinely.

Counterimmune electrophoresis is a sensitive method of detecting some bacterial antigens and aids in the early recognition of bacterial meningitis. Antigen detection tests are commercially available and are equally sensitive. Latex agglutination tests are also available for fungal antigens. The Venereal Disease Research Laboratories (VDRL) and other serologic tests for syphillis remain the methods of choice for diagnosing neurosyphillis.

CSF OF THE PREMATURE AND NEWBORN

Premature infants usually have a xanthochromic CSF and may have as many as 5,000 red blood cells per cubic millimeter. The white blood cell count, glucose concentration, and protein values are greater in premature infants than in older children. The cell count returns to normal within the first 1 to 2 months, and the protein by 6 months. Normal values for premature and term infants are listed in Table 7-6.

SELECTED READINGS

Culter RWP, Spartell RB: Cerebrospinal fluid: a selective review. Ann Neurol 11:1–10, 1982

Fishman RA: Cerebrospinal Fluid in Disease of the Nervous System. WB Saunders, Philadelphia, 1980

Glass JP, Melamed M, Chernik NL, Posner JB: Malignant cells in cerebrospinal fluid (CSF): the meaning of positive CSF cytology. Neurology 29:1369–1375, 1979

Menkes JH: To tap or not to tap. Pediatrics 50:560, 1972

Nerenberg ST, Prasad R, Rothman ME: Cerebrospinal fluid IgG, IgA, IgM, IgD and IgE levels in central nervous system disorders. Neurology 28:988–990, 1978

Petito P, Plum F: The lumbar puncture. N Engl J Med 290:225–226, 1974

Portnoy JM, Olson LC: Normal cerebrospinal fluid values in children: another look. Pediatrics 75:484–487, 1985

Whitaker JN, Lisak RP, Bashir RM et al: Immunoreactive myelin basic protein in the cerebrospinal fluid in neurological disorders. Ann Neurol 7:58–64, 1980

8

PSYCHOLOGICAL TESTING

Psychological testing is the assessment of cognitive, social, and emotional abilities. In the young child one normally measures development, and in the older child intelligence and achievement. Psychological tests are indicated for children who do not develop or perform academically at their appropriate age level. A careful history and neurologic exam are more sensitive tests for detecting organic diseases. The major purpose for obtaining psychological tests is to assess a child's present level of functioning, plan an individual educational program, or evaluate a specific program. This chapter discusses some of the more frequently used tests and their indications. Psychological tests are only as good as the examiner. Not all practicing psychologists have specific training with children or are trained to administer psychological tests to children. In general, it is best to recommend a psychologist who specializes in children.

PSYCHOLOGICAL TESTS

Psychological tests have been standardized for the normal population; therefore there is a bias against children with physical, sensory, or cultural handicaps. Many of the tests have a strong verbal emphasis, and children with language disturbances will test artificially low. One must also consider that the test measures a single point in time in the child's life. Intercurrent illnesses, medications, or emotional disorders may impair the functioning of a child at the time of testing. It is perhaps more accurate to measure different points in time to determine the stability of a test score or the progression or regression of a child's psychological abilities. One must also remember that a test score has a built-in error with a certain variance. This must be considered when comparing repeated tests or tests performed by different examiners.

There are a number of psychological tests that measure different areas of a child's cognitive, behavioral, or social abilities. Those discussed in this chapter are frequently used. One can characterize the tests into several categories. Developmental screening tests are designed for nonpsychologists to screen infants and children for development disorders (Table 8-1). The most widely used test is the Denver Developmental Screening Test. The shortened version, the Denver Prescreening Developmental Questionnaire is a prescreening test administered by interview only. These tests assess development in the four areas of personal/social, language, fine motor coordination, and gross motor skills. Other tests are available for specific areas of development. Many offices routinely screen all

Table 8-1. Developmental Screening Tests

Test	Age Group	Description
General		
Denver Prescreening Developmental Questionnaire	Under 6 years	Rapid prescreening evaluation obtained by interview and used to identify children in of more complete screening
Denver Developmental Screening Test	Under 6 years	Standardized screening exam that assesses personal/social, fine motor adaptable, language, and gross motor development
Academic		
Slocum	Preschool	Preschool academic screening test heavily weighted toward social development
Perceptual		
Developmental Test of Visual-Motor Integration	2–15 years	Visual–motor integration tested by copying geometric forms
Goodenough-Harris Drawing Test	3–15 years	Perceptual test of drawing human figures
Language		
Verbal Language Development Scale		
Receptive-Expressive Emergent Language Scale		
Social behavioral		
Vineland Social Maturity Scale	All ages	Screening test that measures social competency from parental interview
Social Maturity Scale for Blind Preschoolers	All ages	Behavioral scale for independent functioning

children with the initial and subsequent evaluations. Developmental tests do not give an intelligence score or an achievement score but only identify children who are at risk of having developmental disorders. Further testing must be performed to diagnose a developmental or learning disorder. Early diagnosis may facilitate early treatment and ameliorate debilitating handicaps.

There are a number of general intelligence tests that are age specific (Table 8-2). In the infant, the Bayley Scales of Infant Development is the most commonly used test. Infant tests have been standardized for normal infants and there are limitations in interpreting results for children with multiple handicaps. Examiners frequently have to omit items or use substitute items or alternative scoring methods in order to assess the handicapped infant. Long-range predictions must be made cautiously from results of infant testing.

In older children the Weschler series of tests have the most widespread use. These include the Wechsler Preschool and Primary Scale of Intelligence and the Wechsler Intelligence Scale for Children Revised. These tests evaluate the preschool and school age child respectively, and measure specific areas of language and performance skills. Younger children may be evaluated by the Merrill-Palmer Scale of Mental Tests, the Stanford-Binet Intelligence Scale, and the Hiskey-Nebraska Test of Learning Aptitude. The latter is particularly helpful for the hearing-impaired child. The present Stanford-Binet test is weighted toward

Table 8-2. General Tests for Intelligence

Test	Age Group	Description
Bayley Scales of Infant Development	2–30 months	Assessment of early mental and psychomotor development
Merrill-Palmer Scale of Mental Tests	2–4½ years	General intelligence test
Stanford-Binet Intelligence Scale	2–18 years	General intelligence test heavily weighted for language skills
Wechsler Preschool and Primary Scale of Intelligence	4–6½ years	General intelligence test for preschoolers with subtests for verbal and performance skills
Wechsler Intelligence Scale for Children Revised	6–17 years	General intelligence test for school-aged children, with verbal and performance subtests
Columbia Mental Maturity Scale	3½–10 years	General intelligence test which requires no verbalization and little motor response
Hiskey-Nebraska Test of Learning Aptitude	3½–10 years	Learning aptitude test, especially useful for the deaf
McCarthy Scales of Children's Abilities	2½–8½ years	General test of intelligence, particularly good for perceptual and motor skills
Pictorial Test of Intelligence	3–8 years	General test of intelligence, particularly useful for multiply handicapped and retarded children

language abilities and relies on verbal instructions to a great extent. This test is being revised. The Merrill-Palmer test is predominantly performance oriented and is also very useful in the hearing- and language-impaired child.

Tests for the assessment of perception and language abilities are shown in (Table 8-3). The Bender gestalt test is the most commonly used test measuring perceptual abilities. Other such tests include the Frostig Developmental Tests of Visual Perception and the Berry-Buktenica Visual Motor Integration Test. Many of these tests are administered by having the child copy a geometric form. Significant fine motor handicaps may interfere with testing results. The Goodenough-Harris Drawing Test is a relatively simple test in which a child draws

Table 8-3. Psychological Tests of Perceptual and Communication Abilities

Test	Age Group	Description
Perceptual		
Bender Visual Motor Gestalt Test for Children	5–10 years	Geometric form-copying test evaluating visual motor pathways
Frostig Developmental Tests of Visual Perception	3–10 years	Perceptual test of visual–motor performance
Berry-Buktenica Visual Motor Integration Test	2–16 years	Test of visual perceptions and fine motor coordination
Communication		
Illinois Test of Psycholinguistic Abilities	2–9½ years	General test of receptive and expressive language
Peabody Picture Vocabulary Test	2–18 years	Test of receptive language which requires no expressive verbal skills
Wepman Auditory Discrimination Test	5–18 years	Test of auditory discrimination for speech sounds

Table 8-4. Academic Achievement and Other Psychological Tests

Test	Age Group	Description
Academic achievement		
Wide Range Achievement Test	5–16 years	General test of academic ability
Woodcock-Johnson Psycho-educational Battery	3–16 years	General test for academic ability and achievement
Peabody Individual Achievement Test	3–18 years	General test of academic ability
Key Math Diagnostic Arithmetic Test	5–15 years	Specific test of mathematic ability
Metropolital Readiness Test	Preschool	Academic readiness test widely used by school systems
California Achievement Test	School age	Academic achievement test widely used by school systems
Social		
American Association for Mental Deficiency Adaptive Behavior Scale	All ages	Test that measures independent functioning
Neuropsychological		
Halstead-Reitan Test for Children		Complex test used to measure neuropsychological skills

human figures. It is useful for screening purposes but is not a substitute for thorough testing and should not be used to determine intelligence. There are a number of specific language tests available, including the Illinois Test of Psycholinguistic Abilities, the Peabody Picture Vocabulary Test, and the Wepman Auditory Discrimination Test. The advantage of the Peabody Picture Vocabulary Test is that expressive verbal skills are not necessary. The Illinois Test for Psycholinguistic Ability is a more general test measuring all aspects of receptive and expressive language.

Tests for social maturity and abilities include the Vineland Social Maturity Scale, American Association for Mental Deficiency Adaptive Behavior Scale, and the Social Maturity Scale for Blind Preschoolers. These types of tests are very important in assessing a child's adaptive behavior. This is frequently more important than the child's language or cognitive abilities and should be an important part of a general psychological evaluation.

Achievement tests determine what learning a child has retained and primarily assess academic ability. These are listed in Table 8-4. Most of these have specific subtests for different academic areas and give grade-equivalent scores as well as percentile scores.

Neuropsychological tests determine how neurological diseases infringe upon normal cognitive and developmental functioning. These tests evaluate learning strategies as opposed to content. They have limited usefulness because of their complexity and the time it takes to administer them. The Halsted-Reitan Test is the most commonly used.

Behavioral and emotional development is poorly measured by standardized projective tests. The Rorschach and the Children's Apperception Test are the two most commonly used. These tests are particularly difficult for the child who is retarded. They are normally administered by a clinical psychologist.

INTERPRETATION

Psychologists should be able to give an assessment of the child's performance in several areas. It is important to report whether the child was attentive, cooperative, or untestable. The child's behavior during testing obviously influences the results. A general impression of the child's intelligence, the names of the tests administered, and an explanation for scoring, if necessary, should be given. Academic achievement and the child's social and behavior adaptations should be determined and strengths and weaknesses specifically documented. From the results, one can decide if the child needs to be retested at a later date or if specific therapies are indicated by the initial results. The scores do not indicate a specific diagnosis but form the basis for a differential diagnosis. Thus a low intelligent quotient from a psychological test does not determine the cause of mental retardation but only measures it. The identification of cognitive strengths and weaknesses enable educators to design specific therapies for a child with a cognitive disability.

A child who scores low on intelligence, language, and social competence tests probably has mental retardation. Normal intelligence but low achievement test scores may reflect a cultural or language bias or a learning disability. A disparity between verbal and performance skills often suggests a specific learning disability. A child with normal intelligence but poor social adaptive skills may have a behavioral or emotional disorder. Most importantly, testing results can be the key to designing an appropriate treatment plan. Behavioral or social maladaptions may require specific interventions by a clinical psychologist or child psychiatrist.

SELECTED READINGS

Culbertson L, Ferry PC: Learning disabilities. Pediatr Clin N Am 29:121–136, 1982

Frankenburg W, Dodds JB: Denver Developmental Screening Test. J Pediatr 74:181–191, 1967

Magrab PR: A primer for interpreting psychological test results. Pediatr Ann 11:470–479, 1982

Soule AS, Sandley K, Copans SA et al: Clinical uses of Brazelton Neonatal Scale. Pediatrics 54:583–586, 1974

Taylor R, Warren SA: Educational and psychological assessment of children with learning disorders. Pediatr Clin N Am 31:281–296, 1984

SECTION 3

Neurologic Disorders of the Newborn

Neonatal neurology is developing into a subspeciality. Many of the disorders and complications of the neonate are unique to this group of patients. Also, the expression of the nervous system and the methods of examining the nervous system are markedly different from that of older children. These differences become more distinct in the premature infant. The anticipated outcome of every delivery is to produce a healthy child. As methods are developed to treat the many medical complications of the neonate, the integrity of the nervous system should be the measure of successful therapy.

9

NEONATAL ENCEPHALOPATHY

Because of the immature nervous system and the unique susceptibility of newborns to certain disorders, the clinical syndrome of newborn encephalopathy differs from that of older children. Encephalopathy is a relative concept at this age, because newborns, especially premature newborns, spend the majority of their time in either quiet or active sleep and the repertoire of complex behavior is somewhat limited. In this context it implies an alteration in the normal state of somnolence and has the symptoms of decreased arousibility, hyperexcitability, seizures, changes in muscle tone, and alterations in breathing and feeding (Table 9-1). Neurologic deficits tend to be generalized, as opposed to focal, owing to the immaturity of the nervous system. Table 9-2 summarizes the major causes for newborn encephalopathy, some of which will be covered in separate chapters. Seizures, which are the most important neurologic manifestation of encephalopathy, are covered in Chapter 10.

HYPOXIC–ISCHEMIC ENCEPHALOPATHY

Hypoxemia is lack of oxygen and ischemia is decreased blood flow. In the newborn, these usually accompany one another. Hypoxic–ischemic encephalopathy (HIE) is perhaps less well tolerated in the newborn because of the defective autoregulation of the vascular supply to the brain. This may also be a contributing factor to intraventricular hemorrhage (to be discussed later). The majority of infants with HIE have a prenatal onset, whereas only 10 percent are thought to occur after birth. Intrauterine asphyxia is the major cause of HIE and is manifested by abnormalities noted in fetal heart rate monitoring. The longer the duration, the more severe the subsequent encephalopathy. A low Apgar score at birth is another indication of asphyxia and there is a correlation of low Apgar score with the development of encephalopathy. Apgar scores, however, only measure the infant at one point in time. Apgar scores in conjunction with fetal heart rate monitoring and neonatal acid-base data are more predictive of encephalopathy.

The clinical presentation depends upon the severity of the injury (Table 9-3). Brain stem abnormalities with severe asphyxia may be prominent and include abnormalities in ocular motility, sucking, and breathing. The illness peaks at 48 to 72 hours followed by death or recovery. The pathology of HIE shows a variety of abnormalities which account for many of the subsequent neurologic deficits (Table 9-4). The more severe the injury, the longer the period of acute encepha-

Table 9-1. Signs of Neonatal
Encephalopathy

Consciousness
  Excessive sleep
  Stupor
  Coma
Behavior
  High-pitched, persistent cry
  Irritability
  Poor feeding
Muscle tone and activity
  Hypotonia
  Jitteriness
  Opisthotonic posturing
  Repetitive stereotyped movements
Brain stem functions
  Poorly reactive pupils
  Ophthalmoparesis
  Apnea
  Poor suck
Seizures

lopathy. The more rapid the improvement, the better the long-term prognosis. Approximately 10 to 20 percent of infants with HIE die, and of those who survive, approximately 30 to 40 percent have neurologic sequelae such as cerebral palsy, epilepsy, mental retardation, learning disabilities, and behavior disorders.

Treatment of HIE is basically supportive. Adequate blood flow and oxygenation should be maintained and the child prevented from becoming hypoglycemic. Seizures should be treated with anticonvulsant medications. There is some question as to whether efforts to reduce cerebral edema are efficacious in the newborn period. It is reasonable to correct hypovolemia and severe acidosis (pH < 7.10) and to maintain normal electrolytes and other metabolic parameters.

Table 9-2. Etiology of Newborn
Encephalopathy

Hypoxic–ischemic encephalopathy
Intracranial hemorrhage
Infections of the CNS
  Bacterial meningitis and sepsis
  Congenital infections
Metabolic encephalopathies
  Acquired
  Hypoglycemia
  Hypocalcemia
  Hyperbilirubinemia
  Inherited (Ch. 19)
Toxic encephalopathy
Congenital malformations (Ch. 13)
Birth trauma (Ch. 12)
"Near miss" sudden infant death syndrome

Table 9-3. Clinical Features of Hypoxic–Ischemic Encephalopathy

Mild
  State of consciousness: transitory lethargy followed by jitteriness
  Tone: mild head lag on traction
  Convulsions: none
  Time course: symptoms maximal in first 24 hours postpartum
  Prognosis: full recovery
Moderate
  State of consciousness: obtundation progressing to stupor and coma
  Tone: hypotonic posture at rest, depressed traction response
  Convulsions: occurs in some; apnea progressing to multifocal convulsions
  Time course: symptoms maximal at 48–72 hours
  Prognosis: guarded
Severe
  State of consciousness: stupor and coma
  Tone: severe hypotonia at rest and on traction
  Convulsions: a constant feature (if not clinically, then on EEG)
  Time course: symptoms maximal from birth to 72 hours
  Prognosis: invariably poor

(From Fenichel GM: Neonatal Neurology. 2nd Ed. Churchill Livingstone, New York, 1985.)

INTRAVENTRICULAR HEMORRHAGE

It is estimated that about 40 percent of preterm infants weighing less than 1,500 g have an intraventricular hemorrhage (IVH). Intraventricular hemorrhage is unique to the newborn period. It is speculated that because of the hypervascularity of the subependymal regions in the premature brain and defective vascular autoregulation, there is increased perfusion to this area following an episode of ischemia. Transient increases in blood pressure can cause rupture of the thin-walled vessels (Fig. 9-1). There is evidence that the bleeding alters perfusion to the remainder of the hemisphere, compounding the injury. With increasing gestational age and maturation of these structures, the incidence of IVH drops. Rarely a term infant will suffer IVH.

The clinical picture of IVH is quite variable. Infants with mild degrees of bleeding show no detectable clinical signs. Infants with large amounts of bleeding usually experience a catastrophic event within 12 to 24 hours following a hypoxic episode. Other infants may show a saltatory progression. Signs include those typical for encephalopathy listed in Table 9-1 and, in catastrophic bleeding, a bulging fontanelle with a drop in hematocrit. The diagnosis can be made by

Table 9-4. Neuropathologic–Clinical Correlation of Hypoxic–Ischemic Encephalopathy

Pathology	Clinical Signs
Selective neuronal necrosis of cerebral and cerebellar cortices, thalamus, brain stem	Mental retardation, seizures, spastic cerebral palsy, bulbar deficits
Status marmoratus of basal ganglia	Choreoathetosis
Parasagittal cerebral necrosis	Proximal extremity weakness
Periventricular leukomalacia[a]	Spastic diplegia

[a] Premature infants.
(Data from Hill A, Volpe JJ: Seizures, hypoxic-ischemic brain injury, and intraventricular hemorrhage in the newborn. Ann Neurol 10:109–121, 1981.)

PREMATURITY
RESPIRATORY DISTRESS SYNDROME
↓
HYPOXIA & HYPERCARBIA
↓
LOSS OF AUTOREGULATION

APNEA
HANDLING
VOLUME EXPANSION

SYSTEMIC
HYPOTENSION
↓
DECREASED
CEREBRAL BLOOD FLOW
↓
INFARCTION OF
GERMINAL MATRIX
↓
INFARCTION OF PERIVENTRICULAR
WHITE MATTER
↓
PERIVENTRICULAR
HEMORRHAGE

SYSTEMIC
HYPERTENSION
↓
INCREASED
CEREBRAL BLOOD FLOW
↓
GERMINAL MATRIX
HEMORRHAGE
↓
INTRAVENTRICULAR
HEMORRHAGE

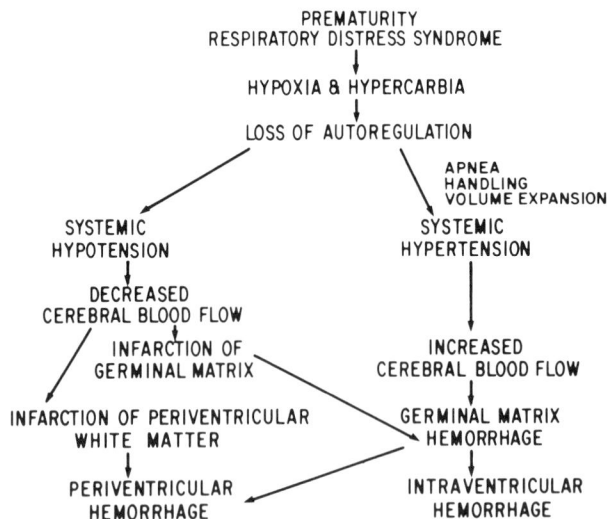

Fig. 9-1. Pathophysiology of periventricular-intraventricular hemorrhage. (From Fenichel GM: Neonatal Neurology. 2nd Ed. Churchill Livingstone, New York, 1985.)

a computed tomography scan or ultrasonography (Fig. 9-2). The severity of hemorrhages can be graded as outlined in Table 9-5. A spinal tap will show bloody cerebrospinal fluid (CSF) with increased protein and often decreased glucose.

The prognosis is related to the severity of hemorrhage. Mild degrees of hemorrhage are associated with little if any morbidity or mortality. Severe hem-

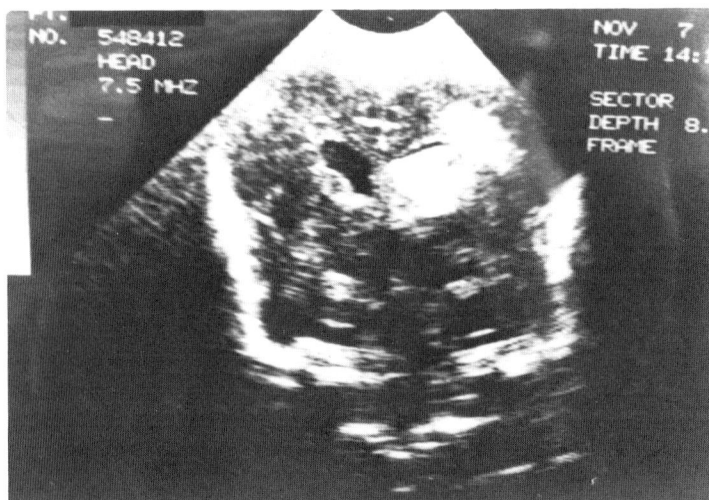

Fig. 9-2. Ultrasonogram of intraventricular hemorrhage.

Table 9-5. Grading of Intraventricular Hemorrhage in the Newborn

Grade	Description
1	Subependymal hemorrhage
2	Intraventricular hemorrhage without ventricular dilation
3	Intraventricular hemorrhage with ventricular dilation
4	Intraventricular hemorrhage with intraparenchymal extension

(Data from Burstein J, Papile LA, Burstein R: Intraventricular hemorrhage and hydrocephalus in premature infants: a prospective study with CT. Am J Radiol 132:427–635, 1979.)

orrhages, however, are associated with a greater than 50 percent mortality and long-term morbidity. Intermediate grades of hemorrhage have an intermediate prognosis. One complication is posthemorrhagic hydrocephalus. It occurs in the majority of patients who have severe hemorrhages and is less likely in the others. Etiology is thought to be secondary to obliterative arachnoiditis in the posterior fossa and subarachnoid system, as well as obstruction of the aqueduct. Ventricular dilatation is frequently present at the time of the bleeding and only later becomes progressive. This may occur initially in the absence of an increasing head size or even a bulging fontanelle. Posthemorrhagic hydrocephalus may resolve spontaneously without therapy.

The treatment of IVH is unsatisfactory. Avoiding excessive swings in blood pressure, such as that which follows rapid bicarbonate or blood infusions and excessive manipulation of the infant, may reduce the likelihood of hemorrhage. Prophylaxis with indomethacin has recently been shown to reduce the incidence of IVH. Specific therapy can lessen the degree of injury once it has occurred by maintaining oxygenation and perfusion, treatment of seizures, and other supportive care. Posthemorrhagic hydrocephalus is somewhat controversial. It can be managed pharmacologically with drugs such as acetazolamide and furosemide to decrease the amount of CSF production, serial lumbar punctures for communicating hydrocephalus, and ventriculoperitoneal shunting (Table 9-6).

BACTERIAL MENINGITIS

Bacterial meningitis may occur as an isolated infection or more commonly as part of generalized sepsis. The most frequent causes are listed in Table 9-7. *Escherichia coli* and group B streptococci are the most common causes of neonatal

Table 9-6. Treatment of Posthemorrhage Hydrocephalus

Therapy	Indications
Pharmacologic	Slowly progressive hydrocephalus
Acetazolamide, 100 mg/kg/day	
Furosemide, 1 mg/kg/day	
Glycerol, 1 mg/kg/day	
CSF drainage	Progressive hydrocephalus
Serial lumbar puncture	Responsive to lumbar puncture[a]
Ventriculostomy	Nonresponsive to lumbar puncture
Ventriculoperitoneal shunt	Greater than 50% ventricular volume, adequate size for permanent shunt

[a] Decrease in ventricular size or intracranial pressure following lumbar puncture.

Table 9-7. Bacteria Associated with Neonatal Sepsis

Organism	Source
Gram-positive bacteria	
Group B streptococci	
Early (sepsis)	Maternal
Late (meningitis)	Nosocomial and maternal
Staphlococcus aureas	Nosocomial
Listeria monocytogenes	
Early (sepsis)	Maternal
Late (meningitis)	Nosocomial and maternal
Streptococcus	
Pneumonocciae	Nosocomial and maternal
Gram-negative bacteria	
Escherichia coli	Maternal and nosocomial
Klebsiella pneumoniae	Nosocomial
Flavobacterium meningoseptum	Nosocomial
Pseudomonas aeruginosa	Nosocomial
Proteus mirabilis	Nosocomial
Citrobacter diversus	Nosocomial
Hemophilus influenzae	Maternal

meningitis. Meningitis in the newborn is acquired in three ways. The first is by inoculation from the infected mother in utero. Often the mother is febrile at the time of delivery or the membranes have been ruptured for more than 24 hours, causing choreoamnionitis. The most frequently cultured organisms are *E. coli* and group B *Streptococcus*. The second mode of inoculation is during passage through the birth canal, and the bacteria are similar. The third mode occurs during the neonatal period and often is due to hospital-acquired organisms such as *Staphylococcus, Pseudomonas,* and other gram-negative organisms, in addition to *E. coli* and group B *Streptococcus*. These infections may occur in epidemics and sometimes are thought to be secondary to the increased instrumentation and exposure of the infant in the neonatal nursery.

The clinical signs of meningitis in the infant are different than in older children and adults. Meningismus, bulging fontanelle, and fever are not reliable signs of meningitis in the newborn. Infants who acquire their infection prior to or at the time of delivery often present with overwhelming sepsis and multiorgan failure and usually die within 24 to 48 hours. Sepsis and meningitis acquired later in the neonatal period present with a variety of signs, some of which are quite subtle, such as a change in behavior, irritability, and poor feeding. Although the lumbar puncture is an important diagnostic test, it can rarely be normal in the neonate in the early stages of meningitis. If abnormal, the findings are similar to those in older children and adults, with increased protein, polymorphonuclear leukocytes, and hypoglycorrhachia. The pathophysiology is also similar to that in older children (see Ch. 33). There is a higher tendency for abscess formation and hemorrhagic necrosis of the brain. *Listeria* may cause microabscesses throughout the brain stem. In addition, ventriculitis is common in newborn meningitis, which complicates the therapy by making it more difficult to irradicate the organism.

The initial treatment of suspected sepsis and meningitis in the newborn is

Table 9-8. Commonly Used Antibiotics for the Treatment of Bacterial Meningitis in the Newborn

| Antibiotic | Daily Dosage and Intervals (Number of Divided Doses/24 hr) | |
	0–7 Days Old	Older Than 7 Days
Amikacin	15 mg/kg (2)	15 (?22.5) mg/kg (2 or ?3)[a]
Ampicillin		
Septicemia	50 mg/kg (2)	75–100 mg/kg/day (3 or 4)
Meningitis	200 mg/kg (2)	300 mg/kg/day (3)
Carbenicillin	200 mg/kg (2)	300–400 mg/kg (3 or 4)
Chloramphenicol	25 mg/kg (1)	50 mg/kg (2)
Gentamicin	5 mg/kg (2)	7.5 mg/kg (3)
Kanamycin	15–20 mg/kg (2)[b]	20–30 mg/kg (2 or 3)[b]
Methicillin		
Septicemia	50–75 mg/kg (2 or 3)	75–100 mg/kg (3 or 4)
Meningitis	100–150 mg/kg (2 or 3)	150–200 mg/kg (3 or 4)
Penicillin G		
Septicemia	50,000 U/kg (2)	75,000 U/kg (3)
Meningitis	100,000–150,000 U/kg (2 or 3)	150,000–250,000 U/kg (3 or 4)
Ticarcillin	150–250 mg/kg (2 or 3)[b]	225–300 mg/kg (3 or 4)[b]
Tobramycin	4 mg/kg (2)	4 (?6) mg/kg (2 or ?3)[a]
Vancomycin	30 mg/kg (2)	45 mg/kg (3)

[a] Additional studies required before larger dose can be recommended.
[b] Smaller dose for infants weighing less than 2,000 g, larger dose for infants weighing more than 2,000 g.
(From McCracken GH: Bacterial and viral infections of the newborn. p. 733. In Avery GB (ed): Neonatology, Pathophysiology and Management of the Newborn. 2nd Ed. JB Lippincott, Philadelphia, 1981.)

a combination of ampicillin and an aminoglycoside. If positive cultures are obtained, then therapy can be directed to the specific antibiotic sensitivities of the bacteria (Table 9-8). A total of 3 weeks of intravenous antibiotics or treatment until 2 weeks after the CSF becomes sterile is recommended. The prognosis of neonatal meningitis is relatively poor. The mortality rate is 30 to 40 percent and the morbidity in survivors is similar. Postinfectious hydrocephalus occurs frequently and must be monitored, as in children with IVH.

NONBACTERIAL INFECTIONS OF THE NERVOUS SYSTEM

The acronym *TORCH* is used to describe a variety of congenital infections which are acquired in utero (*t*oxoplasmosis, *r*ubella, *c*ytomegalovirus, *h*erpes). The clinical presentations of congenital infections are summarized in Table 9-9. There are many common signs and a clinical diagnosis of a specific agent in the newborn period is difficult without laboratory support. Because of maternal transmission, IgG antibodies are not specific in the newborn period and are only helpful if persistently elevated or showing a rising titer; IgM antibodies are much more specific in newborns. Neurologic manifestations of TORCH infections in the newborn period are seizures and encephalitis.

Toxoplasmosis

Toxoplasma gondii is a ubiquitous protozoan. The cat is a natural host for this organism. Infection in the mother usually goes unnoticed or it may cause a mild adenopathy. Transplacental transmission can occur anytime during preg-

Table 9-9. Clinical Features of
Congenital
Infections

Symptomatic infection
  Intrauterine growth retardation
  Rash
  Hepatitis
  Hepatosplenomegaly
  Jaundice
  Anemia
  Encephalitis
  Seizures
  Malformations (rubella)
Late manifestations
  Microcephaly
  Intracranial calcifications
  Chorioretinitis
  Cataracts
  Mental retardation
  Seizures
  Deafness
  Blindness

nancy, and the outcome depends upon the time of infection. Those acquiring the organism in the third trimester of pregnancy are usually asymptomatic. Early in pregnancy, however, the infection can cause severe complications in the fetus, with abortion, stillbirth, or symptomatic infection at birth. Congenital toxoplasmosis does not occur in subsequent children. The neuropathology is one of perivascular inflammation and gliosis. This is followed by cystic formation of necrotic nodules and finally by a deposition of calcium salts. The intracranial calcifications tend to be distributed diffusely. The diagnosis can be made by detection of IgM antibodies to toxoplasma. Therapy with sulfadiazine and pyrimethamine is indicated in older children; however, its use in newborn is an unsettled question.

Congenital Rubella

There has been a remarkable decline in the incidence of congenital rubella since the advent of immunization. The mother may have an asymptomatic infection or a more classic German measles. The virus is transmitted transplacentally and 20 percent of infants infected during the first trimester suffer from the teratogenic effects. The clinical syndrome is characterized by cataracts, hearing loss, congenital heart disease, intrauterine growth retardation, and mental retardation. Diagnosis is made by culturing the virus from the usual sources and by demonstrating IgM-specific antibodies. There is no treatment for this disease other than prevention. The prognosis is poor, with the majority of patients having one or more significant neurologic deficits, the most common being hearing loss. These deficits may progress as the infant ages, and indeed a rubella panen-

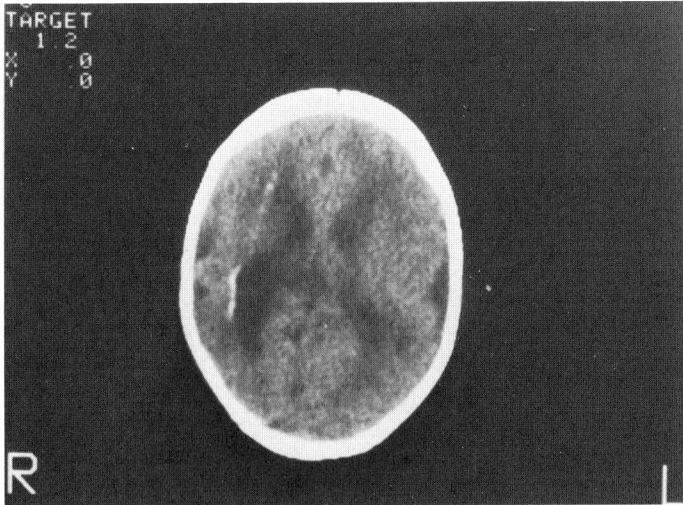

Fig. 9-3. Computed tomography scan of a child with congenital CMV demonstrating periventricular calcification.

cephalitis similar to subacute sclerosing panencephalitis can develop (see Ch. 33).

Cytomegalovirus

Cytomegalovirus (CMV) seldom causes clinical infection except in the medically debilitated, the immunosuppressed, or the fetus. A total of 1 to 2 percent of all healthy newborn have asymptomatic infections, making CMV the most common congenital infection. Of these, about 10% will ultimately demonstrate neurologic complications. A small minority have neonatal manifestations.

The infant can contract the disease in utero, during birth, or after neonatal exposure. Mothers can have subsequent infected infants, probably from a different serotype. Because the infected human may shed the virus in the urine for months to years, it is difficult to determine the time of exposure. Unlike rubella, exposure in the first trimester does not cause embryopathy. Pathologically, the virus has a predilection for ependymal cells, causing ependymitis and gliosis. Calcification is common and is periventricular in location (Figs. 9-3 and 9-4). The diagnosis is made by culturing the virus from the urine and detecting IgM-specific antibodies. There is no therapy and the prognosis is poor for normal development in symptomatic newborn. Seizures, microcephaly, retardation, and hearing and visual loss are common complications.

Herpes

Herpes simplex type II encephalitis is becoming more frequent with the increase of genital herpes in adults. The virus is contracted from an infected birth canal during delivery. The typical clinical presentation is one of vesicular rash

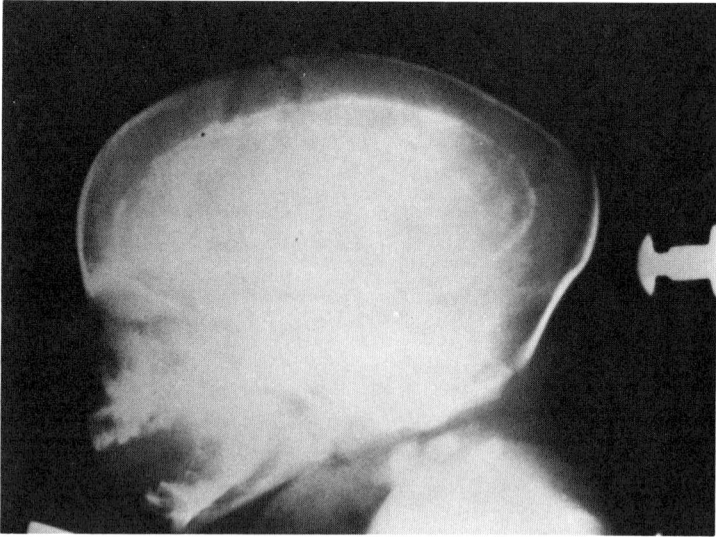

Fig. 9-4. Skull radiographs of a child with congenital CMV demonstrating extensive periventricular calcifications.

2 to 12 days after birth with disseminated, multiorgan infection and signs of sepsis in the newborn. The diagnosis can be made by antibody titers, virus culture from a vesicle, and by demonstrating maternal infection. Approximately 50 percent of neonates with herpes encephalitis die and 50 percent of survivors have severe neurologic deficits. There are no acceptable therapies for neonatal herpes encephalitis, although adenine arabinoside or acyclovir is often used. The best method is prevention because of the 40 percent risk of infection to the infant of an infected mother. Some recommend that a woman with a history of genital herpes have a scheduled cesarean section if there is evidence of infection during the last 6 weeks of pregnancy.

Other Viral Infections

Acquired viral meningoencephalitis is rare in the newborn. Occasionally outbreaks of Coxsackie B encephalomyocarditis occur. This presents as neonatal sepsis with multiorgan involvement, particularly the heart and brain. ECHO virus can cause aseptic meningitis in infants.

Syphilis

Congenital syphilis is caused by *Treponema pallidum* and is the result of transplacental transmission directly into the fetal circulation. The placenta is an effective barrier until approximately 4 months' gestation. Because there is no primary skin inoculation, the clinical manifestations are that of secondary syph-

Table 9-10. Encephalopathies Associated with Acquired Metabolic Disturbances in the Newborn

Disorder	Clinical Features	Etiologies	Treatment
Hypocalcemia <7.0 mg/dl	Muscle twitching Tetany Jitteriness Seizures	Small for gestational age Prematurity Infant of diabetic mother Asphyxia Hyperphosphatemia Hypomagnesemia DiGeorge's syndrome	4 ml (200 mg)/kg calcium gluconate 5% iv
Hypomagnesemia <0.75 mg/dl	Similar to hypocalcemia	Maternal deficiency Infant of diabetic mother Small for gestational age Exchange transfusion with citrated blood Hyperphosphatemia	2 ml (20 mg)/kg MgSO$_4$ 2% iv
Hypermagnesemia >2.0 mg/dl	Hypotonia	Maternal administration for toxemia	Exchange transfusion with citrated blood
Hypoglycemia <30 mg/dl, term <20 mg/dl, premature	Hypotonia Jitteriness Seizures Apnea Stupor	Small for gestational age Infant of diabetic mother	4 ml (1 g)/kg glucose 25% iv
Hyponatremia <125 mEq/L	Seizures Obtundation	Syndrome of inappropriate secretion of antidiuretic hormone (SIADH) with meningitis	Normal saline Fluid restriction

ilis, which has few neurologic signs. About 5 percent of affected infants have an abnormal CSF and will show signs of meningoencephalitis. This presents several weeks after birth with the typical skin rash of secondary syphilis, condylomata, "snuffles," and arthritis. The diagnosis is determined by serologic tests. Positive serology in the mother warrants treatment for both mother and infant. Therapy of suspected disease consists of 50,000 U/kg/day of penicillin G for 10 days.

METABOLIC AND PHARMACOLOGIC ENCEPHALOPATHIES

The most common metabolic encephalopathies in the newborn do not differ significantly from those in older children. Some disorders, such as hypoglycemia, hypocalcemia, and hypomagnesemia, are common in certain populations of

Table 9-11. Drug-Induced Neurologic Disorders in the Newborn

Drug	Neurologic Disorder
Stimulants	
Addiction withdrawal	Jitteriness, irritability, high-pitched cry, seizures
Narcotics	
Barbiturates	
Methylxanthines	Hypertonicity, jitteriness, seizures
Caffeine	
Theophylline	
Phenothiazines	Opisthotonus, tremor, dystonia
Depressants	
Anesthetics	Lethargy, hypotonia
General	
Local	
Narcotics	Respiratory depression, narcosis
Magnesium sulfate	Hypotonia
Lithium carbonate	Hypotonia

newborn, such as those born to diabetic mothers and infants small for gestational age. The long-term prognosis is generally good and is more related to the precipitating cause than to the effects of the metabolic derangement itself. The exception is hypoglycemia. Infants who have symptomatic hypoglycemia have a worse prognosis for normal development than children who are asymptomatic. Inborn errors of metabolism are a rare cause of neonatal encephalopathy and are covered in Chapter 19. Table 9-10 summarizes the common acquired metabolic encephalopathies in the newborn.

Bilirubin encephalopathy is becoming increasingly rare with improved neonatal medicine. In term infants, accepted practice is to maintain the indirect bilirubin concentration below 20 mg/dl, although levels up to 30 mg/dl are probably tolerated. In preterm infants, a general rule sometimes used is to maintain the level below 1 mg/dl per 100 g of weight, although there are no data to support this. Other disorders, such as hypoxia, sepsis, and acidosis, may worsen the risk of bilirubin encephalopathy, although firm data are lacking. Classically, infants with bilirubin encephalopathy go through several phases. The first is one of lethargy, hypotonia, and poor feeding. The second begins at 24 to 48 hours or later, with hyperexcitability, a high-pitched cry, seizures, and irritability. These findings are similar to any encephalopathy in the newborn. This is followed by a return to normal muscle tone for several months. The development of mental retardation and choreoathetosis becomes apparent over the following months. In the early phases, staining of the basal ganglia by bilirubin can be found (kernicterus).

Table 9-11 lists the common pharmacologically induced encephalopathies. These are largely from obstetric usage and secondarily affect the infant. The prognosis is generally good.

SELECTED READINGS

Allen WC, Dransfield DA, Tito AM: Ventricular dilation follow periventricular intraventricular hemorrhage: outcome at age 1 year. Pediatrics 73:158–162, 1984

Giles FH, Jammes JL, Berenberg W: Neonatal meningitis. Arch Neurol 34:560–562, 1977

Gutberlet RL, Cornblath M: Neonatal hypoglycemia revisited 1975. Pediatrics 58:10–17, 1976

Klem JO, Marcy SM: Bacterial sepsis and meningitis. p. 679. In Remington JS, Klein JO (eds): Infectious Diseases of the Fetus and Newborn Infant. 2nd Ed. WB Saunders, Philadelphia, 1983

Kumar ML, Nankervis GA, jacob IB et al: Congenital and postnatally acquired cytomegalovirus infections: long-term follow up. J Pediatr 104:674–679, 1984

Lorber J, Bhat US: Posthaemorrhagic hydrocephalus. Diagnosis, differential diagnosis, treatment, and long-term results. Arch Dis Child 49:751–752, 1974

Mulligan JC, Painter MJ, O'Donoghue PA et al: Neonatal asphyxia II. Neonatal mortality and long-term sequelae. Pediatrics 96:903–907, 1980

Nelson KB, Broman SH: Perinatal risk factors in children with serious motor and mental handicaps. Ann Neurol 2:371–377, 1977

Papile LA, Burstein J, Burstein R, Koffler H: Incidence and evolution of subependymal and intraventriular hemorrhages. A study of infants with birth weights less than 1,500 grams. J Pediatr 92:529–534, 1978

Robertson NRC, Smith MA: Early neonatal hypocalcemia. Arch Dis Child 50:604–609, 1975

Sarff LD, Platt LH, McCracken GH, Jr.: Cerebrospinal fluid evaluation in neonates: a comparison of high risk infants with and without meningitis. J Pediatr 88:473–477, 1976

Sarnat HB, Sarnat MS: Neonatal encephalopathy following fetal distress. Arch Neurol 33:696–705, 1976

Shinnar S, Molteni RA, Gammon K et al: Intraventricular hemorrhage in the premature infant, a changing outlook. N Engl J Med 306:1464–1468, 1982

Van Praagh R: Diagnosis of kernicterus in the neonatal period. Pediatrics 28:870–876, 1961

Williamson WD, Desmond MM, Wilson GS et al: Survival of low birthweight infants with neonatal intraventricular hemorrhage, outcome in the preschool years. Am J Dis Child 137:1181–1184, 1983

Wilson CB, Remington JS, Stagno S, Reynolds DW: Development of adverse sequelae in children born with subclinical congenital toxoplasma infection. Pediatrics 66:767–774, 1980

10

SEIZURES IN THE NEWBORN

The incidence of seizures in the newborn is approximately 0.3 percent and is a common sign of encephalopathy. Neonatal seizures are a poor prognostic sign. Half of the patients will have neurologic handicaps or die from the underlying illness. The prognosis is worse for premature newborn who have seizures.

CLINICAL FEATURES

The clinical characteristics of neonatal seizures are listed in Table 10-1. The CNS of the neonate is immature. Intracortical and descending fiber tracts are incompletely myelinated at birth. A seizure discharge may not be equally expressed in all parts of the brain which can cause seizures in the newborn to be fragmentary or subtle in their clinical appearance. Generalized seizures are similar to those seen in older children, whereas myoclonic seizures are rare in infancy and usually indicate a severe and diffuse brain injury. The type of seizure is not necessarily correlated with the underlying etiology. Movements which may simulate seizures, as well as their underlying etiologies, are listed in Table 10-2.

ETIOLOGY

The most common cause of seizures in the newborn period is perinatal asphyxia. The usual onset is within the first 12 to 24 hours but may continue beyond this period (Table 10-3). In premature infants, intraventricular hemorrhage is also a common cause and occurs on the second or third day after birth. Infections of the nervous system and certain metabolic disorders may occur at any time, whereas seizures associated with malformations of the brain usually occur later. The common etiologies for neonatal seizures are listed in Table 10-4.

EVALUATION

In most cases, the etiology for neonatal seizures can be determined by careful review of the clinical course, maternal and family history, and physical exam. If there is no history of perinatal distress or obvious metabolic predisposition for

Table 10-1. Patterns of Neonatal Seizures

Type	Description
Subtle	Apnea, eye deviations or fluttering, bicycling movements, chewing or sucking, other repetitive stereotyped movements
Multifocal clonic	Migratory focal motor
Partial	Focal clonic
Generalized motor	Generalized clonic or tonic
Myoclonic	Synchronized, brief jerking movements

seizures, then a further evaluation for the etiology is indicated (Table 10-5). Blood glucose and calcium concentrations and an evaluation for sepsis and meningitis must be obtained in every infant with a seizure. Electrolytes are also helpful for the diagnosis of hyponatremia and acidosis, because many inborn errors of metabolism which cause seizures also cause a metabolic acidosis. An increased anion gap alerts the physician to this possibility. Blood and urine amino and organic acids are necessary to diagnose most inborn errors of metabolism. Infants without an explainable metabolic disturbance should have a computed tomography scan or ultrasound of the head to diagnose cerebral trauma, hemorrhage, or cerebral dysgenesis. Drug withdrawal, benign familial neonatal seizures, and pyridoxine dependency may cause seizures in infants with otherwise normal studies.

An EEG is indicated for infants with subtle behaviors for which a seizure diagnosis cannot be made with certainty. The EEG is sufficiently different in infants from that in older children or adults that it should be performed by technologists and interpreted by electroencephalographers who are experienced in infant EEG. Observation of the infant is especially important in interpreting the EEG to determine sleep and active states and to note subtle behaviors which may represent seizures.

The EEG can be abnormal in the newborn because of either abnormal organization of the background or electroconvulsive discharges. Background abnormalities include suppression of activity, lack of variability, and persistence of immature characteristics. Electroconvulsive discharges may be difficult to recognize because of the normal bursting characteristic of the infant EEG, as well

Table 10-2. Nonconvulsive Motor Activity

Abnormality	Description	Etiology
Opisthotonus	Forced extension of the neck	Kernicterus, Gaucher's disease, posterior fossa hematoma
Decerebrate posturing	Forced extension of the extremities	Increased intracranial pressure
Jitteriness	Excessive tremulousness with stimulation	Hypoglycemia, hypocalcemia, drug withdrawal
Tonic neck reflex	"Fencing" position	Normal reflex
Tetany	Muscle spasm	Hypocalcemia, hypomagnesemia
Rigidity	Continuous motor activity	Caffeine intoxication, Isaac's syndrome, phenothiazines
Apnea	Longer than 15 seconds	Nonconvulsive apnea

Table 10-3. Onset of Neonatal Seizures

At 12 hours
   Direct drug effects
   Perinatal asphyxia
   Pyridoxine dependency
At 24 hours
   Bacterial meningitis
   Direct drug effects
   Laceration of tentorium or falx
   Perinatal asphyxia
   Pyridoxine dependency
   Rubella, toxoplasmosis, cytomegalovirus
   Sepsis
At 24–72 hours
   Bacterial meningitis
   Cerebral contusion with subdural hemorrhage
   Cerebral dysgenesis
   Drug withdrawal
   Glycogen synthetase deficiency
   Incontinentia pigmenti
   Intraventricular hemorrhage of the premature
   Nonketotic hyperglycinemia
   Sepsis
   Subarachnoid hemorrhage
   Urea cycle disturbances
At 72 hours
   Benign familial neonatal convulsions
   Cerebral dysgenesis
   Kernicterus
   Ketotic hyperglycinemias
   Nutritional hypocalcemia
   Smith-Lemli-Opitz syndrome
   Urea cycle disturbances
At 1 week
   Cerebral dysgenesis
   Fructose dysmetabolism
   Herpes simplex
   Ketotic hyperglycinemias
   Maple syrup urine disease
   Urea cycle disturbances

(Modified from Fenichel GM: Neonatal Neurology. 2nd Ed. Churchill Livingstone, New York, 1985.)

as the normal spikes and sharp transients present at this age. The most reliable criteria for a convulsive discharge are a repetitive, rhythmic discharge and a persistent discharge from a single focus. A normal EEG does not exclude the diagnosis of a seizure disorder.

TREATMENT

As in any pediatric emergency, the main efforts of treatment should be to maintain adequate ventilation and to support the cardiovascular system. In the presence of adequate oxygenation and blood glucose, brief seizures are unlikely to cause permanent neurologic deficits. Because prolonged convulsions may

Table 10-4. Etiology of Neonatal
Convulsions

Perinatal asphyxia
Birth trauma
Intracranial hemorrhage
Infectious disorders
   Intrauterine
      Rubella
      Toxoplasmosis
      Cytomegalovirus
   Perinatal
      Herpes simplex
      Bacterial meningitis
      Sepsis
Metabolic
   Hypoglycemia
   Hypocalcemia
   Hyponatremia
   Hypomagnesemia
   Kernicterus
Inborn errors of metabolism
   Maple syrup urine disease
   Nonketotic hyperglycinemia
   Ketotic hyperglycinemias
   Urea cycle disorders
Other genetic defects
   Pyridoxine dependency
   Incontinentia pigmenti
   Smith-Lemli-Opitz syndrome
   Disorders of ganglioside metabolism
Drugs
   Withdrawal
   Intoxications
Cerebral dysgenesis
Benign familial neonatal convulsions

(Modified from Fenichel GM: Neonatal
Neurology. 2nd Ed. Churchill Livingstone,
New York, 1985.)

Table 10-5. Evaluation for Neonatal Seizures

Initial evaluation
   Blood glucose, calcium, magnesium, and electrolytes
   Cerebrospinal fluid examination for glucose, protein, and cell count
   Complete blood count
   Culture of blood, cerebrospinal fluid, urine
Further evaluation
   Computed tomography or ultrasonography of the head
   Blood ammonia, liver enzymes and lactate
   Blood and urine amino and organic acids
   Urine-reducing substances
   Therapeutic trial with pyridoxine
   TORCH antibody determinations

Table 10-6. Anticonvulsants for the Treatment of Seizures in the Newborn

Drug	Dosage for Status Epilepticus	Maintenance Dose (Schedule)
Phenobarbital	20 mg/kg iv	4 mg/kg/day (bid)
Phenytoin	20 mg/kg iv	5 mg/kg/day (bid)
Diazepam	0.3 mg/kg iv	
Paraldehyde	2 ml per rectum (50% solution with mineral oil)	
Primidone		15 mg/kg/day (tid)
Valproic acid		30 mg/kg/day (tid)

cause brain injury, treatment is indicated. Fragmentary seizures which are not causing direct injury to the child can be approached more conservatively. If an underlying cause such as drug withdrawal, electrolyte disturbance, or a treatable underlying metabolic disorder can be diagnosed, then the treatment should obviously be directed toward its correction. When anticonvulsive therapy is indicated, it should be administered promptly and in appropriate dosages (Table 10-6).

Phenobarbital is the most commonly used anticonvulsant in the newborn. It can be administered intravenously or orally and is generally well tolerated. Phenytoin is also an effective anticonvulsant in the newborn. It is difficult to maintain adequate phenytoin blood levels with oral administration in neonates, so intravenous administration must be continued as long as the child is on the medication. Intramuscular administration should be avoided because of poor absorption and the possibility of creating a sterile abcess at the site of injection. Both phenobarbital and phenytoin are the initial drugs of choice for the treatment of status epilepticus in the newborn. Other drugs that are used to treat status in infants are diazepam, paraldehyde, and valproic acid.

The treatment of intractable seizures which do not respond to phenytoin or phenobarbital becomes difficult. Primidone and valproic acid are alternative therapies, although there is no extensive experience in infants and prematures. Drug levels in the blood should be monitored regularly to ensure therapeutic dosages and to avoid toxicity. In general, if the child has seizures associated with an identifiable acute encephalopathy, there should be coverage for the seizures during the encephalopathic period. If the encephalopathy resolves and there are no further seizures, then it is not necessary to continue therapy after discharge.

SELECTED READINGS

Bergmann I, Painter MJ, Crumrine PK: Neonatal seizures. Semin Perinat 6:54–67, 1982

Cockburn E, Brown JK, Belton NR, Forfar JO: Neonatal convulsions associated with primary disturbances of calcium, phosphorus, and magnesium metabolism. Arch Dis Child 48:99–108, 1973

Holden KR, Mellitis ED, Freeman JM: Neonatal seizures: I. Correlation of prenatal and perinatal events with outcomes. Pediatrics 70:165–176, 1982

Mellits ED, Kenton RH, Freeman JM: Neonatal seizures: II. A multivariate analysis of factors associated with outcome. Pediatrics 70:177–185, 1982

Tibbles JAR: Dominant benign neonatal seizures. Dev Med Child Neurol 22:664–667, 1980

Volpe JJ: Neonatal seizures. N Engl J Med 289:413–416, 1973

11

THE FLOPPY INFANT

Hypotonia is the loss of muscle tone and is usually, but not necessarily, associated with loss of muscle strength. Hypotonia, muscle weakness, or both cause the common clinical picture in the neonatal period of the floppy infant. In the newborn period the diverse causes of hypotonia present very similar clinical pictures. Thus a careful history, physical examination, and selected laboratory tests are necessary to differentiate the various causes of this disorder.

Hypotonia can result from dysfunction of any part of the motor system, which includes the motor cortex and pyramidal tracts, extrapyramidal and cerebral systems, and the motor unit (anterior horn cell, peripheral nerve, neuromuscular junction, and muscle fibers. See Ch. 24). This forms the basis for the differential diagnosis of hypotonia in the newborn. Table 11-1 summarizes the various categories of hypotonia and their etiologies.

PHYSICAL FINDINGS

Hypotonia refers to the resting muscle tone of the muscle and is best observed in those muscles which support the body against gravity. In the supine position, the hypotonic infant shows a loss of fetal posturing and assumes the characteristic "frog leg" position (Fig. 11-1). Vertical suspension (Fig. 11-2) and horizontal suspension (Fig. 11-3) demonstrate the infant's inability to maintain normal posture against gravity. The most sensitive test for muscle strength is the traction test, which involves pulling the infant upright from the supine position by traction on the hands. The normal response is flexion of the neck, lifting the head, and a reflex pulling of the arms. Head lag and lack of grasping or pulling in the arms is an indication of decreased strength (Fig. 11-4).

Certain parts of the physical examination should be highlighted. Aside from hypotonia, muscle weakness can present in the newborn with respiratory distress and swallowing difficulties. The deep tendon reflexes are helpful only if they are present or exaggerated. If so, they exclude a diagnosis of anterior horn cell disease or a neuropathy. The absence of reflexes does not exclude any specific diagnosis. Ophthalmoplegia and ptosis in the alert child is always indicative of an underlying disorder of the motor unit. Joint deformities, especially multiple joint contractures (arthrogryposis multiplex congenita), indicate a long-standing state of hypotonia or immobility (Table 11-2). Abnormal primitive reflexes such as persistent tonic neck response or scissoring with vertical suspension are signs of upper motor neuron injury. Dysmorphic features can suggest a specific syn-

Table 11-1. Classification and Etiologies of Infantile Hypotonia

Category	Etiology
Cerebral hypotonia	Acute perinatal encephalopathy Chronic encephalopathy
Myelopathy	Trauma Malformations
Spinal muscular atrophy	Werdnig-Hoffmann disease (infantile spinal muscular atrophy) Neurogenic arthrogryposis
Polyneuropathy	Congenital hypomyelinating polyneuropathy, hereditary sensory neuropathy Familial dysautonomia (Riley-Day syndrome)
Myasthenia disorders	Transitory neonatal myasthenia gravis, congenital myasthenias Infantile botulism
Myopathies	Myotonic dystrophy, congenital muscular dystrophy Congenital myopathies with fiber-type disproportion Metabolic myopathies

drome or chromosome abnormality, both of which are associated with hypotonia.

CEREBRAL HYPOTONIA

Any acute or chronic insult to the cerebrum or the extrapyramidal system can cause hypotonia. In children with systemic illnesses or evidence of perinatal disease the diagnosis is not difficult because of the altered consciousness and other evidence of encephalopathy. In others in which the sensorium appears to be intact, congenital malformations of the brain, chromosomal disorders, dysmorphic syndromes, and the rare degenerative diseases must be considered.

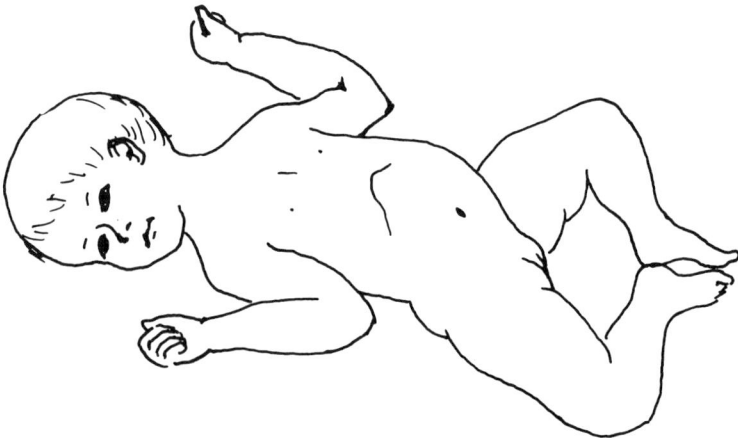

Fig. 11-1. Frog-leg position of the hypotonic infant.

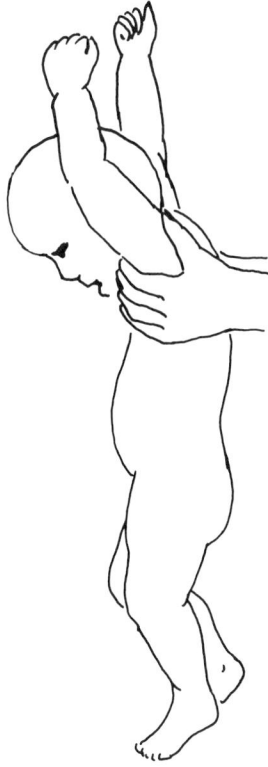

Fig. 11-2. Abnormal vertical suspension.

Physical findings often demonstrate severe hypotonia, preserved reflexes, and normal strength on reflex movement. A number of infants with hypotonia will later develop cerebral palsy but many may be normal. Marked, persistent hypotonia is often indicative of an extrapyramidal form of cerebral palsy, particularly those associated with ataxia. In many such cases there will be a malformation of the cerebellum. In general, the most common causes of cerebral hypotonia in the newborn period are perinatal distress from any cause and genetic defects. Table 11-3 summarizes some of the more common causes for cerebral hypotonia. Some of these syndromes also affect the motor unit as well.

MYELOPATHY

The connections of the upper motor neuron system to the lower motor neuron can be disrupted by trauma to the cervical spinal cord during a complicated delivery. High cervical cord trauma, which is more common in rotational injuries to the neck, presents with failure to initiate respirations, flaccid quadriparesis, and conscious sensation of pain restricted to the head. Lower cervical cord trauma is more often associated with hyperextension of the neck and often

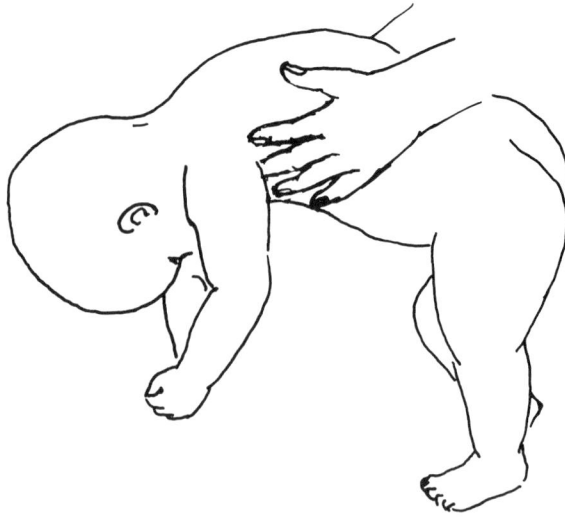

Fig. 11-3. Abnormal horizontal suspension.

associated with breech delivery. Respiration, as well as some voluntary movement of the upper extremities, is usually preserved. In either case hypotonia,
particularly of the lower portions of the body, is marked owing to the spinal
shock. In time, some segmental reflexes will return, which can cause confusion
in the differential diagnosis. The diagnosis can be made, however, by showing
indifference to pain by lack of crying or facial grimaces when the lower legs are
stimulated.

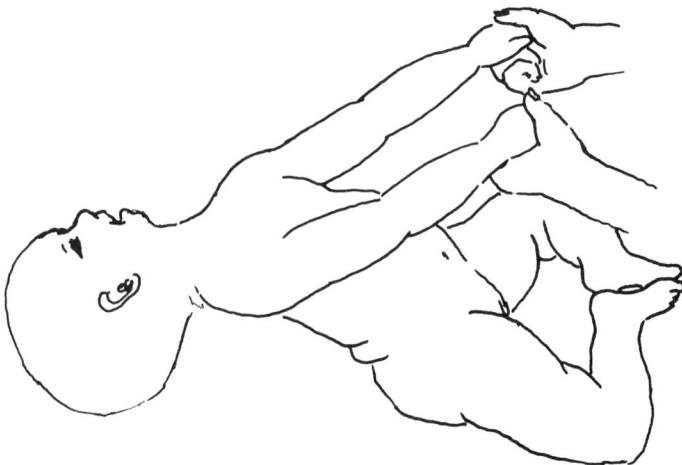

Fig. 11-4. Abnormal traction test.

Table 11-2. Disorders Associated with Arthrogryposis
Multiplex Congenita

Neuromuscular
  Congenital fiber-type disproportion
  Congenital muscular dystrophy
  Spinal muscular atrophy and other neurogenic causes
  Myotonic dystrophy
  Vertebral segmental dysplasia, caudal regression syndrome
  Spina bifida
Other
  Oligohydramnios
  Fetal crowding (bicornuate uterus, fibroid, etc.)
  Renal agenesis
  Larsen syndrome (arthrogryposis, minor dysmorphic features)
  Idiopathic

Meningomyelocele is apparent at birth and causes a flaccid paraparesis in the lower extremities if the lesion is low. Occasionally there will be no apparent malformation externally, but paraparesis can exist with occult dysrhaphic malformations of the neural tube. The tethered cord usually presents later in childhood, but those associated with lipomas and intra-abdominal myeloceles may present earlier. The diagnosis is suggested by finding spina bifida on radiographs and confirming it by myelography. Surgical excision and repair are necessary.

Table 11-3. Cerebral Hypotonia

Disorder	Predominant Signs	Etiologies
Acute encephalopathy	Seizures, altered consciousness	Perinatal asphyxia Sepsis and meningitis Acquired metabolic disturbances of glucose, calcium, electrolytes Inborn errors of metabolism Birth trauma Intracranial hemorrhage Intoxications, drug withdrawal

Chronic encephalopathy	Dysmorphism, malformations, microcephaly	Neural tube defects
		Microcephaly
		Cerebral and cerebellar malformations
		Chromosomal disorders
		Congenital infections
		Dysmorphic syndromes
		  Prader-Willi (hypotonia, micropenis, obesity, mental retardation)
		  Cohen (hypotonia, obesity, mental retardation, multiple minor dysmorphic features)
		  Zellweger (cerebrohepatorenal: hypotonia, hepatomegaly, multiple minor dysmorphic features, polycystic kidneys)
		  Lowe (oculocerebrorenal: hyporeflexia, cataracts, glaucoma, renal tubule dysfunction

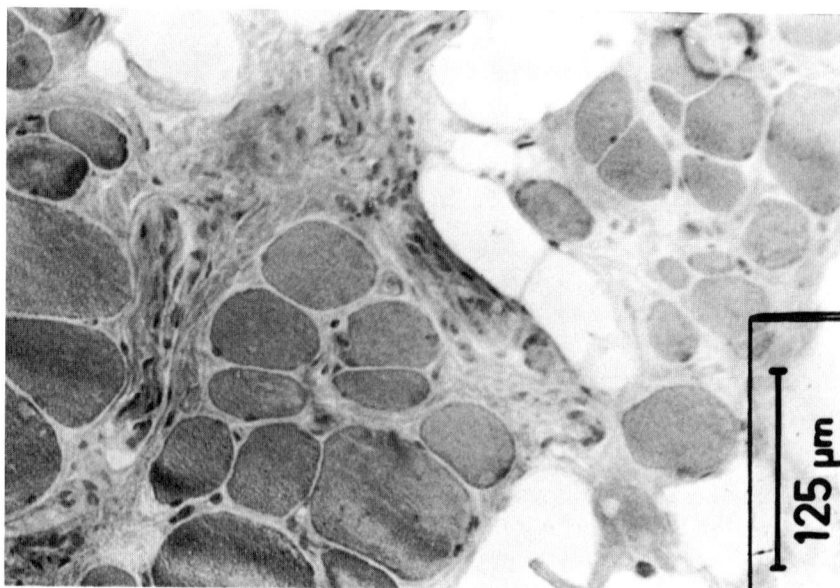

Fig. 11-5. Photomicrograph of congenital muscular dystrophy.

SPINAL MUSCULAR ATROPHIES

Infantile spinal muscular atrophy (Werdnig-Hoffmann disease) is a progressive degeneration of lower motor neurons. The most common onset is in the first 6 months of life; rarely will it cause hypotonia in the newborn period. In some cases severe weakness is present at birth and frequently there is a history of decreased fetal movements. Some of these children will have arthrogryposis multiplex congenita. The pertinent clinical findings are diffuse hypotonia and muscle weakness, absence of deep tendon reflexes, and fasciculations of the tongue. Electromyography shows the typical picture of large-amplitude polyphasic potentials, a reduced interference pattern, fasciculations, and fibrillations. The muscle biopsy demonstrates groups of fiber atrophy, fiber-type grouping, and histochemical evidence of denervation (see Fig. 25-1). Children with the onset of spinal muscular atrophy in the first few months have a very poor prognosis. There is no treatment.

POLYNEUROPATHY

Polyneuropathy is rare in the newborn period. Familial hypomyelinating polyneuropathy is a disorder in which there is a deficiency in the production of peripheral nervous system myelin. The infants are severely weak and often succumb to their illness in the newborn period. Familial dysautonomia, or the Riley-Day syndrome, is another neuropathy which may present as infantile hypotonia. In this disease there is evidence of dysfunction of the autonomic system, with temperature instability, failure to thrive, disorders of sweating and cardiac arrhythmias, inability to tear, and absent fugiform papillae on the tongue. The diagnosis of polyneuropathy is made by showing slowed motor or sensory nerve conduction velocities. The electromyogram may show denervation. A nerve biopsy shows a marked reduction in myelin. The Riley-Day syndrome can be diagnosed by performing a histamine test which shows the absence of a flare surrounding the wheal.

DISEASE OF THE NEUROMUSCULAR JUNCTION

Myasthenic syndromes occur in three major syndromes in infancy. Transitory neonatal myasthenia is a disorder acquired from the mother who has myasthenia gravis. This is an autoimmune disease mediated by IgG antibodies which are directed at the acetylcholine receptor of the skeletal muscle that are passively transferred across the placenta and cause a myasthenic disorder in the infant. The mother may be in remission at the time the infant is affected. The most frequent manifestations in addition to hypotonia are swallowing difficulties and respiratory distress. The diagnosis is made by performing a Tensilon test (1 mg iv), which improves weakness within 10 to 15 minutes. Treatment is intramuscular neostigmine injection (0.1 mg) prior to feeding. Usually the infant needs no therapy except at feeding time; however, in severe cases the condition may require plasmapheresis or exchange transfusion. Electrodiagnostic tests show a decremental response to repetitive stimulation.

The second myasthenic syndrome in the newborn period is congenital myasthenia. This causes ophthalmoplegia and rarely hypotonia. The third group consists of the familial infantile myasthenias, which present with marked weakness and respiratory distress. The etiology is thought to be presynaptic and associated with deficiencies in the production or degradation of acetylcholine or acetylcholinesterase or the physiologic effects of acetylcholine on the receptor. These are rare, recessively inherited disorders and may or may not respond to acetylcholinesterase inhibitors. Diagnosis is contingent upon the absence of myasthenia gravis in the mother, the lack of circulating antireceptor antibodies in the mother or infant, and the demonstration of biochemical or physiologic abnormalities by muscle biopsy.

Infantile botulism is very rare in the newborn period, although it has been reported. Botulinum toxin is a potent inhibitor of acetylcholine release. Infants affected with this disease frequently have swallowing difficulties and bulbar weakness in addition to hypotonia. Unlike adults and older children with botulism, in infancy the organism can frequently be recovered from the stool. Thus a culture of *Clostridium botulinum* or biologic assay for the botulinum toxin makes the diagnosis. Treatment is directed at supporting the infant, frequently with assisted ventilation, until recovery.

MYOPATHIES

Diseases of the muscle which are present at birth are termed congenital myopathies. These disorders are not easily distinguishable clinically in the newborn period and all require a muscle biopsy for precise diagnosis. Many of the

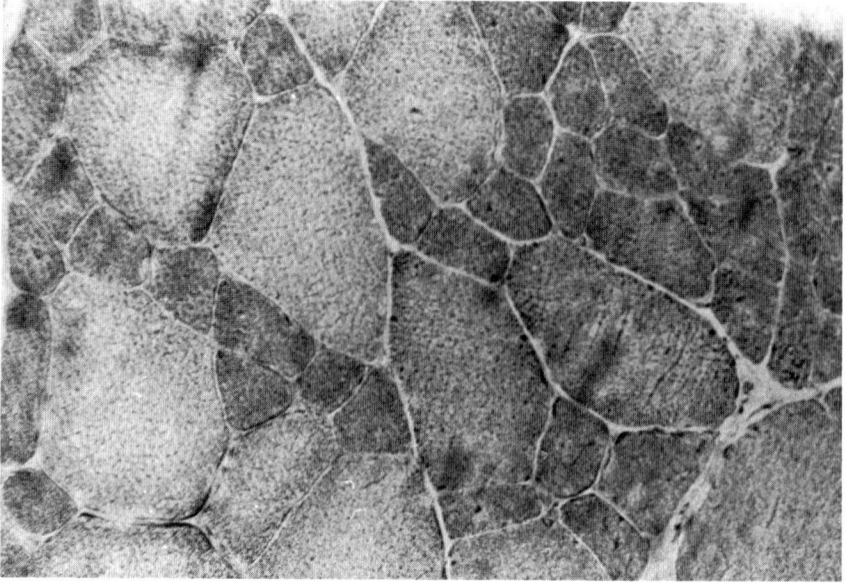

Fig. 11-6. Photomicrograph of congenital fiber-type disproportion.

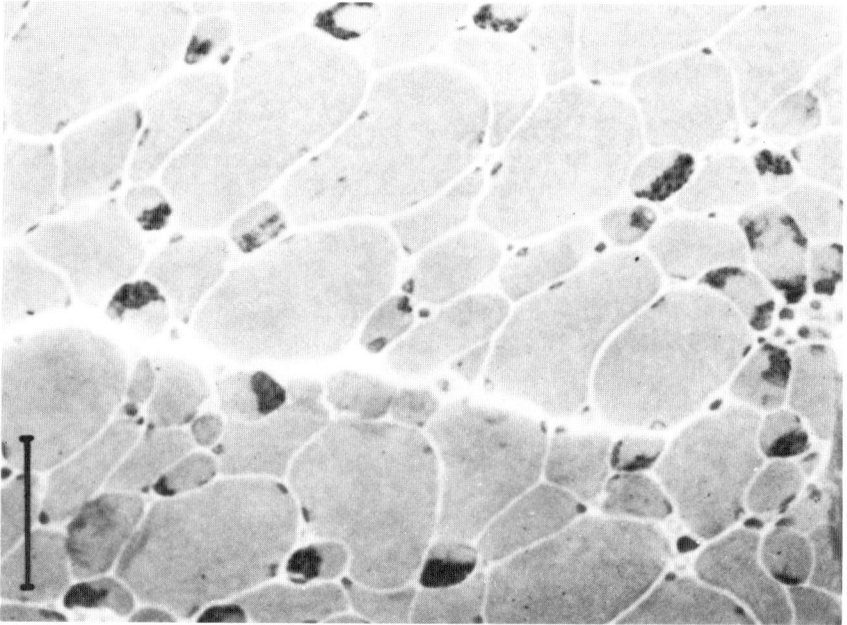

Fig. 11-7. Photomicrograph of nemaline rod myopathy.

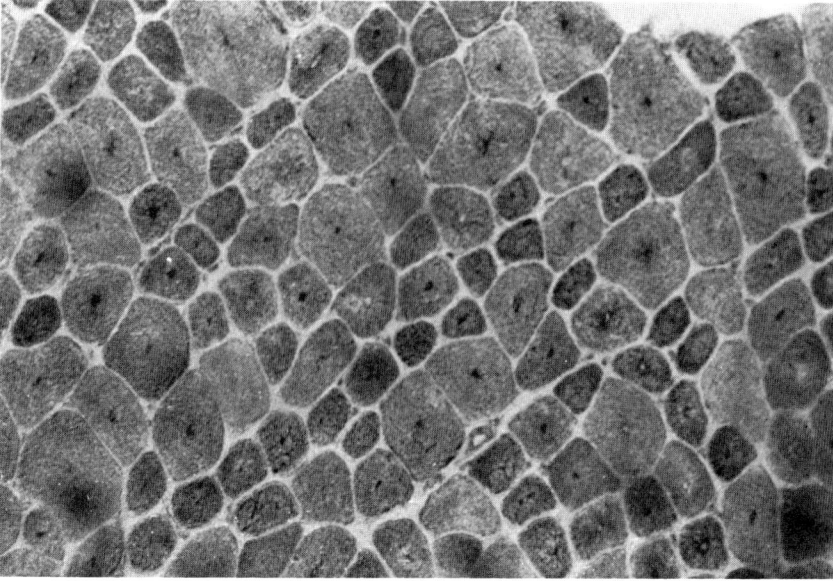

Fig. 11-8. Photomicrograph of myotubular myopathy.

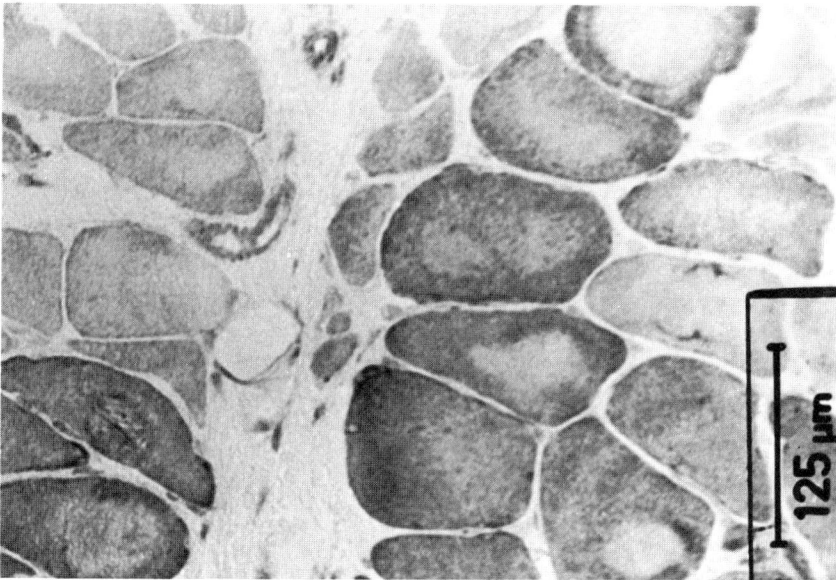

Fig. 11-9. Photomicrograph of central core myopathy.

Table 11-4. Disorders of the Motor Unit that Cause Infantile Hypotonia

Structure and Disorder	Signs	Electrodiagnostic Findings	Muscle Biopsy	Other
Anterior horn cell				
Spinal muscular atrophy	Areflexia, fasciculations	Neuropathic electromyography, fasciculations	Fiber atrophy Fascicular atrophy	Fiber-type grouping
Peripheral nerve				
Neuropathy	Areflexia	Slowed nerve conduction velocities	Neurogenic atrophy	Abnormal nerve biopsy
Dysautonomia	Autonomic disturbances, failure to thrive		Normal	Positive histamine test
Neuromuscular junction				
Transistory neonatal myasthenia	Bulbar weakness	Abnormal repetitive stimulation	Normal	Positive Tensilon test Antireceptor titer
Congenital myasthenia	Prosis ophthalmoplegia	Abnormal repetitive stimulation	Normal	Positive tensilon test
Botulism	Bulbar weakness, constipation	Posttetanic facilitation	Normal	Fecal culture, detection of toxin
Muscle				
Congenital muscular dystrophy	Joint deformities	Myopathic electromyography	Dystrophic	
Myotonic dystrophy	Bulbar weakness, joint deformities	Myotonia	Type 1 atrophy	
Fiber-type disproportions	Deformities	Myopathic electromyography	Fiber-type disproportion	Nemaline rods, myotubes, central cores may be found in biopsy
Nemaline rod				
Myotubular				
Central core				
Multicore				
Congenital fiber-type disproportion				
Metabolic myopathies	Weakness	Myopathic electromyography	Vacuolar myopathy	Glycogen and lipid storage, abnormal mitochondria

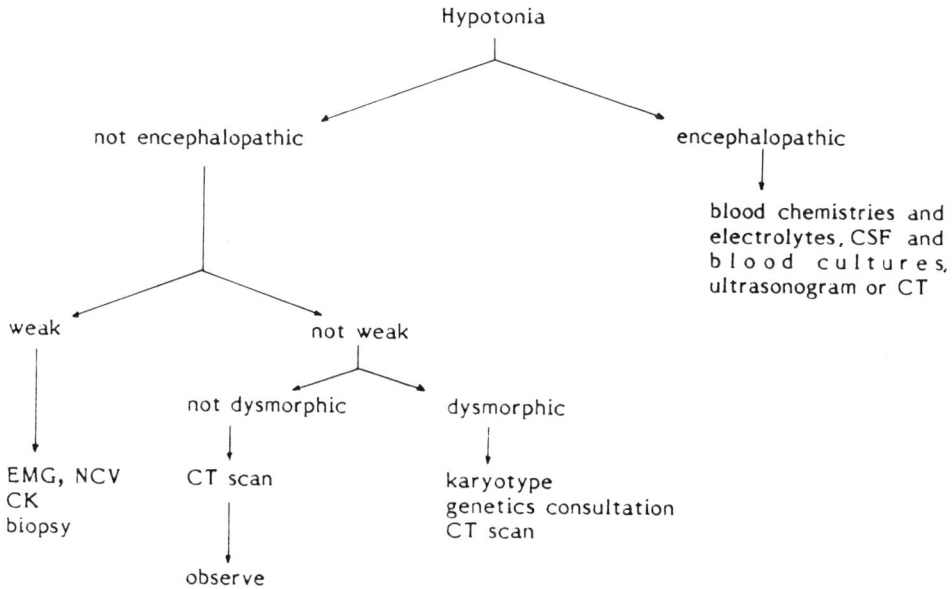

Fig. 11-10. Diagnostic approach to infantile hypotonia.

affected infants will have joint contractures and some will have dysmorphic features. These myopathies can be divided into four basic groups: congenital muscular dystrophy, myotonic dystrophy, congenital fiber-type disproportions, and the metabolic myopathies.

Congenital muscular dystrophy is a recessively inherited disorder characterized by joint contractures and weakness at birth. There may be an elevated creatinine kinase. Electromyography usually shows myopathic abnormalities and the biopsy shows a markedly dystrophic muscle with fatty infiltration and connective tissue proliferation (Fig. 11-5). There is some confusion about the long-term prognosis of such infants. Many have a very slowly progressive or static course, whereas others worsen more rapidly.

Myotonic dystrophy is a dominantly inherited disorder. Infants who are symptomatic have mothers, rather than fathers, with the disorder. Myotonia may be difficult to elicit clinically but is present on electromyography in the newborn period. The infants frequently present with respiratory distress, feeding difficulties, and generalized hypotonia. The diagnosis may be made by muscle biopsy and a very careful family history. Often the parent is unaware of the disorder.

A large group of congenital myopathies are characterized by fiber-type disproportion (Fig. 11-6). These are diagnosed on the muscle biopsy by the abnormal distribution, size, and relative proportions of the fiber types. Normally there is a random distribution of type I, type IIA, and type IIB muscle fibers in roughly equal proportions. In the fiber-type disproportions, however, there are numerous small type I fibers and few large type II fibers. There may be other pathologic characteristics, such as myotubes with central nuclei, central cores or multicores, and nemaline rods (Figs. 11-7 through 11-9). These added features furnish the characteristic names for these disorders: nemaline rod myopathy, central core disease, myotubular myopathy, and congenital fiber-type disproportion. Most of these disorders are inherited recessively; however, there have been a few occasions of X-linked and dominant inheritance as well. Diagnosis can only be made by muscle biopsy. The metabolic myopathies rarely present in the neonatal period and are discussed in Chapter 28. The mitochondrial myopathies can present with severe hypotonia, lactic acidosis, and failure to thrive.

Table 11-4 summarizes the diseases of the motor unit. It should be emphasized that these infants present very similar clinical pictures. The studies needed to make the diagnosis include electrodiagnostic tests (electromyography and measurement of the nerve conduction velocities), blood creatinine kinase, and a muscle biopsy. Histochemical analysis of the biopsy is necessary to make the diagnosis of many of these diseases. Figure 11-10 outlines a general approach to the evaluation of infantile hypotonia.

SELECTED READINGS

Amick LD, Johnson WW, Smith HL: Electromyographic and histopathologic correlations in arthrogryposis. Arch Neurol 16:512–513, 1967

Argov Z, Gardner-Medwin D, Johnson MA, Mastaglia FL: Patterns of muscle fiber-type disproportion in hypotonic infants. Arch Neurol 41:53–57, 1984

Bell DB, Smith DW: Myotonic dystrophy in the neonate. Pediatrics 81:83–86, 1972

Dubowitz V: Evaluation and differential diagnosis of the hypotonic infant. Pediatr Rev 6:237–243, 1985

Fenichel, GM: Clinical syndromes of myasthenia in infancy and childhood: a review. Arch Neurol 35:97–103, 1978

Karch SB, Urich H: Infantile polyneuropathy with defective myelination: an autopsy study. Dev Med Child Neurol 17:504–511, 1975

Lazaro RP, Fenichel GM, Kilroy AW: Congenital muscular dystrophy: case reports and reappraisal. Muscle Nerve, 2:349–355, 1979

McKee KT, Jr., Kilroy AW, Harrison WW, Schaffner W: Botulism in infancy. Report of a case. Am J Dis Child, 131:857–859, 1977

Melins RB, Hays AP, Gold AP et al: Respiratory distress as the initial manifestation of Werdnig-Hoffmann disease. Pediatrics 53:33–40, 1974

Packer RJ, Brown MJ, Berman PH: The diagnostic value of electromyography in infantile hypotonia. Am J Dis Child 136:1057–1059, 1982

12

BIRTH INJURIES

Birth injuries almost always occur as a complication of a difficult delivery. They are particularly more likely in children delivered vaginally in the breech position. The significant nervous system injuries are those to the cranium, spinal cord, and peripheral nerves. Often multiple injuries occur and rarely a predisposing disorder, such as congenital hypotonia or hydrocephalus, is present which makes the child more susceptible to birth injuries. Finally, asphyxia can also complicate a difficult delivery. Asphyxia is most likely to be confused with intracranial hemorrhage because of the brain swelling. With hemorrhage, the fontanelle bulges earlier and early focal neurologic deficits may appear that are not usually seen with asphyxia.

INJURIES TO THE CRANIUM

Figure 12-1 demonstrates the relationships of the soft tissues, bone, meninges, and underlying brain in the newborn infant and the site of frequent injuries. Injuries to the skull and scalp present as a local swelling on the head. Caput succedaneum is due to edema of the presenting part of head in the pelvic canal. It is very common and has no associated complications. Subgaleal hemorrhage is a more significant injury in that large amounts of blood can accumulate to the extent that the child can become hypovolemic. The subgaleal hemorrhage is more likely to occur with cephalopelvic disproportion and a difficult forceps-assisted vaginal delivery. Cephalohematoma is a collection of blood beneath the periosteum. It differs from the former two injuries in that it does not extend past the midline. The most common location is the parietal area and in some infants an underlying skull fracture can be demonstrated. In general, these injuries are benign and, unless complicated by a skull fracture, no therapy is indicated.

Skull fractures are relatively uncommon and occur most frequently with difficult forceps extractions. The fracture is usually beneath the application point of the forceps. Both linear and depressed skull fractures occur. Unless the fracture is depressed by more than 5 mm, no therapy is indicated. More than this degree of depression, however, may cause cerebral irritation or injury that requires surgical elevation. Patients with skull fractures should be followed because of the possibility of developing a leptomeningeal cyst which develops when the leptomeninges herniate through the fracture sight, causing a "growing fracture."

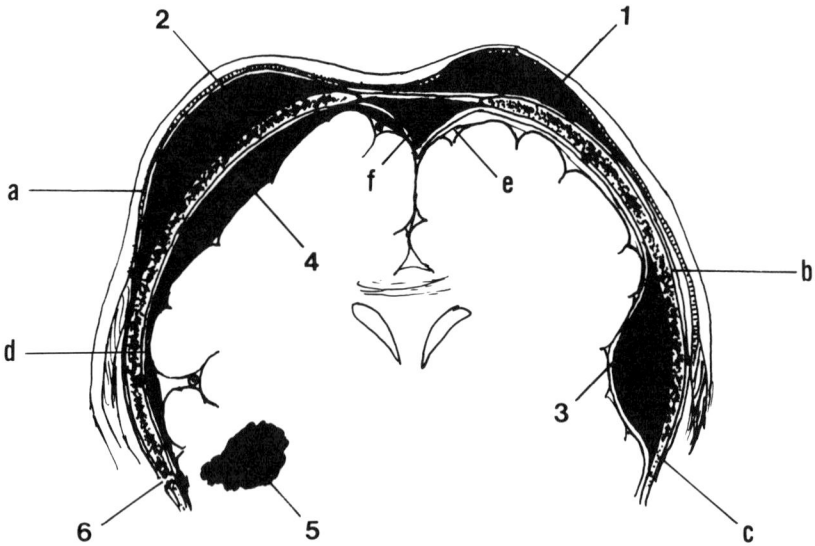

Fig. 12-1. Traumatic cranial birth injuries: (*1*) subgaleal hemorrhages, (*2*) cephalohematoma, (*3*) epidural hemorrhage, (*4*)subdural hemorrhage, (*5*) intracerebral hemorrhages, (*6*) skull fracture [(*a*) galeum, (*b*) periosteum, (*c*) skull, (*d*) dura mater, (*e*) arachnoid mater, (*f*) dural sinus].

Diastasis of the occipital suture occurs with difficult breech extraction and is often associated with intercranial hemorrhages in the posterior fossa.

INTRACRANIAL HEMORRHAGES

A number of structures are capable of causing intracranial bleeding from trauma (Table 12-1). Epidural hemorrhage is uncommon because the middle meningeal artery is not encased in bone as in older children and adults. Separation of the dura from the skull can cause tearing of meningeal arteries. Rapid hemorrhage into this space causes significant increased intercranial pressure and if untreated, death.

Subdural hemorrhages are due to shearing forces on the bridging veins between the brain and dura (Fig. 12-2). Infants present with a bulging fontanelle and signs of increased intracranial pressure. The most common site is over the cerebral convexities, but subdural hemorrhages can also occur in the posterior

Table 12-1. Sources of Intracranial Hemorrhage

Location	Type of Hemorrhage
Meningeal arteries	Epidural hemorrhage
Dural sinuses	Subarachnoid hemorrhage
Bridging veins	Subdural and subarachnoid hemorrhage
Cortical vessel	Intracerebral hematoma

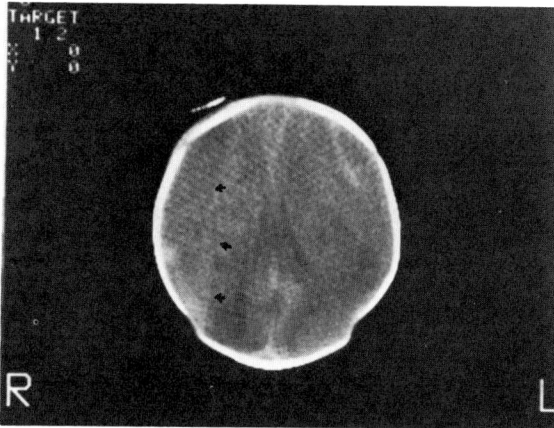

Fig. 12-2. Computed tomography scan of a subdural hematoma.

fossa, which is rare in older children and adults. Often there is an associated fracture or diastasis of the sutures in that area. Tears of the dural sinuses, such as the tentorium or falx, occur with excessive rotational forces or vertical molding. Signs of increased intracranial pressure may develop several days following the injury. Almost all infants with subdural hemorrhages will have retinal hemorrhages, but 20 percent of normal infants delivered vaginally have retinal hemorrhages as well. Finally, contusion of the brain can occur, causing intracerebral hemorrhage, particularly if there is a depressed skull fracture or other evidence of external trauma.

Regardless of the cause, traumatic intracranial hemorrhages produce similar signs which usually follows the injury by several hours or days with venous bleeding. The most common signs are listed in Table 12-2. In many cases asphyxia coexists, which can make the diagnosis difficult. The most reliable method of diagnosis is by computed tomography, because ultrasound is less sensitive in recognizing abnormalities in the posterior fossa and subdural spaces. Lumbar puncture should be deferred but, if performed, usually shows bloody fluid.

Table 12-2. Signs of Brain Injury
in the Newborn

Progressive decline of consciousness
Bulging fontanelle
Retinal hemorrhages
Enlarging head size
Separation of sutures
Focal motor deficits
Cranial nerve palsies
Apnea
Vomiting
Seizures

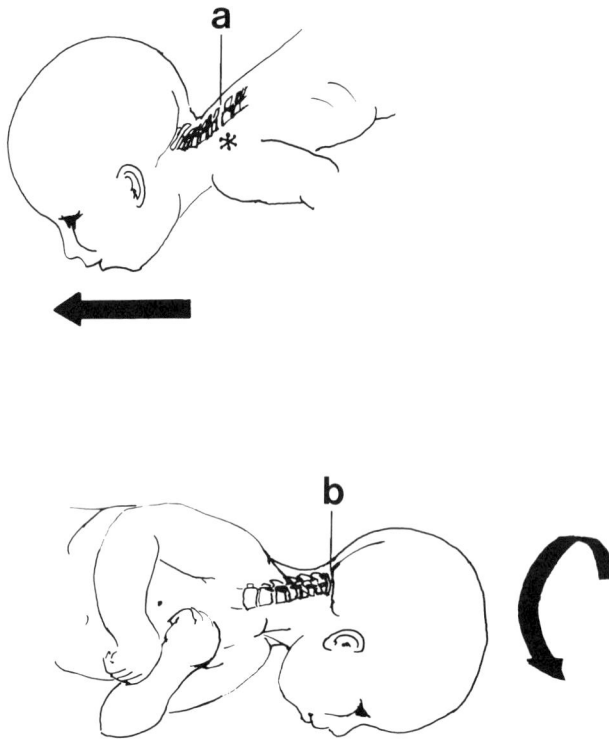

Fig. 12-3. Traumatic injury to the spinal cord. The heavy arrows indicate the forces applied to the spine. (*a*) Hyperextension injury and (*b*) rotation injury.

The treatment of intracranial hemorrhage is evacuation of the blood. This should not be performed unless there is definite increased intracranial pressure and the blood is easily accessible. Subdural blood can be removed by subdural puncture through the anterior fontanelle. Indications by subdural puncture are signs of increased intracranial pressure, rapidly enlarging head circumference, or signs of a mass effect, such as seizure, focal neurologic deficits, and a midline shift on computed tomography scan. Epidural and posterior fossa hemorrhages require surgical intervention. Intracerebral blood requires surgical aspiration if there is a mass effect and increased intracranial pressure.

SPINAL CORD INJURIES

Spinal cord injuries are associated with a difficult delivery, although they are becoming rare with improved obstetric care. Two types of injuries occur (Fig. 12-3). Breech extraction is associated with excessive stretching of the spinal cord, particularly if the infant's neck is hyperextended. The injury may be minimal, with swelling of the cord, or severe, with hemorrhage into the cord. The most frequent site of injury is in the lower cervical and upper thoracic regions.

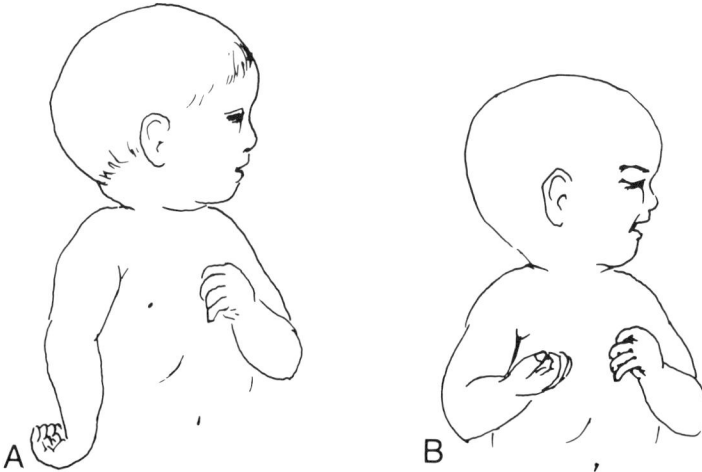

Fig. 12-4. Brachial plexus injury. (A) Upper cervical cord injury. (B) Lower cervical cord injury.

The major symptom is paraparesis below the level of injury, although there may be intact spinal cord reflexes, such as withdrawal. There is no conscious awareness of pain with complete injury and there is absence of sweating below the lesion, with loss of sphincter control. The patient usually has some movement of the arms and preserved respirations.

The second type of cord injury is associated with midforceps rotation for an occiput posterior presentation. Injury occurs with rotation of the head without the body. This is more likely if there is oligohydramnios or if the membranes have been ruptured for some time. The rotation injures the upper cervical portions of the spinal cord and the most severe lesion is complete dislocation of the atlas from the occiput, with transection of the cord. Infants born with this injury are flaccid from the neck down with no appreciation of pain but do have intact facial and eye movements and facial sensation. Respirations and sphincter control are lost.

Spinal radiographs may not demonstrate traction injuries but may show dislocation with rotational injury. The treatment of spinal cord injuries is immobilization as soon as the diagnosis is suspected. When the patient is an acceptable surgical risk, fixation of an unstable fracture is indicated to prevent further injury.

PERIPHERAL NERVOUS SYSTEM INJURIES

Facial nerve injury is caused by forceps pressure on the nerve extracranially or by pressure of the facial nerve against the bony structure of the pelvis. Facial nerve palsies cause a unilateral paralysis of facial motility, with both the upper and lower parts of the face flaccid. The child is unable to close the eye, has an expressionless face on that side, and drools. It may not be readily apparent until the child cries. The prognosis is good for full recovery. Congenital absence of the depressor anguli oris can mimic a partial facial nerve palsy.

Brachial plexus injuries can be divided into two types, those of the upper brachial plexus, or Erb's palsy, and those in the lower brachial plexus, Klumpke's palsy. In fact, there are very few clear-cut cases of the latter and the injuries are either upper plexus injury or total paralysis. Upper brachial plexus injury usually occurs with shoulder dystocia with excessive traction applied to the neck. The upper cervical segments are involved, causing injury to the C5–C6 innervated musculature. These roots innervate shoulder abduction, elbow flexion, and supination of the arm. Weakness of these muscles gives rise to the typical "waiter's tip" position (Fig. 12-4A). Horner's syndrome (ipsilateral ptosis, pupillary constriction, and absent facial sweating) may accompany the injury. Injuries of the lower cervical brachial plexus are rare. Excessive traction on the extended arm injures the lower cervical and upper thoracic roots, causing the arm to be flexed and supinated (Fig. 12-4B). Brachial plexus injuries usually resolve with time. Rarely the actual roots are evulsed, which can cause permanent injury. There is no indication that surgery or other therapies will alter the outcome of this disease, in which 90 percent recover by 1 year of age.

SELECTED READINGS

Eng GD: Brachial plexus palsy in newborn infants. Pediatrics, 48:18–28, 1971

Gordon M, Rich H, Deutschberger J, Green M: The immediate and long-term outcome of obstetric birth trauma. Am J Obstet Gynecol 117:51–56, 1973

Haldeman S, Fowler GW, Ashwal S, Schneider S: Acute flaccid neonatal paraplegia: a case report. Neurology 33:93–95, 1983

Molnar G: Brachial plexus injury in the newborn. Pediatr Rev 6:110–115, 1984

Nelson KB, Eng GD: Congenital hypoplasia of the depressor angulia oris muscle: differentiation from congenital facial palsy. J Pediatr 81:16–20, 1972

Plauche WC: Subgaleal hematoma: a complication of instrumental delivery. JAMA 244:1597–1598, 1980

Serfontein GL, Rom S, Stein S: Posterior fossa subdural hemorrhage in the newborn. Pediatrics 65:40–43, 1980

Shulman ST, Madden JD, Esterly JR, Shanklin DR: Transection of spinal cord. Arch Dis Child 46:291–293, 1971

Towbin A: Central nervous system damage in the human fetus and newborn infant. Am J Dis Child 119:529–542, 1970

Yasunaga S, Rivera R: Cephalohematoma in the newborn: observations based on a review of 139 infants. Clin Pediatr 13:256–260, 1974

13

CONGENITAL MALFORMATIONS

Ontogenesis is the predetermined pattern of events which causes the normal morphologic development of the CNS. Deviations from the proper sequencing of these events cause malformations. It is estimated that approximately 75 percent of fetal deaths are due to severe neurologic malformations, and about 1 to 5 in 1,000 live births have neurologic malformations. Survivors with CNS system malformations usually have significant physical, mental, and emotional handicaps. This chapter reviews the morphologic development of the CNS and the more common congenital malformations.

EMBRYOLOGY

The development of the CNS is divided into embryogenesis and histogenesis. Embryogenesis is the induction of the basic morphology of the CNS. The primitive neural plate is formed by 2 weeks of gestation and separated from the primitive endoderm by the notochord. Neural folds appear at 3 weeks and the formation of the neural tube (neurolation) begins at the future location of the medulla. Neurulation progresses in the anterior and posterior directions and closes at the anterior and posterior neuropores by 4 weeks. The primitive neural tube consists of neuroectoderm and a primitive canal which will be the future ventricular system and central canal. The apexes of the neural folds develop separately into neural crest tissue. Prosencephalization is the process of segmentation of the anterior neural tube to form the forebrain. The cephalic flexure appears at approximately 4 weeks. The anterior primitive canal distends to form the third ventricle at approximately 8 weeks. Surrounding this is the primitive diencephalon and rhinal lobes. Lateral extensions of the third ventricle forms the primitive lateral ventricles and surrounding limbic lobes and telencephalon (Fig. 13-1). The gross morphology of the brain is recognizable by 4 months' gestation. Table 13-1 summarizes the gross development of the brain, listing defects which occur when these processes are disrupted.

Histogenesis is the process of cellular proliferation and differentiation. Glioblasts and neuroblasts can be identified by 3 weeks of gestation. Histogenesis begins at approximately 6 to 8 weeks and continues until approximately 30 weeks, except for the cerebellum, which may continue until birth or shortly thereafter. Disruption of cellular proliferation causes microcephaly. Between 10 and 18 weeks there is intense neuronal proliferation at the subependymal germinal matrix. Between 12 and 24 weeks take place a series of migrations of

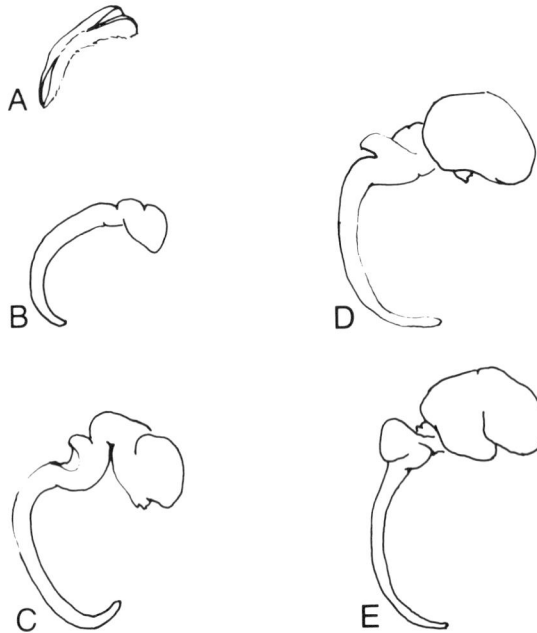

Fig. 13-1. Representative illustrations of CNS embryogenesis: (A) closure of neural folds (4 weeks), (B) segmentation (5 weeks), (C) prosencephalization (10 weeks), (D) telencephalization (12 weeks), (E) fissure formation (16 weeks).

these cells to the cortical area. The first cells migrate to and settle in the deeper layers of the cortex; later migrating cells pass through these to assume the more superficial layers. Interruption of neuronal migration causes heterotopias or islands of gray matter within the white matter. During histogenesis neuronal and glial structures attain proper alignment and orientation, axonal and dendritic processes are elaborated, and synaptic contacts are established. Finally, the proliferation of glial cells and their differentiation induce the formation of myelin, as well as cellular support for blood vessels and other structures and formation of the functional blood–brain barrier. The fissurization of the cerebral cortex occurs because of the more rapid growth of the outer layers of the cerebral cortex

Table 13-1. Summary of Morphogenesis of the Cerebral Nervous System

Process	Gestation	Malformation	Definition
Neurulation	1 month	Dysrhaphia	Incomplete closure of the neural tube
Prosencephalization	2–3 months	Holoprosencephaly	Failure of forebrain cleavage
		Agenesis of the corpus callosum	Failure of commissural plate
Histogenesis	2–3 months	Microcephaly	Loss of neurons and glial cells
Migration	4 months	Heterotopia	Incomplete migration of neurons
Fissurization	4–6 months	Lissencephaly	Absence of gyri
		Pachygyria	Reduced gyral number

Table 13-2. Classification of CNS Malformation

Neurulation	Prosencephalization
Dysrhaphia	Holoprosencephaly
Rachischisis	Holotelencephaly
Cranioschisis	Arhinencephalia
Anencephaly	Agenesis of the corpus callosum
Exencephaly	Aicardi syndrome
Encephalocele	Septo-optic dysplasia
Meningocele	Segmentation
Congenital sinus tract	Klippel-Feil anomaly
Spina bifida	Basilar impression
Cystica	
Meningocele	**Histogenesis**
Meningomyelocele	Microcephaly vera
Occulta	Lissencephaly
Congenital sinus tract	Pachygyria
Congenital tumors	Cerebellar aplasias
Lipoma	Heterotopias
Dermoid	
Thickened filum terminale	**Other**
Ventral dysrhaphia	Hydrocephalus
Sacral meningocele	Aqueductal stenosis
Neuroentercyst	Dandy-Walker malformation
Diastematomyelia/diplomyelia	Syringomyelia, syringobulbia
Caudal regression syndrome	Hydranencephaly
Sacral agenesis	Porencephalia
Arnold-Chiari malformation	Craniosynostosis

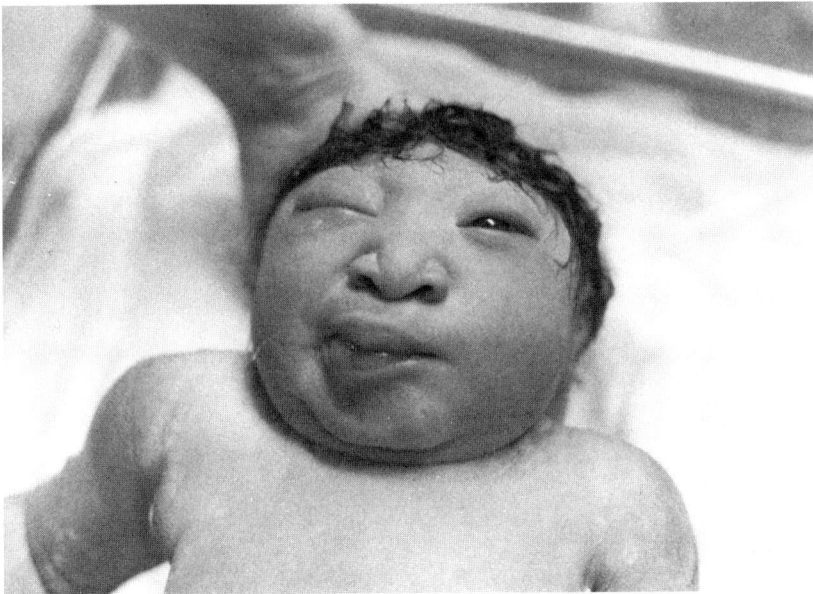

Fig. 13-2. Anencephaly.

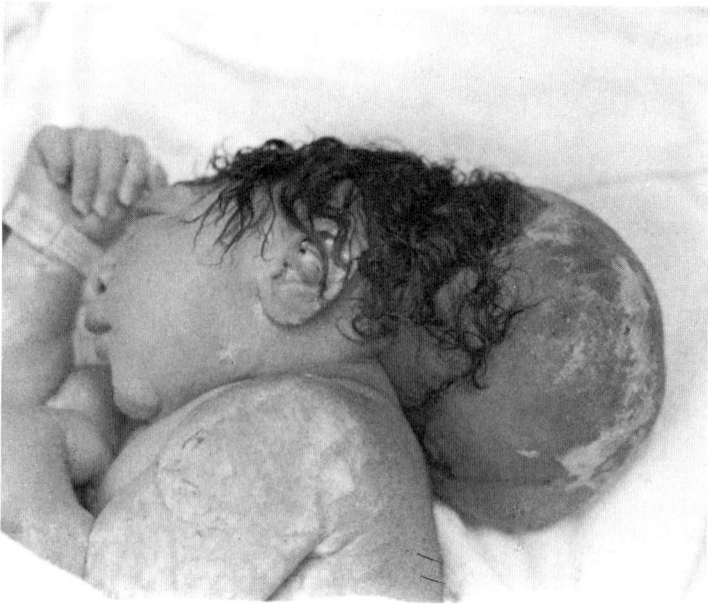

Fig. 13-3. Encephalocele.

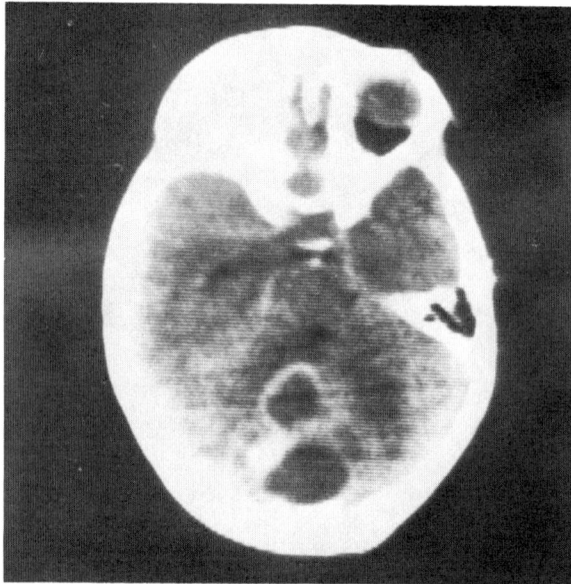

Fig. 13-4. Computed tomography scan of a dermoid tumor in the posterior fossa.

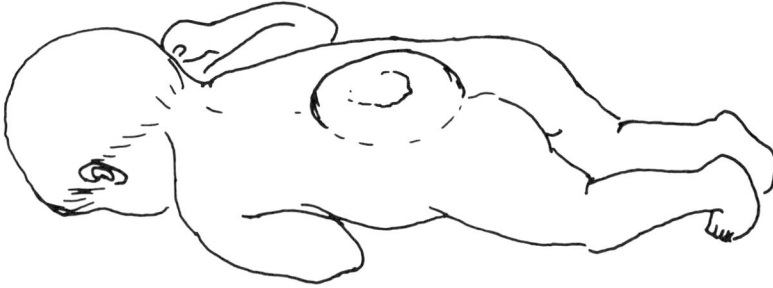

Fig. 13-5. Meningomyelocele.

along with the physical constants of the calvaria. The primary fissures are completed at approximately 4 months' gestation, the secondary fissues at 6 months' gestation, and tertiary fissures at birth. Abnormalities of fissurization are associated with a number of developmental abnormalities, including lissencephaly (lack of sulci) and pachygyria.

CONGENITAL MALFORMATION

Table 13-2 summarizes the major malformations of the CNS. One can classify these into those disorders associated with defects of neurulation, prosencephalization, and histogenesis.

Disorders of Neurulation

Neural tube defects are the most common of the CNS malformations present at birth, occurring in approximately every 1 per 1,000 live births. The prevailing theory for dysrhaphic defects is that they are due to lack of closure of the neural folds. The most severe defect is anencephaly, in which there is no closure of the

Table 13-3. Clinical Features of the Tethered Cord Syndrome

Clinical Features	Percentage of Patients
Abnormal spinal radiographs	84
Back lesion (hair, macula, dimple)	77
Incontinence	45
Foot deformities	36
Leg weakness	29
Diminished reflexes	25
Leg numbness	23
Pain or stiffness in back or legs	19

(Adapted from Anderson FM: Occult spinal dysrhaphism: a series of 73 cases. Pediatrics 55:826–835. Reproduced by permission of Pediatrics. Copyright 1975.)

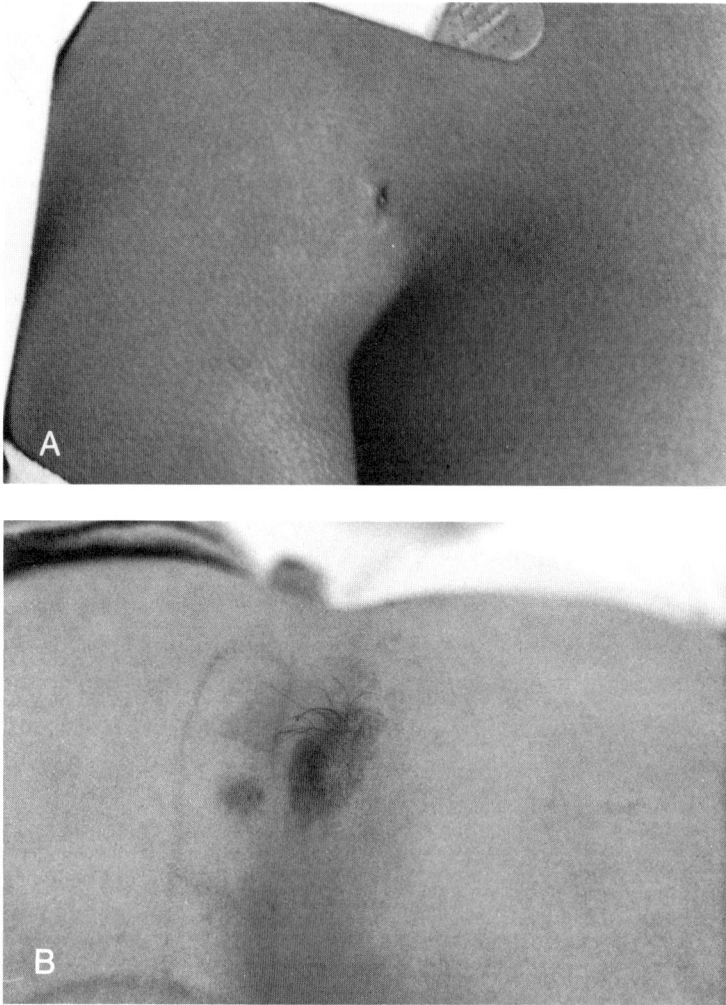

Fig. 13-6. Skin lesion associated with tethered cord syndrome. (A) Sacral dimple. (B) Hair patch.

anterior neuropore (cranium bifidum) (Fig. 13-2). Encephalocele is a less severe form of failure of anterior closure (Fig. 13-3). The cyst is usually located on the occiput but can occur in the frontal areas. These masses may be purely cystic or contain brain tissue. Meckel's syndrome is an encephalocele with other somatic malformations and is inherited as a recessive trait. The least serious disorder of anterior closure is a dermal sinus. These are most commonly located in the occipital region and often have a recognizable dimple or birthmark in the area. Dermal sinuses may end blindly or can communicate with the CNS. At times a formed cyst can mimic a posterior fossa tumor in older children and can

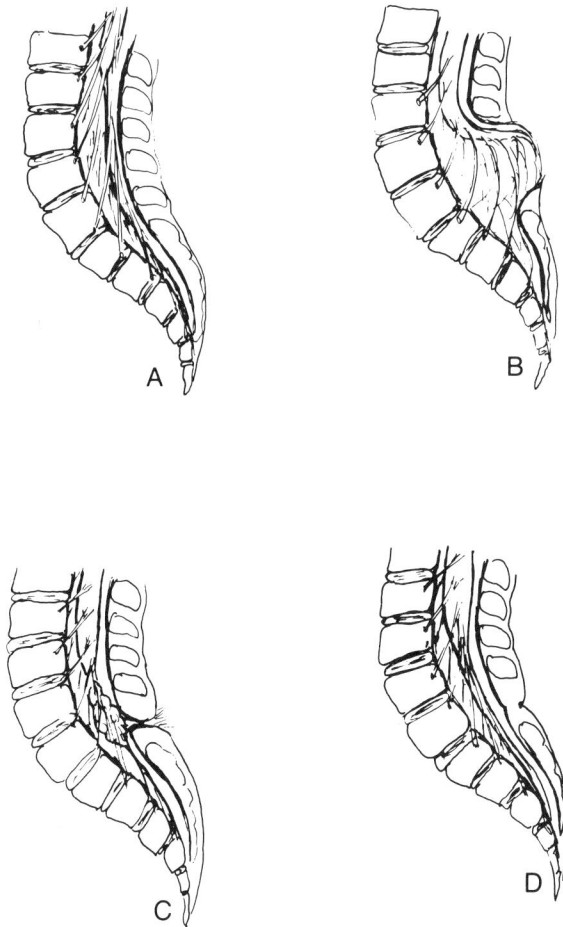

Fig. 13-7. Tethered cord syndrome. (A) Normal anatomy showing the conus above L2. (B) Meningomyelocele. (C) Dermoid tumor. (D) Thickened filum terminale.

cause recurrent chemical meningitis or act as the portal for recurrent septic meningitis (Fig. 13-4).

Spina bifida is the most common congenital neurologic malformation. Because dermal development and neural tube development are closely influenced by one another, malformation of the spinal cord usually accompanies malformation of the skin, vertebrae, and soft tissues. The most severe abnormality is craniorachischisis totalis, which is a totally open nervous system. Meningomyelocele (spina bifida cystica) is characterized by herniation of meningeal and neural tissue through an open spine (Fig. 13-5). The usual location is the lumbosacral region, but it can occur in the thoracic and cervical areas. A fibrous membrane or skin covers this defect. Children are paraplegic below the level of the defect, which may extend over 1 to 10 segments. The pattern of neurologic

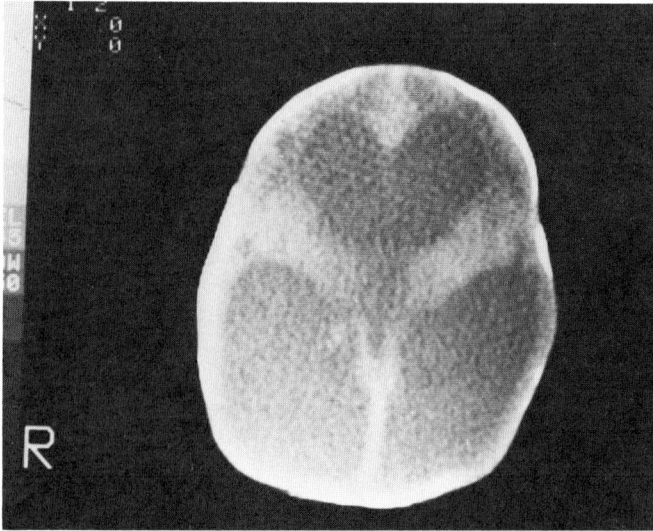

Fig. 13-8. Computed tomography scan of congenital aqueductal stenosis and hydrocephalus.

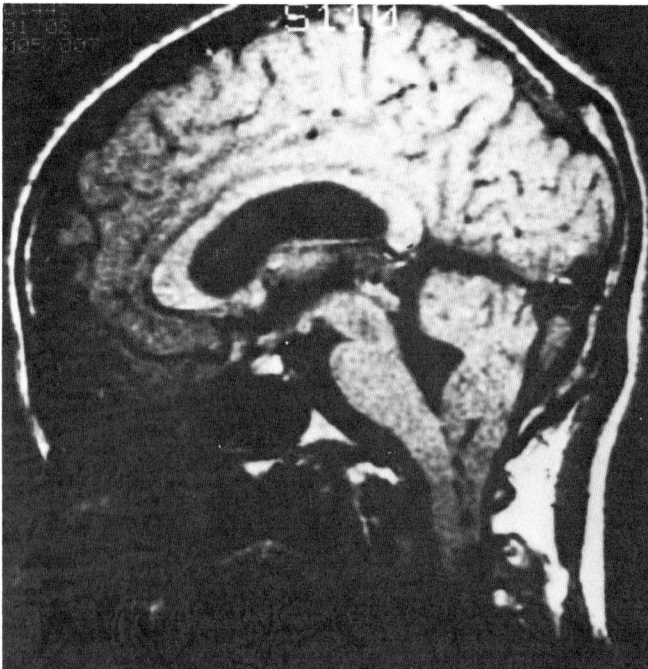

Fig. 13-9. Nuclear magnetic resonance scan of a type II Arnold–Chiari malformation. Note the cerebellar tonsils in the cervical canal.

Table 13-4. Arnold-Chiari Malformations

Type I	Displacement of cerebellar tonsils, posterior lobe of cerebellum, and caudal medulla into cervical canal
Type II	Same as type I, but more extensive and commonly associated with meningomyelocele, hydrocephalus, and other defects
Type III	Displacement of the cerebellum, fourth ventricle, and brain stem through a cervical vertebral defect
Type IV	Hypoplasia of the cerebellar vermis and cystic dilatation of the fourth ventricle (Dandy-Walker malformation)

(Data from Icenogle DA, Kaplan AM: A review of congenital neurologic malformations. Clin Pediatr 20:565–576, 1981.)

deficits depends entirely upon the extent and location of the lesion. Voluntary movement, sphincter control, and sensation are lost distal to the lesion. Isolated cord reflexes may persist in islands of intact tissue. A meningocele refers to just herniation of dural membranes without neural components and may or may not have skin closure. These children have normal neurologic function. Rarely an anterior meningomyelocele or neuroenteric cyst occurs in the sacral region. Sacral agenesis occurs most frequently in infants of diabetic mothers. There is usually some degree of sacral cord involvement.

Other disorders of neural tube closure are less serious and present later. The most common clinical presentation is that of the tethered cord syndrome. There is an abnormal attachment of the spinal cord to mesodermal structures, causing dysfunction of the conus medullaris or cauda equina. The clinical presentation may be quite subtle and only apparent in later years, after the child begins to grow. The majority of patients are diagnosed between 5 and 15 years, following about 1 year of symptoms. The clinical features are summarized in Table 13-3. Occult spinal malformations are often suggested by an abnormal skin lesion, dimple, or hair patch in the lower back (Fig. 13-6). Radiographs show spina bifida occulta, widened spinal canal, or other abnormalities in almost all patients. The most common causes for the tethered cord syndrome are a tight or thickened filum terminale, dermal sinus, dermoid tumor, diastematomyelia, meningocele, and lipoma (Fig. 13-7).

Many patients with neural tube defects also have hydrocephalus and the Arnold-Chiari malformation. Hydrocephalus occurs in 70 percent of children with meningomyelocele. Hydrocephalus may be caused by aqueductal stenosis or a complication of the Arnold-Chiari malformation (Fig. 13-8). This latter malformation consists of herniation of the cerebellar tonsils and medulla through the foramen magnum and kinking of the brain stem (Fig. 13-9). Arnold-Chiari malformations are classified into four types (Table 13-4). Signs arise in the newborn period because of compression and traction of the brain stem and cranial nerves. Apnea, poor swallowing, and cranial nerve paresis are common. The Arnold-Chiari malformation often presents later in life as neck pain and progressive long tract signs. Other malformations associated with Arnold-Chiari malformations are basilar impression and Sprengel's deformity.

Congenital hydrocephalus occurs in a variety of settings, both acquired and inherited. Aqueductal stenosis can be secondary to malformations or masses

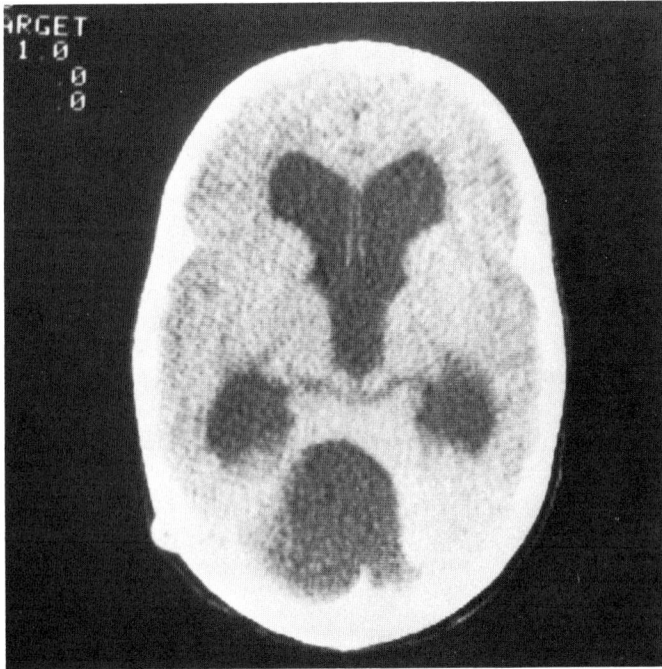

Fig. 13-10. Computed tomography scan of a Dandy-Walker malformation.

which compress the aqueduct or inflammation which obstructs cerebrospinal fluid flow. Abnormal formation of the aqueduct with secondary hydrocephalus can be inherited as an X-linked trait (Fig. 13-8). The Dandy-Walker malformation is characterized by agenesis of the cerebellar vermis and cystic dilatation of the fourth ventricle (Fig. 13-10). There may or may not be obstruction of the outlets of the fourth ventricle and associated hydrocephalus. Some have aqueductal stenosis, agenesis of brain stem structures, and cerebral heterotopias. All children with Dandy-Walker malformation are retarded.

Disorders of Prosencephalization

Disorders of prosencephalization are characterized by defects in cleavage of the anterior neural tube. The most severe defect is holoprosencephaly (Fig. 13-11), in which there is a single ventricle with little or no surrounding neural structures. Holotelencephaly has an intact third ventricle and diencephalic nuclei with little forebrain. Arhinencephalia is common to all prosencephalic disorders and is characterized by absence of the olfactory bulbs and lobes. Defects in prosencephalization often accompany chromosomal abnormalities, including trisomy 13 and 21 and deletion syndromes of 18 and 13. Patients with these disorders frequently have abnormal facial features. The more severe the disorder, the more severe the facial abnormalities, which can range from a cyclopean

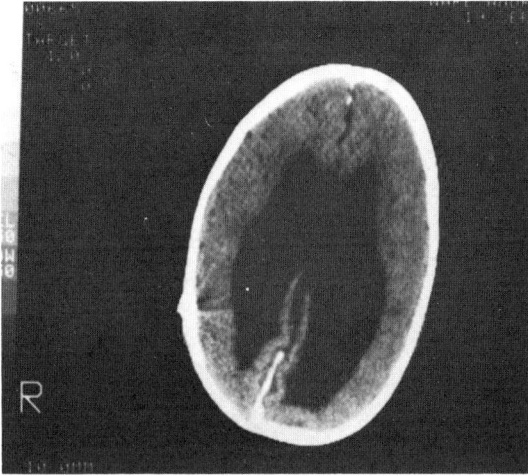

Fig. 13-11. Computed tomography scan of holotelencephaly. Note the absence of any midline structures.

appearance to a simple cleft lip or palate. Often associated with disorders of prosencephalation are abnormal connections between the hemispheres. The most common is agenesis of the corpus callosum, which can occur as an isolated defect or as a component of multiple defects. One association is infantile spasms, retinal colobomas, and agenesis of the corpus callosum (Aicardi syndrome).

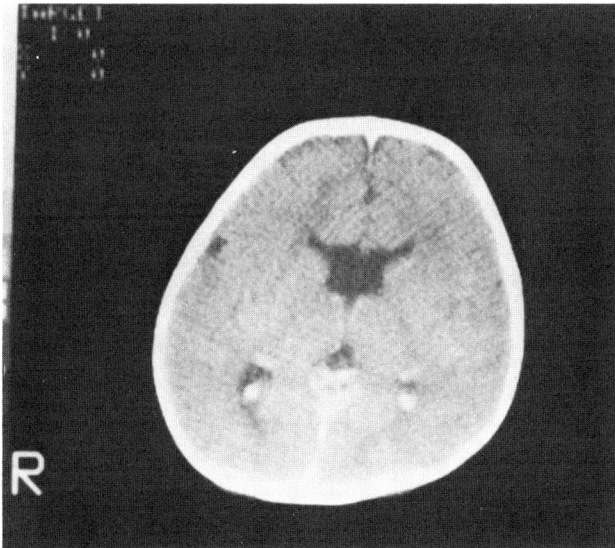

Fig. 13-12. Computed tomography scan showing agenesis of the corpus callosum.

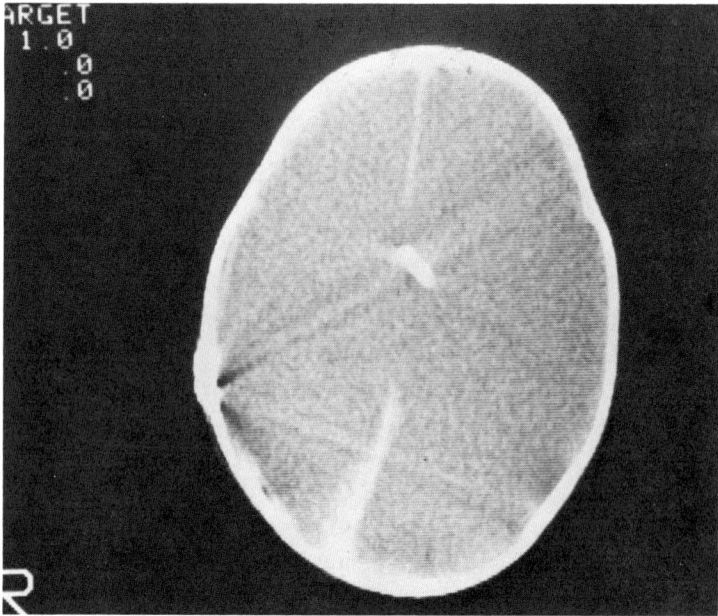

Fig. 13-13. Computed tomography scan of hydranencephaly.

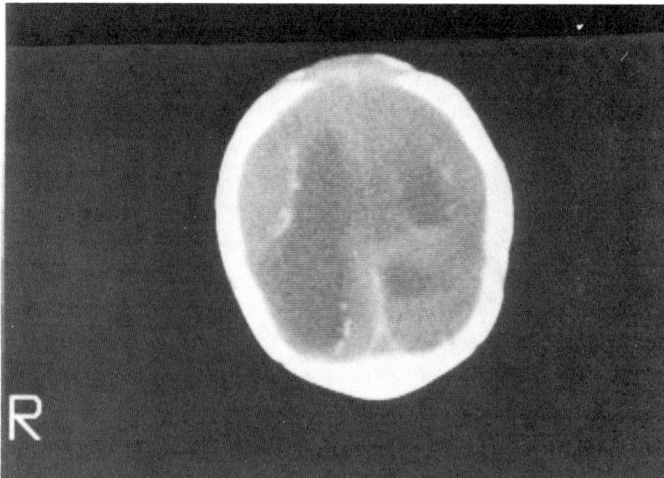

Fig. 13-14. Computed tomography scan of porencephalia.

Table 13-5. Risk Factors for Congenital Neurologic Defects

Previous stillbirths or repeated abortions
Previous child with congenital defect
First-trimester viral infection
Rapid or discordant growth
Family history of congenital neurologic defects
Age greater than 40 years
First-trimester hemorrhage
Parent with neurotube defect or multiple vertebral anomalies

Agenesis of the corpus callosum gives a characteristic "bat wing" appearance on computed tomography (CT) (Fig. 13-12).

Disorders of Histogenesis

Disorders of histogenesis are secondary to abnormal cellular proliferation and migration. Schizencephaly is a severe disorder of migration and proliferation such that there is little if any recognizable cellular architecture. In common, many of these disorders have heterotopias caused by failure of migration. Lissencephaly refers to failure of gyral formation, resulting in a smooth brain surface pattern. Pachygyria is the presence of large but few gyri, and micropolygyria is an overabundance of very small gyri. The most severe of the disorders of histogenesis is microcephaly vera. There is a marked reduction of cerebral cortex, particularly over the frontal lobes. Microcephaly is apparent at birth and infants have the characteristic appearance of prominent facies but a very small cranial vault. All of these conditions are associated with severe retardation.

Other Malformations

The Möbius syndrome is due to absence of cranial nerve nuclei. Usually 6 to 12, but not 8, cranial nerve nuclei are absent, causing a masklike facial appearance and internal squint. One can also have isolated agenesis of single cranial

Table 13-6. Causes of False-Positive α-Fetoprotein Elevation in Amniotic Fluid

Omphalocele
Congenital nephrosis
Cystic hygroma
Duodenal or esophageal atresia
Multiple fetuses
Fetal bleeding or death
Severe erythroblastosis
Maternal liver disease
Incorrect gestational dates
Threatened abortion
Neural tube defects
Sacrococcygeal teratoma
Turner syndrome

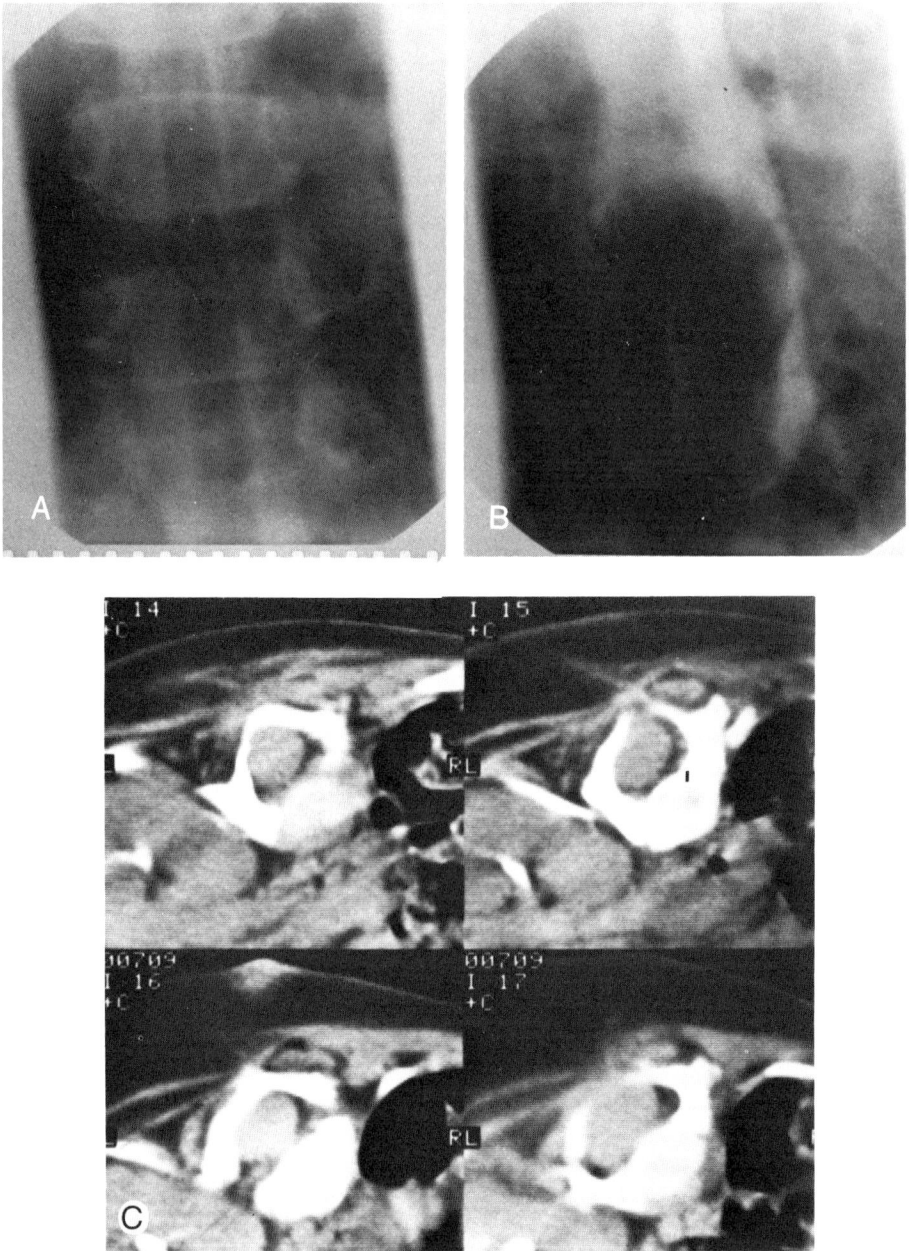

Fig. 13-15. Radiographic abnormalities of the tethered cord syndrome. (A) Myelography showing low position of conus. (B) Myelography showing congenital lipoma. (C) Computed tomography scan showing spina bifida occulta and a congenital dermoid tumor.

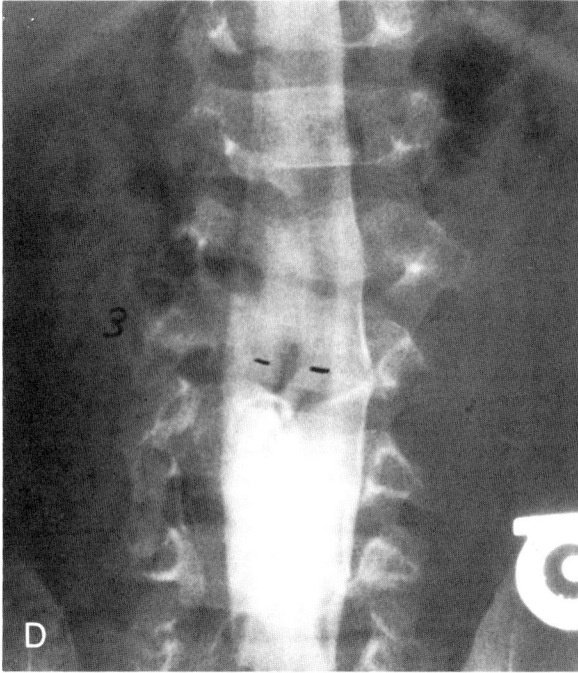

Fig. 13-15. (*continued*). (D) Myelography showing diastematomyelia.

nerve nuclei. Septo-optic dysplasia is a disorder of hypothalamic and pituitary dysfunction and optic hypoplasia.

Hydranencephaly and porencephaly are caused by tissue destruction. Hydranencephaly is thought to be an acquired, in utero disorder secondary to severe hydrocephalus with secondary tissue destruction (Fig. 13-13). Alternatively, hydranencephaly may be caused by a severe ischemic event and necrosis of the entire cortex. Congenital porencephalia is thought to be caused by a cerebrovascular accident occurring within the first trimester with secondary dilatation of the ventricle into the resorbed brain (Fig. 13-14). Children with hydranencephaly are severely disabled and frequently die within the first year. Porencephalia presents with variable clinical symptoms, depending upon severity, but seizures, retardation, and hemiplegic cerebral palsy are common. Syringomyelia is abnormal cavitation of the spinal cord, usually in the cervical region and often associated with Arnold-Chiari malformation or spinal tumors. Craniosynostosis does not cause neurologic disease unless there is pansynostosis with brain compression or if it is associated with another dysmorphic syndrome and mental retardation.

DETECTION, DIAGNOSIS, AND TREATMENT

The most reliable method of prenatal detection is screening the population of pregnant females at risk (Table 13-5). For those in whom screening is indicated, a combination of the measurement of α-fetoprotein and fetal ultrasound are the most useful methods of detection. α-Fetoprotein, a fetal protein similar to albumin, is detectable at 4 weeks' gestation and peaks at 32 weeks in the fetus and maternal serum and at 14 weeks in amniotic fluid. Until the neural folds close, α-fetoprotein is elaborated in the cerebrospinal fluid, circulates in the amniotic fluid, and is absorbed by the placental circulation. It is also passed in the urine and through unkeratinized skin. Failure of neural fold closure causes persistent and markedly elevated α-fetoprotein and is therefore a useful diagnostic procedure in patients at risk. A fivefold elevation of α-fetoprotein levels in the amniotic fluid is highly suggestive of a neurotube defect; however, a number of factors can cause false elevations (Table 13-6). Fetal ultrasonography has been very helpful in recognizing a number of congenital anomalies, particularly hydrocephalus, hydranencephaly, porencephalia, anencephaly, meningomyelocele, and encephalocele.

The diagnosis of neurotube defects, microcephaly, congenital hydrocephalus, and severe disorders of prosencephalization is usually apparent at birth because of the typical appearance. The CT scan will confirm the diagnosis. Hydranencephaly and porencephalia often present with early seizures and motor signs such as spasticity or hypotonia. Often the diagnosis is not made until months after delivery, when there is failure of development. The CT scan will determine the diagnosis. It may be difficult at times to differentiate hydranencephaly from severe hydrocephalus.

Patients with suspected Arnold-Chiari malformations are best diagnosed by nuclear magnetic resonance scanning (Fig. 13-9). The Dandy-Walker syndrome is also apparent on CT scanning (Fig. 13-10). The tethered cord syndrome and related disorders are identified by abnormal radiographs of the spine and myelography which demonstrates the conus below L1 and a thickened filum or tumor (Fig. 13-15).

The treatment of these disorders is largely neurosurgical and rehabilitative. The surgically correctable disorders include hydrocephalus and meningomyelocele. Any child, regardless of prognosis, should have ventriculoperitoneal shunting if progressive hydrocephalus is present. Untreated hydrocephalus is very disfiguring and makes nursing and parenting difficult. An open spine defect needs to be closed to reduce the possibility of infection, which is the major cause of mortality. Encephaloceles and similar disorders should be treated on an individual basis determined by the amount of neural tissue present in the mass. In general, they are repaired as in spinal defects. Tethered cord repair often improved neurologic function and reduces pain.

Rehabilitative therapy is often extensive, although the yield can be discouraging. Most children are at risk for mental retardation and most have multiple handicaps. It is beyond the scope of this book to discuss rehabilitation in depth. In general, one should prevent the treatable medical surgical complications such as urinary tract obstruction and infections; work toward ambulation with physical therapy, bracing, and if necessary orthopedic surgery; provide for adequate education and training; and, most importantly, support the family.

SELECTED READINGS

Anderson FM: Occult spinal dysraphism: a series of 73 cases. Pediatrics 55:826–835, 1975

Chi, JG, Dooling EC, Gilles FH: Gyral development of the human brain. Ann Neurol 1:86–93, 1977

Daube JR, Chou SM: Lissencephaly: two cases. Neurology 16:179–191, 1966

DeMyer W: The medial cleft face syndrome. Neurology 17:961–971, 1967

DeMyer W: Megalencephaly in children. Neurology 22:634–643, 1972

Emergy JL: Deformity of the aqueduct of Sylvius in children with hydrocephalus and myelomeningocele. Dev Med Child Neurol 32:40–48, 1974

Haslam RHA, Smith DW: Autosomal dominant microcephaly. J Pediatr 95:701–705, 1979

Holmes LB, Nash A, ZuRhein GM et al: X-Linked aqueductal stenosis: clinical and neuropathological findings in two families. Pediatrics 51:697–704, 1973

James CCM, Lassman LP: Diastematomyelia: a clinical survey of 24 cases submitted to laminectomy. Arch Dis Child 39:125–30, 1964

Lemire RJ, Graham CB, Beckwith JB: Skin-covered sacrococcygeal masses in infants and children. J Pediatr 79:948–954, 1971

McLone DG: Results of treatment of children born with a myelomeningocele. p. 407. In Weiss ME (ed): Clinical Neurosurgery.Vol. 30. Williams & Wilkins, Baltimore, 1983

Matson DD, Ingraham FD: Intracranial complications of congenital dermal sinuses. Pediatrics 8:463–474, 1951

Milunsky A: Prenatal detection of neural tube defects. JAMA 244:2731–2735, 1980

Parrish ML, Rosessman U, Levinsohn MW: Agenesis of the corpus callosum: a study of the frequency of associated malformations. Ann Neurol 6:349–354, 1979

Stark GD, Drummond M: The spinal cord lesion in the myelomeningocele. Dev Med Child Neurol, suppl. 25:1–14, 1971

Tal Y, Freigang B, Dunn HG et al: Dandy-Walker syndrome: analysis of 21 cases. Dev Med Child Neurol 22:189–201, 1980

SECTION 4

Developmental Disorders

Developmental disorders are some of the most common problems in pediatrics. The decreasing tendency to institutionalize severe handicapped children makes it more likely that primary care physicians will increasingly encounter these children in practice. Mildly handicapping disorders and behavior disturbances have always been prevalent, yet most physicians are relatively untrained in the diagnosis and management of these disorders. With the new education legislations that make provisions for the public education of handicapped children, physicians must be involved in the identification and management of developmental disorders. This section discusses the major handicapping conditions of children. The magnitude of the problem can be judged from the prevalence of chronic handicapping disorders*:

Mental retardation	25/1,000
Cerebral palsy	4/1,000
Blindness	2/1,000
Profound congenital hearing loss	1.5/1,000
Developmental speech/language disorders	1/1,000
Moderate to severe behavior problems	7/1,000

---

* From Kaminer R, Jedrysek E: Early identification of developmental disabilities. Pediatr Ann 11:427–437, 1982.

14

MENTAL RETARDATION

The American Association of Mental Deficiency defines *mental retardation* as a disorder of "significantly subaverage general intellectual functioning existing concurrently with deficits in adaptive behavior and manifested during the developmental period." This implies that the symptoms arise in childhood and are characterized by delayed development and impairment of learning, social adjustment, and economic productivity. Mental retardation is a dynamic disorder in the developing child because development, both intellectual and neurologic, continues until maturation even in the brain-injured child. In the mature individual, mental retardation is a static disorder. Dementia, a progressive loss of intellectual abilities, will be discussed elsewhere. Mental deficiency is any impairment in intellectual functioning. The prevalence of mental retardation is approximately 2 to 3 percent of the United States population; more than 100,000 children are born each year with mental retardation. Approximately 0.3 percent of live births will be mild to moderately retarded and 0.1 percent severely retarded.

Mental retardation is part of a syndrome complex and is associated with a number of acquired and congenital disorders. Developmental delay is only a symptom of mental retardation and other disorders. Many causes of developmental delay may be reversible and not necessarily associated with mental retardation, particularly if the delay is in an isolated area of development such as language or motor development. Global delay in all areas of development suggests mental retardation. Developmental delay may also be an early symptom of a progressive disorder.

CLASSIFICATION

Table 14-1 classifies mental retardation by performance on psychological testing. The average IQ, by definition, is 100, with a standard deviation of 16; the normal population will be within 2 standard deviations of the mean, or 68 to 132. Children testing between 68 and 80 are classified as borderline. Table 14-2 shows the functional capabilities of mentally retarded children. About 7 percent of mentally retarded children are in the mild to borderline range.

ETIOLOGY

The causes for mental retardation are diverse and our knowledge of these causes is growing as newer diagnostic methods become available. For practical purposes one can characterize the etiologies into prenatal, perinatal, and post-

Table 14-1. Classification of Mental
Retardation

Classification	IQ
Borderline	68–80
Mild	62–67
Moderate	36–51
Severe	20–35
Profound	Under 19

(Modified from Grossman HJ (ed): The
Manual on Terminology and Classification in
Mental Retardation, American Association of
Mental Deficiency, Washington, DC. Rev. Ed.
1977.)

natal injuries to brain development. For a sizable percentage the cause is unknown. Most cases of mild mental retardation are environmental in origin,
whereas most severe cases are due to prenatal causes.

Prenatal causes include chromosomal abnormalities, congenital dysmorphic
syndrome, inherited retardations, and intrauterine injuries to the fetus. Table
14-3 outlines the major chromosomopathies associated with mental retardation.
Table 14-4 lists the major dysmorphic syndromes for which at the present time
there are no known etiologies. Many of the less common syndromes have been
omitted. Metabolic disorders (e.g., hypothyroidism and phenylketonuria) associated with mental deficiency are discussed in Section 5.

There are many inherited causes of mental deficiency. Some of the most
common are the X-linked mental retardations as listed in Table 14-5. The "fragile
X" syndrome can be diagnosed by karyotyping. X-Linked "dominant" disorders
are not genetic in terms of familial disease but occur in females only and are
sporadic and probably lethal in the male. Dominant transmission of chromosomal anomalies can occur if a parent has a balanced translocation. Dominant
mental retardation also occurs without chromosomopathy. In such cases, the
degree of retardation is usually mild and variable and the inheritance polyge-
netic. Recessive retardation occurs and is the most common mode of transmission for metabolic diseases.

Fetal injuries and complications of pregnancy are listed in Table 14-6. Also
included are conditions associated with pregnancy in which there is a higher
than normal incidence of mental retardation, although a specific cause has not
been established. Perinatal causes for mental retardation are listed in Table 14-
7. Medical records of the neonatal period should be obtained in every child
suspected of having mental retardation, because a clue to the etiology may be
found. It must be remembered that children with prenatal insults or congenital
disorders have a higher percentage of birth complications and prematurity,
which can be additive to the primary brain injury. Unless there is evidence for
neonatal encephalopathy, perinatal complications probably do not cause
retardation.

Postnatal causes for mental retardation are outlined in Table 14-8. Most of
these disorders will be discussed in detail in other chapters of this manual.

Table 14-2. Expected Functional Abilities of the Mentally Retarded

Levels	Academic Potential	Activities of Daily Living	Travel Capability	Vocational Ability
Borderline	Educable, with potential up to about 6th grade level	Fully independent	Independent	Employable without special help, though may need vocational training for competitive employment
Mild	Educable to 4th or 5th grade level (or less). Capable of reading and writing	Relatively independent in all areas, some training might be required	May require travel training to use public transportation	Employable, but often needs some special training if competitive employment is feasible
Moderate	May read or write but very limited (1st or 2nd grade level)	Trainable for all ADL Can dress, be toilet trained, prepare food	Travel only with special training Usually requires special transport	No real competitive employment except in restricted setting, sheltered employment likely with specialized training
Severe	Very unlikely to read or write	Partially trainable Should acquire most ADL skills, is toilet trainable, can dress but may require assistance	Very limited independent travel potential	Sheltered employment only, special training required
Profound	None	May sometimes be toilet trained and dress with assistance Generally very dependent	May or may not be ambulatory Requires special transport	Very limited trainability for vocational functions

(From Cohen HJ: Mental retardation: introduction. Pediatr Ann 11:424–426, 1982.)

Table 14-3. Chromosomopathies Associated with Mental Retardation

Disorder	Characteristics
Trisomies	Moderate retardation, mild dysmorphic appearance
8	Thick lips, deep-set eyes, prominent ears, camptodactyly
9	Microcephaly, micrognathia, prominent nose
13	Holoprosencephaly, cleft palate, polydactyly
18	Failure to thrive, clenched hands, short sternum
21	Hypotonia, flat facies, slanted palpebral fissures
22	Microcephaly, microphthalmia, micrognathia
Triploidy	Syndactyly, low-set malformed ears
Partial trisomies	Moderate to severe retardation, microcephaly, dysmorphic appearance
p+: 2, 4, 5, 8, 9, 10, 12	
q+:2, 3, 4, 7, 8, 10, 11, 13, 14, 15, 22	
Partial monosomies	Moderate to severe retardation, microcephaly, dysmorphic appearance
p-: 4, 5, 9, 12, 18	
q-:11, 12, 18, 21, 22	
Sex chromosomes	Normal to mild retardation
45, X (Turner's)	Short stature, webbed neck, ovarian failure
47, XXY (Klinefelter's)	Tall stature, testicular failure
47, XXY	Tall stature
47, XXX	None
fragile X	Macrocheilia

DIAGNOSIS AND EVALUATION

The diagnosis of a child with mental retardation begins with identification of risk factors, which one obtains from a good history and physical examination during routine well-child care. Significant risk factors include a positive family history and low birth weight. Physical findings of microcephaly, any neurologic deficit, and stigmas of neurocutaneous disorders are also high-risk factors. Developmental progress should be tested using one of the standardized developmental screening tests available. It should be emphasized that although motor development is the most easily measured mode of development, it is perhaps the least predictive of ultimate intellectual outcome. If the screening test is abnormal, then referral should be made to a psychologist for more formal testing. The reader is referred to Chapter 8 for a discussion of psychological testing.

There is no single specific test that should be performed to diagnose the etiology of mental retardation. Emphasis should be placed on tests for treatable disorders and for those having genetic transmission. From the history one should determine if any significant prenatal, perinatal, or postnatal event occurred which was likely to contribute to the brain injury. In those cases in which such history is positive, there is seldom need for further laboratory investigation, unless there is an associated complication such as hydrocephalus, environmental deprivation, uncontrolled seizures, drug intoxication, or other acquired disorders. Also, from the history one should be able to determine whether the condition is static or progressive. If the child has a progressive disorders, then specific

Table 14-4. Dysmorphic Syndromes Associated with Mental Retardation

Syndrome	Degree of Retardation	Description
De Lange	+ + +	Synophrys, micromelia, down-turning upper lip
Rubinstein-Taybi	+ +	Broad thumbs and great toes, slanted palpebral fissures
Dubowitz	+ +	Eczema, small stature, microcephaly
De Sanctis-Cacchione	+ +	Xeroderma pigmentosa, microcephaly, hypogonadism
Johnson-Blizzard	+ + +	Hypoplastic alae nasae, hypothyroidism, deafness
Seckel	+ + +	Short stature, microcephaly, prominent nose (bird-headed dwarf)
Smith-Lemli-Opitz	+ +	Syndactyly, hypospadias, cryptorchidism, ptosis
Sotos	+	Macrosomia, macrocephaly
Beckwith-Wiedemann	+	Macrosomia, macroglossia, omphalocele
Sjögren-Larssen	+ +	Icthyosis, spasticity
Prader-Willi	+ +	Hypotonia, obesity, micropenis
Laurence-Moon-Biedl	+	Retinal pigmentation, obesity, polydactyly
Marinesco-Sjögren	+	Ataxia, hypotonia, cataracts
Cockayne's	+ +	Retinal degeneration, deafness, photosensitivity
Menkes'	+ +	Seizures, twisted fractured hair
Lowe's	+ +	Hypotonia, cataracts, renal tubular defects
Möbius	+	Cranial nerve deficits
Orofaciodigital	+ +	Oral frenula and clefts, hypoplasia of alae nasae, digital asymmetry

Table 14-5. X-Linked Conditions Associated with Mental Deficiency

X-Linked recessive mental retardation
    Isolated mental retardation (Renpenning's syndrome)
    With hydrocephalus
    With microcephaly
    With macro-orchidism (fragile X syndrome)
X-Linked recessive metabolic and degenerative disorders associated with mental deficiency
    Lesch-Nyhan
    Hunter's mucopolysaccharidosis
    Menkes' kinky hair syndrome
    Ornithine transcarbamylase deficiency
    Pelizaeus-Merzbacher
X-Linked "dominant" disorders
    Aicardi syndrome
    Rett syndrome
    Incontinentia pigmenti

Table 14-6. Prenatal Complications and Disorders Associated
with Mental Retardation

Developmental malformations
   Disorders of prosencephalization (holoprosencephaly, arhinence-
     phalia, etc.)
   Disorders of cell migration (lissencephaly, pachygyria, etc.)
   Dysrhaphia (encephalocele, cranial bifida)
   Porencephalia
   Hydranencephaly
   Hydrocephalus
   Microcephaly
Fetal infections
   Rubella
   Toxoplasmosis
   Cytomegalovirus
   Syphilis
Toxins
   Alcohol
   Anticonvulsants
   Aminopterin
   Warfarin
Obstetric complications
   Toxemia
   Malnutrition
   Bleeding
   Trauma
Risk factors
   Maternal age: under 16 years and over 40 years
   Low birth weight
   Breech presentation
   Multiparous pregnancy
   Diabetes
   Family history of mental retardation

Table 14-7. Perinatal Complications and Risk
Factors Associated with Mental
Retardation

Birth trauma
Asphyxia, any cause
Hypoxia, any cause
Acquired metabolic disorder
   Hypoglycemia
   Severe jaundice
Infections
   Bacterial meningitis, sepsis
   Congenital infections
Intraventricular hemorrhage
Multiple congenital deformities
Neonatal seizures

Table 14-8. Postnatal Acquired Disorders
Associated with Mental
Deficiency

Infections and inflammatory disorders
  Meningitis
  Encephalitis
  Postinfectious leukoencephalitis
  Immunization-associated encephalopathy
Head trauma
Intoxications
  Lead encephalopathy
  Chronic anticonvulsant intoxication
Environmental
  Abuse
  Neglect
  Deprivation
Other
  Asphyxia, any cause
  Reye's syndrome
  Brain tumor

tests for degenerative, structural, psychiatric, or metabolic disorder should be pursued as outlined in Chapter 30. The mentally retarded patient with no obvious etiology established from the history or physical examination should be evaluated in an attempt to diagnose treatable and genetically transmitted disorders. Table 14-9 outlines an evaluation plan. In most instances, when the diagnosis does not reveal a treatable or preventable condition, it is nevertheless helpful for the parents to have an explanation of their child's condition. Table 14-10 provides a differential diagnosis for mental retardation.

Table 14-9. Investigations to Be Considered in
the Child with Idiopathic Mental
Retardation

Thyroid function tests
Psychologic testing
Assessment of hearing and vision
EEG (in awake and sleep states)
Blood lead level, free erythrocyte protoporphyrin
  (FEP)
Chromosome analysis
TORCH antibody titers in blood
Skull X-rays
Cranial CT scan
Blood and urine for amino acids, urine for organic
  acids
Urine for mucopolysaccharides
Lysosomal enzyme analysis in blood
Serum uric acid

(From Herskowitz J, Rossman NP: Pediatrics, Neurology, and Psychiatry—Common Ground. © 1982 by Macmillan Publishing Co., New York.)

Table 14-10. Differential Diagnosis of Mental Retardation

Normal variation in development
Cerebral palsy affecting motor and speech functions
Seizure disorder or excessive anticonvulsant medi-
cation depressing development
Hearing deficit
Visual impairment
Degenerative disease
Dull facial appearance
Depression
Specific learning disability

(From Herskowitz J, Rossman NP: Pediatrics, Neurology, and Psychiatry—Common Ground. © 1982 by Macmillan Publishing Co., New York.)

TREATMENT

Treatable causes for mental deficiency will be covered in other sections of the manual dealing specifically with these disorders. The IQ measures the degree of mental retardation in the child or adult. Table 14-2 indicates that patients with borderline and mild retardation are usually functionally independent while requiring some supervision. Children with moderate to severe mental retardation usually require sheltered or even custodial care. Therapy includes providing general health care for the child, treating associated disorders such as epilepsy, and managing or alleviating other handicaps such as vision or hearing deficits and behavioral problems. It is important to encourage parents to let the child pursue those activities in which he can participate. There is controversy as to whether early stimulation programs benefit the child beyond what normal parenting can provide. Mental retardation cannot be cured. Appropriate education can effectively teach all but the profoundly retarded basic social and self-help skills ("survival skills").

Family support is crucial. Parents react with various degrees of intensity to the realization of having a handicapped child by grieving over the loss of the expected normal child. Identifying the etiology and planning a treatment program help the parent work through the grief process. Many parents experience exceptional guilt which can cripple the family unit. Professional counseling may benefit both parent and child. Finally, genetic counseling is an important part of the treatment plan when indicated.

SELECTED READINGS

Herskowitz J, Rossman NP: Pediatrics, Neurology, Psychiatry—Common Ground. Macmillan, New York, 1982

Nelson RP, Crocker AC: The medical care of mentally retarded persons in public residential facilities. N Engl J Med 299:1039–1044, 1978

Rogers MG: The early recognition of handicapping disorders in childhood. Dev Med Child Neurol 13:90, 1971

Schor EL, Smalky KA, Neff JM: Primary care of previously institutionalized children. Pediatrics 67:536–540, 1981

Smith DW, Bostian KE: Congenital anomalies associated with idiopathic mental retardation. J Pediatr 65:189–196, 1964

Smith DW, Simons FER: Rational diagnostic evaluation of the child with mental deficiency. Am J Dis Child 129:1285–1290, 1975

Starrow S, Zigler E: Evaluation of patterning treatment for retarded children. Pediatrics 62:137–150, 1978

15

CEREBRAL PALSY

Cerebral palsy is a disorder of muscle movement or posture caused by a static, nonprogressive disease of the brain. This is not to imply that the clinical course is unchanging. Indeed, the child may go through a variety of stages before the static nature of his clinical syndrome is established. In most cases the condition is congenital; however, acquired injuries of the brain during infancy are included. The incidence of the cerebral palsy is approximately 2 to 4 per 1,000. This incidence has remained relatively constant, although the incidences of specific types of cerebral palsy have shown some changes.

ETIOLOGY

The etiologies for cerebral palsy are diverse. They include prenatal, perinatal, and postnatal insults to the brain (Table 15-1). The prenatal causes are largely due to complications of pregnancy such as congenital infections and fetal distress from a number of obstetric complications. Some causes are inherited and may be associated with malformations of the brain or chromosomal abnormalities. Asphyxia continues to be one of the major causes of cerebral palsy in term infants. Intracranial hemorrhage, perinatal infections, and, less commonly, acquired metabolic disturbances such as hyperbilirubinemia cause cerebral palsy in the neonate. Many of the postnatal causes are due to injuries and infections of the CNS. In over 50 percent of cases, however, there is no specific etiology that can be determined.

CLASSIFICATION

There are a number of classifications of cerebral palsy. Table 15-2 is one classification system. It must be remembered that there will be many patients who will not fit a typical pattern and that many children cannot be accurately classified into a specific cerebral palsy syndrome until after their first year.

Spastic hemiplegia occurs in approximately 40 percent of all patients with cerebral palsy. The right side is more commonly affected than the left. Because many movements of the newborn are basically subcortical reflexes, it may be difficult to make a diagnosis of hemiplegia before the age of 4 to 6 months. Asymmetries in the examination before this age are frequently caused by peripheral nerve injury. As the child matures and cortical influences come to bear

159

Table 15-1. Etiologies of Cerebral Palsy

Prenatal
  Congenital infections
    Toxoplasmosis
    Rubella
    Cytomegalovirus
    Herpes
    Syphilis
  Teratogenic substances
  Obstetric complications
    Toxemia
    Placenta previa, abruptio placentae
    Malnutrition
    Substance abuse
  Hereditary
    Chromosomal abnormalities
    Family history of cerebral palsy

Perinatal
  Prematurity
    Intracranial hemorrhage
    Hypoxia
  Complicated delivery
    Asphyxia
    Cerebral trauma
  Infections
    Bacterial sepsis, meningitis
    Herpes
  Metabolic
    Hyperbilirubinemia
    Hypoglycemia

Postnatal
  Cerebral trauma
  Infections
    Meningitis
    Abscess
    Encephalitis
  Cerebrovascular accident
    Intracranial hemorrhage
    Stroke
  Acquired encephalopathies
    Toxic, e.g., lead
    Metabolic, e.g., Reye's syndrome
    Hypoxic–ischemic, e.g., near-drowning

Idiopathic

on movement, then asymmetries become more noticeable. Early signs of hemiplegia include a persistent asymmetric tonic neck response and persistent fisting; later the parachute reaction may show asymmetry. Early handedness, which is abnormal before the age of 12 months, may be noted by the parents. The muscle tone may be decreased initially but as the child matures it increases and develops into spasticity with hyperreflexia. The hemiplegic child shows more weakness in the arm and face and then in the leg and has a typical posture (Fig. 15-1). Complications of hemiplegic cerebral palsy include corticosensory disturbances on the affected side with undergrowth of the affected limbs and partial seizures.

Table 15-2. Classification of Cerebral Palsy

Spastic
  Hemiplegia
  Double hemiplegia
  Diplegia
  Quadriplegia
Extrapyramidal
  Choreoathetosis
  Tremor
  Rigidity
  Atonia
  Ataxia
Mixed

Spastic double hemiplegia occurs in approximately 20 percent of patients with cerebral palsy. There is a higher incidence of severe perinatal complications. The infant may remain hypotonic for several months before increased tone gradually becomes apparent. Some children remain flaccid, however. Persistence of primitive reflexes and abnormal posturing are common early findings, with scissoring in the lower extremities and flexor posturing in the upper extremities (Fig. 15-2). Many children will have marked hyperextension and opisthotonus in the supine position. Prone positions favor a flexor posture. In severe cases, contractures develop as the child matures. Global cerebral dysfunction with mental retardation, seizures, and microcephaly frequently complicates the motor deficit.

Approximately 5 to 10 percent of patients with cerebral palsy have spastic diplegia. This condition is more frequently associated with premature birth and the motor signs are more marked in the lower extremities than in the upper extremities. Lower extremity hypotonia and persistent steppage and placing reflexes are early findings. The children frequently bear weight at a much earlier age than normal and also tend to toe-point. The classic posture is one of scissoring on vertical suspension (Fig. 15-3). The upper extremities may be markedly involved as well (spastic quadriplegia). In mild cases there may be no abnormality other than toe-walking.

Older literature refers to spastic monoplegias, triplegias, or other combinations. Most of these children, when examined closely, will be found to have

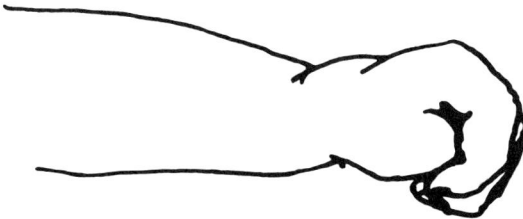

Fig. 15-1. Fisting.

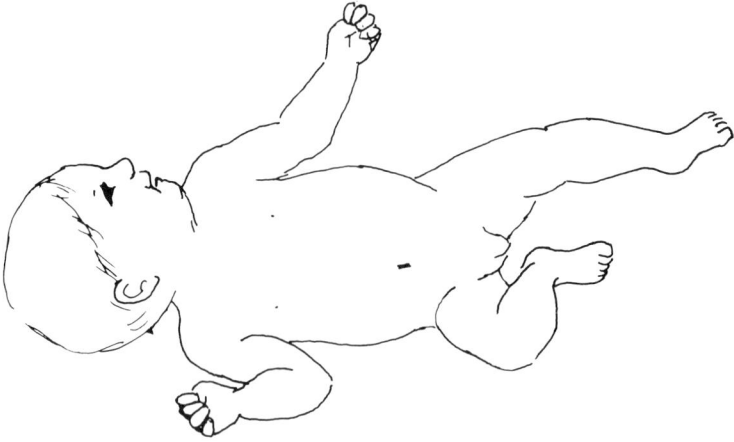

Fig. 15-2. Persistent asymmetric tonic neck response.

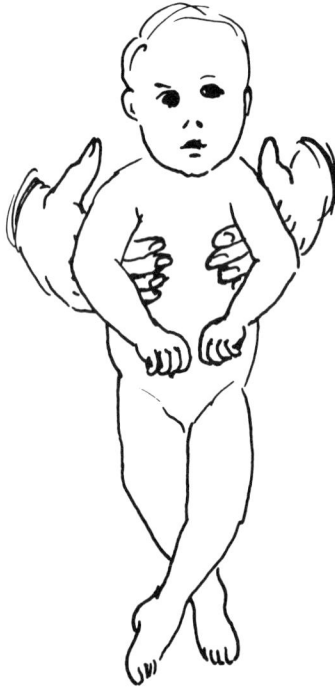

Fig. 15-3. Scissoring.

variations of diplegia, hemiplegia, or bilateral hemiplegia. Many children with spastic cerebral palsy have involuntary movements as well.

The extrapyramidal cerebral palsies include those with predominant dystonia and those with predominant ataxia. The incidence of athetoid cerebral palsy has decreased somewhat since the advent of the adequate prevention and therapy for hyperbilirubinemia. Children with kernicterus usually have a latent phase of several months during which they have decreased movement and hypotonia. Following this phase there is progressive increase in muscle tone but not of the spastic type. There is usually persistence of primitive reflexes and marked difficulty in chewing and swallowing. Involuntary movements become increasingly common, particularly in the second year. At the present time approximately 5 to 10 percent of children with cerebral palsy will have the athetoid type, and of these the majority are due to perinatal asphyxia. Fewer are caused by congenital malformation of the brain and rarely by neonatal jaundice. Other cerebral palsy syndromes with major abnormalities in posture are those with atonia, rigidity, and tremor.

Approximately 5 percent of patients with cerebral palsy have ataxic cerebral palsy. These can be divided into children with both spastic diplegia and ataxia and those with ataxia alone. The former group is more likely to be caused by perinatal injuries, whereas the latter is often caused by cerebellar malformations. Recessive inheritance is common in the latter as well and some authors subgroup these into the disequilibrium syndrome. In general, patients with ataxic cerebral palsy have fewer neurologic complications than other types.

DIAGNOSIS

The diagnosis of cerebral palsy is difficult to make in the immature infant. It is only after myelinization is completed that the full deficit can be determined. For this reason many neonates are sent home with no apparent motor deficit only to return at a later age with cerebral palsy. The most common symptom leading to a diagnosis is delayed motor milestones, particularly at age 6 months when the child has not begun to sit and later, of course, when the child does not stand or attempt to walk. Physicians frequently suspect abnormalities when there is persistence of primitive reflexes such as the asymmetric tonic neck reflex. Early diagnosis can also be established by observation in the older child showing asymmetry in movements or tone, involuntary movements, and early establishment of handedness. Table 15-3 summarizes some of the early findings of cerebral palsy (see Figs. 15-1 to 15-3). In the older child the diagnosis is usually self-evident.

There are a number of conditions included in the differential diagnosis of cerebral palsy that must be excluded (Table 15-4). Because this is predominantly a motor systems disease, the neuromuscular disorders are particularly misdiagnosed as cerebral palsy. In the newborn, marked asymmetry of the motor activity usually implies a peripheral nervous system disorder, particularly peripheral nerve injuries. Congenital neuromuscular diseases are a very common

Table 15-3. Early Signs of Cerebral Palsy

Alterations in muscle tone
  Hypotonia
  Scissoring
  Fisting
  Opisthotonic posturing
  Passive resistance to stretch
Persistence of primitive reflexes
  Obligatory asymmetric tonic neck reflex
  Crossed extensor reflex
Asymmetric neurologic signs
  Tone
  Parachute reflex
  Handedness before 12 months
  Deep tendon reflexes
Deep tendon reflexes
  Sustained clonus
  Persistent crossed adductor reflex

cause of the hypotonic infant. Special studies, including measurements of creatinine kinase, electromyography, and a muscle biopsy, are frequently necessary to differentiate these patients from those who have cerebral causes for their hypotonia. The course of cerebral palsy is one of initial change becoming static with maturity; most neuromuscular disorders are progressive. Children who have spinal dysrhaphia may also present with undergrowth of a limb, paraparesis or paraplegia, or other signs suggestive of cerebral palsy. Spinal radiographs and careful examination of the back as well as a detailed neurologic examination will usually separate these from children who have cerebral palsy. In the newborn period, arthrogryposis is often confused with cerebral palsy. This condition is almost always due to fetal immobility secondary to either confinement or a neuromuscular disorder. In older children, mental retardation frequently causes a delay in the acquisition of motor skills and may not represent a specific motor systems disorder. Finally, the degenerative diseases of childhood such as Friedreich's ataxia, familial spastic paraparesis, and some of the metabolic disorders such as metachromatic leukodystrophy and other storage diseases may present with predominantly motor systems dysfunction early in the course. Their progressive nature differentiates these disorders from cerebral palsy. The approach to determining the etiology begins with a careful history. Perinatal causes can be implicated if there is a history of fetal distress from monitoring data, low Apgar scores, acidosis, and an abnormal neonatal course with neurologic complications. Selected laboratory tests may be necessary in the child with no discernable etiology from history and physical exam. In general, the evaluation is similar to that for mental retardation (see Table 14-9).

Although cerebral palsy is a motor system disorder, it usually occurs in the context of a syndrome of multiple problems. Table 15-5 lists the complications which are frequently seen with cerebral palsy. Approximately 50 percent of the patients have mental retardation or other cognitive defects which will significantly impair their ability to perform in the classroom or at home. A total of 45

Table 15-4. Differential Diagnosis of Cerebral Palsy

Neuromuscular
  Congenital
    Myopathies
    Myasthenia gravis
    Hypomyelinating neuropathies
    Spinal muscular atrophy
  Postnatal
    Muscular dystrophies
    Familial polyneuropathies
    Myasthenia gravis
    Spinal muscular atrophy

Degenerative
  Familiar spastic paraparesis
  Friedreich's ataxia and other spinocerebellar degeneration
  Childhood Huntington's disease

Metabolic
  Lysosomal storage disease
  Aminoacidurias
  Pyruvate dysmetabolism
  Metabolic myopathies
  Wilson's disease
  Many others

Bone and joint deformities
  Arthrogryposis multiplex congenita
  Equinovarus deformities

Disorders of involuntary movement
  Tics/Tourette's syndrome
  Dystonia musculorum deformans
  Torsion dystonia
  Sydenham's chorea
  Spasmus nutans
  Continuous motor activity (Isaac's, stiff-man syndrome)

Myelopathies
  Spinal dysrhaphia
  Diastematomyelia
  Tethered cord syndrome
  Spinal cord tumor, arteriovenous malformation
  Malformation of the brain

percent have ocular abnormalities, including significant visual loss, refractive errors, and most frequently strabismus. Seizures occur in approximately one-third of patients. Seizures are less common in the extrapyramidal forms of cerebral palsy. Hearing is affected in 15 percent. Growth disturbances, either unilaterally or generalized, are common. The more severely affected an extremity, the more likely it will be atrophied. A majority of the patients have problems with communication due to either mental retardation, hearing deficit, or poor articulation.

The overall prognosis for cerebral palsy is relatively poor and is proportional to the severity of the dysfunction. In large series only 5 percent attain independent functioning. The majority require some type of sheltered environment and a sizable minority require custodial care. Children with mental retardation have

Table 15-5. Medical Complications
Associated with Cerebral
Palsy

Cognitive
  Mental retardation
  Learning disabilities
  Attention deficit disorder
Ocular
  Strabismus
  Refractive errors
  Visual field deficit
Communicative
  Hearing loss
  Dysarthria
  Aphasia
Epilepsy
Orthopedic
  Joint contracture, subluxation
  Scoliosis
Growth
  Small stature
  Hemiatrophy

the worst prognosis. Some children with cerebral palsy have normal intelligence but will still require a sheltered environment because of their severe motor disabilities. There is approximately a 10 percent mortality due to respiratory infections, status epilepticus, and other complications.

THERAPY

Although there is no cure for cerebral palsy, there are therapies which can improve function. For cerebral palsy itself, the two specific therapies which are most widely used are physiotherapy and orthopedic intervention. There is debate as to the exact value of physiotherapy. Many physical therapists and centers which treat a large number of patients use the system developed by the Bobaths or a modification thereof. The therapeutic strategy is to modify abnormal reflexes to enhance a specific function. A prone position enhances a flexor movement whereas a supine position enhances extensor tone. Variations on reinforcing or extinguishing these reflexes are used to try to improve the child's function. There is considerable debate as to how much this actually affects long-term outcome. Traditional physiotherapy involves passive stretching of muscles and has some benefit in the prevention of contractures in patients who have spasticity.

Orthopedic intervention is frequently used when the child has stabilized and is rarely indicated before the age of 4 or 5 years. It is specifically helpful in releasing contracted muscles and the bracing of weak extremities, particularly in the legs. This will enable the child to have better standing balance and often will help the child learn to walk. Orthopedic intervention may also improve nursing care of a spastic child, particularly toileting and perineal care. Marked contractures of the knees, ankles, and hips can also make it difficult to transport children. In general, surgery should only be performed for a specific achievable goal.

Seizures should be managed by a physician competent in treating such disorders. Ophthalmologic and audiometric evaluations should be made in most children. Some will benefit from corrective lenses or hearing aids, and most with squints need surgical correction to prevent permanent loss of vision. Medical treatment of spasticity has met with mixed results. Diazepam is probably the best spasmolytic agent available; however, it frequently causes significant impairment of higher cortical function at doses necessary to relieve the spasticity. Dantrium and baclofen are also used for spasticity, but no persistent efficacy has been shown. Older children and adults often benefit from occupational therapy. There have been a number of devices that have been designed specifically for handicapped children, which can enhance their self-care. In addition, an occupational therapist is invaluable in prescribing a variety of equipment for optimal care of the child in such routine tasks as bathing, feeding, transporting, and sitting.

Because of the nature of this syndrome and its many complications, a team approach is usually advocated in the treatment of these disorders. Facilities that can bring together the different specialists needed to optimally treat these children are of obvious benefit; however, a pediatrician can usually organize and direct the child through the various subspecialties if a referral center is not available. Parents should be cautioned about therapies which do not have proven efficacy in the treatment of cerebral palsy. These therapies frequently require the involvement of a number of family members as well as extensive time for the exercises and other activities involved. The excessive time or effort required may distract from the family unit and cause problems in and of itself.

A child with cerebral palsy needs attention and care just as a normal child does. The pediatrician or primary care physician can be particularly helpful in giving the parents an opportunity to ventilate their feelings about having a handicapped child. The comments concerning parental counseling in Chapter 14 on mental retardation are equally applicable here.

SELECTED READINGS

Bax MC: Terminology and classification of cerebral palsy. Dev Med Child Neurol 6:295, 1964

Kanthor H, Pless B, Satterwhite B, Myers G: Areas of responsibility in the health care of multiple handicapped children. Pediatrics 54:779–785, 1974

Kudvjavcev T, Schoenberg BS, Kurland LT et al: Cerebral palsy: survival rates, associated handicaps, and distribution by clinical subtype (Rochester, MN, 1950–1976). Neurology 35:900–905, 1985

Nelson KB, Ellenberg JH: Apgar scores as predictors of chronic neurological disability. Pediatrics 68:36–44, 1981

Nelson KB, Ellenberg JH: Children who "outgrew" cerebral palsy. Pediatrics 69:529, 1982

Nelson KB, Ellenberg JH: Antecedents of cerebral palsy. Am J Dis Child 139:1031–1038, 1985

Taft LT: Cerebral palsy. Pediatr Rev 6:35–45, 1984

Task Force on Joint Assessment of Prenatal and Perinatal Factors Associated with Brain Disorders: National Institutes of Health Report on Causes of Mental Retardation and Cerebral Palsy. Pediatrics 76:457–458, 1985

16

LEARNING DISABILITIES

Public Law 94-142 ensures the right of handicapped children, including those with learning disorders, to a free and appropriate public education. The role of the physician in the program was not clearly defined, and, indeed, the medical model in the management of handicapped children has been largely supplanted by an educational model. This was an appropriate shift in emphasis because of the very nature of the problem and the treatment methods. Nevertheless, the physician continues to play an important role in the identification and management of learning disorders. This is especially true for the pediatrician, who may have the earliest professional contact with the child.

LEARNING DISABILITIES

The process of learning is not fully understood. Much of what is known has been derived from localization of higher cortical functions following isolated destructive lesions of the brain and the computer model of learning. The temporal cortex is related to auditory processing, the occipital cortex to visual processing, the anterior parietal cortex to somatosensory processing, and the posterofrontal cortex to motor output programming. Cerebral hemispheric specialization has been clearly identified: The left pertains primarily to linguistic skills and the right to visual spacial skills. The computer model provides a basis for observing the steps in the learning process. These steps include input, integration, memory, and output. In human learning the input is primarily visual and auditory perceptions, although other sensory perceptions are also important. Integration involves sequencing, association, and abstraction. Memory can be divided into three categories: immediate, which is usually a function of consciousness; recent, or the ability to make new memories; and remote, which involves the process of retrieving previously stored information. Output usually involves talking, writing, and motor performance.

A specific learning disability can be defined as a disorder in one or more of the basic psychological processes involved in understanding or using spoken or written language. One method of classification is summarized in Table 16-1. Descriptive terms used for these disorders have been *minimal brain dysfunction, perceptual handicaps, dyslexia,* and *developmental aphasia,* among others. The disability is usually manifested by difficulties in listening, thinking, and communication. Other disorders can present with learning problems and the differential diagnosis of specific learning disabilities is summarized in Table 16-2.

169

Table 16-1. Classification of Learning Disabilities

Disorders of verbal and nonverbal learning
  Verbal disabilities
    Oral language comprehension
    Oral language usage
    Reading
    Writing
  Nonverbal disabilities
    Time orientation
    Spatial orientation
    Directionality
    Picture interpretation
    Social perception

Disorders of input and output
  Input
    Oral language comprehension
    Reading
  Output
    Oral language usage
    Writing

Disorders within specific learning modalities
  Disorders of perception
    Visual
    Auditory
    Haptic
  Disorders of memory
    Short-term storage
    Long-term storage
    Retrieval
    Sequencing
  Disorders of thinking
    Categorization
    Associations among objects
    Concept formation
  Disorders in perceptual motor learning

(Data from Culbertson JL, Ferry PL: Learning disabilities. Pediatr Clin North Am 31:121–136, 1982.)

Table 16-2. Differential Diagnosis of Learning Disabilities

Mild mental retardation
Behavior disorders
Primary psychiatric disorders
Developmental dysphasia and other language disorders
Primary sensory impairments
  Deafness
  Blindness
Cultural deprivation
Neurologic disorders
  Epilepsy
  Degenerative disease
  Intoxications
Substance abuse

Table 16-3. Causes of Hearing Loss in Childhood

Etiology	Approximate Incidence (%)
Genetic	50
Deafness only	
Other deficits	
Prenatal	10
Congenital malformations	
Congenital infection	
Perinatal	15
Meningitis	
Associated with cerebral palsy	
Aminoglycoside therapy	
Postnatal	25
Chronic middle ear disease	
Meningitis	
Trauma	
Ototoxic drugs	

(Adapted from Fraser GR: The causes of profound deafness in childhood. p. 5. In Wosten Holme GE, Knight J (eds): Sensorineural Hearing Loss. J & A Churchill, London, 1970.)

Children with disordered consciousness usually present early for medical attention. This often presents as acute (e.g., seizures) or subacute (e.g., intoxication) alterations in wakefulness. However, a child with partial or absence seizures may go undetected unless a physician asks specifically about symptoms of these seizures. Often these children are accused of daydreaming or being inattentive and may have difficulty completing tasks.

Adequate sensation is crucial for learning in the classroom. A physician should suspect a hearing loss in the child with delayed or poor speech development or in the older child who constantly increases the television volume or exhibits other characteristics of the hearing impaired. Visually impaired children often fail to notice small objects, sit close to the television, squint, and have other characteristics of visual impairment. Early diagnosis of these potentially treatable disorders is obviously important. Causes for hearing and visual loss are listed in Tables 16-3 and 16-4.

Attention requires the ability to filter sensory input and assign priorities to perceptions. The child with an attention deficit disorder is unable to filter sensory input such that most or all inputs compete for full attention. This disability leads to distractability and shortening of the attention span and is usually associated with hyperkinetic behavior. A child with difficulty filtering internal stimuli shows disinhibition and impulsive behavior. The child with a thought disorder (psychosis) has difficulty discerning external from internal stimuli. Behavior problems are discussed in Chapter 17.

The physician should suspect mental retardation in the child with global developmental delay or in the child at risk for having mental retardation (e.g., cerebral palsy). Children with mental retardation improve with age, although at a slower rate than normal. A rare cause of learning problems is a progressive neurologic disorder. Often the earliest manifestation of a degenerative disease is a deterioration in cognitive skills associated with a personality change. It is

Table 16-4. Causes of Blindness in Children

Etiology	Incidence (%)
Retrolental fibroplasia	19
Congenital cataracts	18
Optic atrophy	17
Leber's congenital amaurosis	8
Retinoblastoma	5
Congenital glaucoma	5
Albinism	3
Retinitis pigmentosa	3
Severe myopia	2
Other	20

(Modified with permission from Friedman AC: Severe visual defects in educable children. p. 174. In Nawratzki I, Merin S (eds): Impaired Vision in Childhood. Copyright, 1977 Pergamon Press, Ltd. New York.

important to recognize a past history of normal or near-normal development with a period of stagnation in learning new skills followed by a period of deterioration. By and large, these disorders are not treatable but should be diagnosed.

Language disorders are frequently confused with learning disabilities. Failure to use specific words by 18 months or phrases by 2 years and unintelligible, echolalic, or inappropriate speech suggest a language disturbance. Table 16-5 lists the major causes for language disturbance. The most common cause for language delay is mental retardation. Developmental dysphasia is a primary disorder that is not necessarily associated with other cognitive, neurologic, hearing, or behavioral deficits. Acquired aphasias usually result from injury to the dominant hemisphere. One interesting syndrome of acquired aphasia is associated with temporal lobe epileptiform discharges. Convulsions may occur at the onset. Failure of language development by 4 years results in a poor prognosis for developing speech.

EVALUATION

One can approach the child with learning problems using neurologic, psychological, and educational prerequisites for learning as outlined in Table 16-6. Using the definition of a specific learning disability above, the precise diagnosis

Table 16-5. Disorders of Language Development

Primary dysphasic syndrome
  Verbal auditory agnosia (word deafness)
  Mixed receptive and expressive dysphasia (poor verbal and comprehension)
  Expressive dysphasia (impaired verbal language)
Secondary
  Mental retardation
  Autism
  Deafness
  Acquired injury to language area of the brain (aphasia)
  Acquired aphasia with convulsions

Table 16-6. Prerequisites for Learning

Neurologic
  Consciousness
  Adequate visual and auditory sensation
  Attention
  Adequate intelligence and cerebral maturation
Psychological
  Perception
  Adequate integration, processing, and sequencing skills
  Adequate memory
Education and social
  Adequate motivation
  Adequate instruction
  Adequate mechanism for performance and its evaluation

will be made by appropriate psychological tests. Other causes of learning problems should be excluded by neurologic, educational, and social evaluations. Because the treatment of specific learning disabilities is largely educational, this chapter will discuss the neurologic causes of learning problems.

The evaluation begins with a complete history of the problem and an academic history of performance and testing. Documentation of the chronicity or progression of symptoms is important. The past medical history is explored for risk factors associated with past medical illnesses and injuries. These include perinatal complications, CNS infection or trauma, seizures, drug treatment, and behavior problems. A family history is often positive for other members having similar problems. A screening history should be obtained for common presenting signs of learning disabilities (Table 16-7). One must consider the age and stage of development of the child and the fact that no single item will be a positive screen; the disorder will present as a constellation of these signs and symptoms.

Table 16-7. Academic Characteristics of Learning
Disabilities

Spelling
  Incorrect letter order
  Difficulty in associating letters to sounds
  Letter and word reversals
Writing
  Inability to stay on line
  Slow writing production
  Inability to copy
  Inappropriate mixing of upper and lower case
Reading
  Word repetition, omission, or addition
  Poor fluency
  Word/letter similarity (visual or sound) confusion
  Reading dislike
Math
  Difficulty with association of number with symbol
  Poor recall or comprehension of math facts
  Confusion with columns and spacing

(Data from Culbertson JC, Ferry P: Learning disabilities.
Pediatr Clin North Am 29:121–136, 1982.)

Development must be assessed by recording milestones. Standardized developmental screening tests, such as the Denver Developmental Screening Test, are available for more formal screening.

Physical and screening neurologic examinations are necessary to exclude physical or neurologic handicapping conditions that may impede learning. Hearing and vision must be estimated by screening techniques and recorded. If the initial evaluation raises suspicions, the physician should proceed to exclude disorders which affect consciousness, sensation, attention, and development as listed in Table 16-6.

There is no typical examination finding or laboratory test that differentiates the learning-disabled child from the normal child. So-called soft signs have relatively little meaning in the evaluation of a child with a school problem. These signs, such as clumsiness, posturing, right–left disorientation, fine choreiform movements, and mirror movements, are not reproducible and usually represent only neurologic immaturity. The point at which they become abnormal is not well standardized. Also, studies have shown that the presence or absence of these soft signs cannot be related to school performance.

Signs of focal or diffuse neurologic deficits warrant further evaluation for neurologic disease. After the appropriate screening procedures, specific tests such as the EEG and hearing tests may aid in the diagnosis of medical disorders. It should be noted that these ancillary tests are not screening procedures but are used to evaluate a specific problem. For example, the EEG is used for the suspected diagnosis of a seizure disorder.

TREATMENT

The treatment for learning disabilities lies within the classroom. The preschool child with a learning disorder may not have access to public education unless this resource has been legislated. Within the community there may be a variety of private and public institutions to which the child may be referred for services, including educational stimulation, speech and language training, and behavior modification. The physician should be aware of these resources or have access to a social services agency for making appropriate referrals. Medical intervention is indicated for children with disorders of consciousness, attention, sensation, and behavior. After appropriate diagnostic evaluation the child is treated with modalities specific for his disorder.

Drugs are useful in the treatment of seizures and some behavioral and psychiatric disorders. The most controversy has developed around the use of stimulants in children with hyperkinesis. This is because hyperkinesis is a sign and not a diagnosis in itself. It may represent a primary constitutional or genetic hyperactivity or can be secondary to behavioral or emotional problems. The Diagnostic and Statistical Manual of the American Psychiatric Association has revised terminology for minimal brain dysfunction. The term *attention deficit disorder* will be used for children with specific diagnostic criteria for hyperactivity, inattention, impulsivity, and epidemiologic data. This definition is useful in the approach to the hyperkinetic child (see Ch. 17).

Most CNS stimulants increase attention and therefore are indicated in some children with attention deficit disorder. Drugs, however, should be used sparingly and only after other diagnoses have been eliminated and other treatment programs, such as behavior modification, attempted. The typical child with this syndrome has a history of overactivity dating since long before school years. These children are of normal intelligence, but approximately 60 percent have an associated specific learning disability. Treating the hyperactivity does not treat the learning disability. Without concomitant educational therapy the child cannot be expected to learn any better than he did prior to treatment. Therapy will improve the child's classroom behavior and therefore have a secondary effect on his learning. Children with hyperkinetic behavior secondary to emotional problems normally present with behavior problems after starting school. They are unlikely to respond to psychostimulants and need to have their primary disorder treated appropriately.

The physician must often assume responsibility for managing the secondary emotional problems which frequently occur. The child may react to school failure in a number of ways. These include regressive behavior, depression, acting out, and antisocial behavior. The behavior problems often complicate and may even overshadow the learning disability. The physician should either manage these problems himself or refer them to appropriate private or public facilities. Often explaining the problem in simple terms can calm parental anxiety.

Other noneducational approaches to the treatment of children with learning disabilities or disorders should be approached with skepticism. Patterning exercises, special diets, orthomolecular treatments, and optometric exercises have not undergone objective scientific evaluation for efficacy. Educators are ultimately responsible for the design and provision of treatment for specific learning disabilities and the physician makes little useful contribution. Whether the child is treated in a full-time special school, a self-contained classroom, or a resource room or receives aid from itinerant specialists is an educational decision. The physician's role should be that of advising the educators of medical disorders, the effects of medications, and the classroom management of medical problems.

SELECTED READINGS

Culbertson JL, Ferry PC: Learning disabilities. Pediatr Clin North Am 29:121–136, 1982

Garrard SD: Role of the pediatrician in the management of learning disorders. Pediatr Clin North Am 201:737–754, 1973

Kandt RS: Neurologic examination of children with learning disorders. Pediatr Clin North Am 31:297–316, 1984

Nelson LB: The visually handicapped child. Pediatr Rev 6:173–182, 1984

Resnick TJ, Allen DA, Rapin I: Disorders of language development. Diagnosis and intervention. Pediatr Rev 6:85–92, 1984

Shaywitz SE, Shaywitz BA, McGraw K et al: Current status of the neuromaturational examination as an index of learning disability. J Pediatr 104:819–825, 1984

Taylor R, Warren SA: Educational and psychological assessment of children with learning disorders. Pediatr Clin North Am 31:281–296, 1984

Wolffe HC: Children with communication problems. How does one evaluate them? Clin Pediatr 6:635–640, 1967

17

BEHAVIOR DISORDERS

A behavior disorder is one in which the observed behavior does not meet expectations for the child's age. Behavior disorders vary considerably, not only by the primary dysfunction, whether it be in thought, emotions, or conduct, but also with the expectations of the family, community, and culture. Many behavior disorders are an exaggeration of normal behaviors, and many are a persistence of behaviors which were more appropriate for a younger age. The most severe behavior disorders are those which are caused by disorders of thinking and conduct. This chapter reviews those behavioral disorders which are frequently confused with neurologic disease and cause neurologic consultation. Most children with behavior disorders do not have evidence of neurologic injury although injuries to the nervous system may make a child more susceptible to the usual stresses of childhood that precipitate behavioral problems.

BREATH-HOLDING SPELLS

The onset of breath-holding spells (BHSs) is approximately 6 to 18 months. Twenty percent have the onset before 6 months and about that many go beyond the age of 18 months. The prevalence is 2 to 4 percent of normal children, with a male preponderance, and there is a family history in 25 percent of cases. Clinically, one can divide BHS cases into two groups. The cyanotic BHS accounts for approximately two-thirds of patients and can be characterized as self-asphyxiation following an adverse emotional encounter. Other behaviors in these children include temper tantrums, negativism, and aggression. Typically, children with cyanotic BHS are angered, frustrated, or injured. Following a brief period of vigorous crying the child stops breathing, becomes cyanotic, and loses consciousness. The child may have a brief period of hypertonia, or there may be clonic movements toward the end of the unconscious period. After 15 to 30 seconds the child gradually returns to consciousness. The cyanotic BHS may appear similar to the generalized motor seizure. The differential diagnosis between these disorders is shown in Table 17-1.

The pallid BHS differs from the cyanotic BHS in that the trigger of the event is usually a minimal injury or sudden fright. Particularly common is an injury to the head. The child cries momentarily and then lapses into unconsciousness, frequently associated with pallor. Studies have shown that such children have a hyperactive vagal reflex and are very sensitive to ocular compression. Asystole for greater than 2 seconds is suggestive of the diagnosis. Children who have

Table 17-1. Differential Diagnosis Between Generalized Motor Seizures and Breath-Holding Spells

Features	Generalized Motor Seizure	Breath-Holding Spells
Age of onset	Usually after 1 year	Usually before 1 year
Family history	Negative or positive for epilepsy	May be positive for BHS or fainting
Precipitating factors	Nonspecific stress (fever, etc.)	Specific emotional or nociceptive stimuli
Occurrence during sleep	Common	Never
Motor sequence	Tonic/clonic limpness	Limpness and tonic or clonic movement
Duration	Usually more than 1 minute	Usually less than 1 minute
Incontinence	Common	Uncommon
Interictal EEG	Usually abnormal	Usually normal

(Modified from Lombroso CT, Lerman P: Breathholding spells (cyanotic and pallid infantile syncope). Pediatrics 39:563–581. Copyright American Academy of Pediatrics 1967.)

been monitored during these events show asystole during the initial part of unconsciousness and if this persists longer than 10 seconds, a brief hypoxic seizure may follow.

Essential to the diagnosis of BHS of either type is the relationship to emotional stimulation. Regardless of the type of BHS, the prognosis is excellent. There is no significant association with later development of epilepsy, mental retardation, or behavior disorders. Almost no children have spells beyond the age of 6 years. Children with pallid BHS have a 17 percent chance of later developing syncope. There is no specific treatment for cyanotic BHS other than behavior modifications. Pallid BHs, if frequent or severe, may respond to low doses of atropine.

HEAD ROLLING AND HEAD BANGING

Head banging or head rolling has the onset at approximately 8 months, with a range of 5 to 11 months. It is extremely rare after 3 years. It is said to occur in anywhere from 2 to 5 percent of all children and is three times more common in males than in females. The activity has a very repetitive quality and can be confused with a rhythmic movement disorder or rarely a seizure. Because the child often indulges in this activity for no apparent reason, it may be confused with the self-stimulatory activity observed in autistic children. Long-term follow-up studies show no significant association between head-rolling or head-banging activity and later development of behavior problems. This is a benign condition and there is no specific therapy.

ATTENTION DEFICIT DISORDER

Attention deficit disorder (ADD) is the most common pediatric behavior disorder. Prevalence rates range from 1.2 percent to 20 percent, depending upon the author, criteria, and population studied. Of the clinical syndromes of ADD,

Table 17-2. Criteria for Attention Deficit
Disorder

Inattention (at least three of the following)
  Fails to finish tasks
  Poor listening
  Easily distracted
  Difficulty concentrating
  Difficulty persisting to play activities
Impulsivity (at least three of the following)
  Acts before thinking
  Shifts activities excessively
  Difficulty organizing tasks
  Needs excessive supervision
  Frequently speaks out of turn
  Difficulty awaiting turns
Hyperactivity (at least two of the following)
  Runs or climbs excessively
  Difficulty sitting still
  Difficulty staying seated
  Moves excessively during sleep
  Persistent, excessive activity

(Data from DSM-III. American Psychiatric Association, Washington, DC.)

that associated with hyperactivity is the most common, especially in younger children. There is a marked male predominance of approximately 6:1. The etiology of ADD is obscure. There is no significant association with birth injury or postnatal encephalopathy. There is relatively good evidence to suggest that ADD syndromes are related to genetic factors. There is a higher incidence of hyperactivity in parents of children with ADD than in parents of children without this disorder. There is also a much higher concordance in monozygotic twins compared to dizygotic twins.

The key to the diagnosis of ADD rests on the triad of inattention, impulsivity, and hyperactivity (Table 17-2). The onset is before 7 years of age. The history must show that the behavior abnormality if pervasive both at home and at school and not centered around particular situations. The history should also attempt to exclude evidence for a degenerative disease, seizures, and severe mental retardation, although hyperactivity can occur in such conditions.

The neurologic and physical examination shows no specific findings to identify the child with ADD. Although there are some who believe that the neuromaturational signs (Table 17-3), often called soft signs, have clinical significance in this disorder, many of these signs can be found in normal children. There is no other specific laboratory tests that will confirm the diagnosis of ADD. Psychometric testing may be helpful in some instances. The arithmetic, coding, information, and memory span subtests of the Wechsler Intelligence Scale for Children Revised are sensitive to deficits in attention, concentration, and alertness, and low scores may reflect ADD. Children's Personal Data Inventory and the Teacher's Behavior Rating Scale are frequently used screening tests for ADD. The diagnosis is ultimately a clinical one, based upon the criteria listed in Table 17-2. Exclusion criteria for the diagnosis of ADD include organic diseases that

Table 17-3. Borderline, Equivocal, or "Soft" Neurologic Signs in Children

Clumsiness in tasks requiring fine motor coordination (tying shoelaces or doing buttons)
Choreiform movements
Mild dysphasias
Associated movements
Borderline hyperreflexia and reflex asymmetry
Finger agnosia
Dysdiadochokinesis
Ocular apraxia and endpoint nystagmus
Tremor
Graphesthesias
Whirling
Extinction to double simultaneous tactile stimulation
Pupillary inequalities
Mixed laterality and disturbances of right–left discrimination
Unilateral winking defect
Awkward gait
Avoiding response in outstretched hands

(From Shain RJ: Neurology of Childhood Learning Disabilities. 2nd Ed. © 1977 The Williams & Wilkins Co., Baltimore.)

impair vision or hearing or interfere significantly with thinking and reasoning, such as severe mental retardation or intoxications, or severe thought disorder such as autism or schizophrenia. Many of these children will have hyperactivity as an epiphenomenon to their disorder.

Seventy to eighty percent of children treated with stimulant medication (methylphenidate, dextroamphetamine, pemoline) have a favorable response. Stimulant medication works primarily on improving attention and perhaps improving fine motor coordination. The dose of methylphenidate is about 5 to 10 mg given just before the child goes to school and at noon. Its use should be in conjunction with appropriate school placement to maximize a favorable response and should also be used in conjunction with standard behavioral techniques. Most authors recommend using stimulant medications on school days only unless the behavior is disruptive enough to interfere with family functions. Many side effects of stimulant medications are transient, including appetite suppression and insomnia. There is potential for reduced growth if used over long periods of time. For this reason drug holidays over summer vacation and weekends are recommended. Rarely stimulant medication can precipitate tics as seen in Tourette syndrome.

The prognosis for hyperactivity is relatively good in that the hyperkinesis usually abates with age. Associated problems with impulsiveness and inattentiveness, however, may continue to adulthood. If ADD is associated with learning disabilities, however, the prognosis may be worse for future job satisfaction and educational achievement. At present there are no objective data to show that there are any dietary influences on hyperactivity or that specific diets or vitamins improve ADD.

CHILDHOOD DEPRESSION

A change in school performance and a change in personality are the two important characteristics of childhood depression. These are also important symptoms in degenerative disease of the nervous system. Depression occurs in

Table 17-4. Diagnostic Criteria for Major Depressive Episode

A. Dysphoric mood or loss of interest or pleasure in all or almost all usual activities and pastimes. The dysphoric mood is characterized by symptoms such as the following: depressed, sad, blue, hopeless, low, down in the dumps, irritable. The mood disturbance must be prominent and relatively persistent, but not necessarily the most dominant symptom. It does not include momentary shifts from one dysphoric turmoil. (For children under six, dysphoric mood may have to be inferred from a persistently sad facial expression.)

B. At least four of the following symptoms have each been present nearly every day for a period of at least two weeks (in children under six, at least three of the first four).
  1. Poor appetite or significant weight loss (when not dieting) or increased appetite or significant weight gain (in children under six consider failure to make expected weight gains).
  2. Insomnia or hypersomnia.
  3. Psychomotor agitation or retardation (but not merely subjective feelings of restlessness or being slowed down) (in children under six, hypoactivity).
  4. Loss of interest or pleasure in usual activities, or decrease in sexual drive not limited to a period when delusional or hallucinating (in children under six, signs of apathy).
  5. Loss of energy; fatigue.
  6. Feelings of worthlessness, self-reproach, or excessive or inappropriate guilt (either may be delusional).
  7. Complaints or evidence of diminished ability to think or concentrate, such as slowed thinking or indecisiveness not associated with marked loosening of associations or incoherence.
  8. Recurrent thoughts of death, suicidal ideation, wishes to be dead, or suicide attempts.

C. Neither of the following dominate the clinical picture when the affective syndrome (i.e., criteria A and B above) is not present, that is, before it developed or after it has remitted:
  1. Preoccupation with a mood-incongruent delusion or hallucination (see definition below).
  2. Bizarre behavior.

D. Not superimposed on either schizophrenia, schizophreniform disorder, or a paranoid disorder.

E. Not due to any organic mental disorder or complicated bereavement.

(From Diagnostic and Statistical Manual of Mental Disorders, Third Edition. Washington, DC, American Psychiatric Association, copyright 1980. Used with permission.)

approximately 1 to 2 in every 1,000 children, whereas transient episodes of sadness are much more common. Depression frequently accompanies a loss of self-esteem due to a variety of primary developmental disorders, such as learning disabilities, or it may be a reaction to a personal loss, such as death in a family. Endogenous depression is relatively rare in children.

The diagnosis of childhood depression primarily rests on alteration in affect and mood. Table 17-4 lists one criteria for the diagnosis of depression. Many of these criteria are similar to those found in adults. Although depressed children frequently become quite and withdrawn, occasionally they may be angry or hostile or become aggressive and antisocial. The major differences between depression and organic causes for a personality change and decline in school performance are the vegetative signs. These include changes in appetite, sleep disturbances, fatigue, as well as the loss of self-esteem and pathologic guilt. The neurologic examination is normal in childhood depression; however, the mental status examination may suggest sadness, guilt, or thought of suicide.

The diagnosis of depression includes the exclusion of organic diseases such as substance abuse, intoxications, hypothyroidism, anemia, chronic infections, degenerative neurologic disorders, and other illnesses. Psychiatric evaluation is usually indicated for severe depression. Recently the dexamethasone suppression test has been shown to be abnormal in a high percentage of children with depression. A 0.5-mg dose of dexamethasone is given at 11 p.m. and serial cortisol determinations are made the following day. Cortisol levels of 5.0 mg/dl or greater indicate nonsuppression and are abnormal.

Treatment of childhood depression is a combination of psychotherapy and antidepressive medication. Presently the antidepressant amitriptyline is the most frequently used. The dose is approximately 1 to 5 mg/kg/day in divided dosages.

PERVASIVE DEVELOPMENTAL DISORDERS

Pervasive developmental disorders are severe distortions in multiple areas of psychological development. Autism and what was previously called childhood schizophrenia are the primary disorders. The major symptoms are a lack of development of social and language skills caused by disturbances in reality testing, attention, perception, and rational thinking. Autistic children usually present with severe developmental and behavioral problems, whereas children with other pervasive developmental disorders may present with deterioration of school performance and obvious personality changes. Organic brain disease is often a consideration in both.

Autism is characterized by a disturbance in social interaction, language, and behavior with an onset before 3 years. The incidence is about 50 in 100,000 and there is a 4:1 male predominance. The majority of children are retarded and a sizable majority have seizures by the time they reach adolescence. Autism is probably not a single entity but caused by many factors. Organic brain disease and autism may coexist and be caused by similar injuries. Children with infantile autism are frequently referred for neurologic evaluation because of a failure to progress developmentally. Children may have an initial period of relatively normal development, but language development always fails to progress and there is a minimum of language usage. Children who have autism without retardation still have a severe impairment of language function. About 50 percent never achieve language function and the prognosis is especially bad if the child has none by the age of 5 years. Many of these patients have poor social development to the point that other persons are little more than inanimate objects. There may be stereotyped repetitive activities which are self-stimulatory in nature and so extensive as to interfere with normal activity. Poor eye contact and superficial relationships, if any, are common. The clinical features of infantile autism are listed in Table 17-5.

Other pervasive developmental disorders are characterized by severe disturbances in social relationships, excessive anxieties, inappropriate affect, resistance to change, and other disturbances (Table 17-6). The course is chronic and the prognosis is poor for independent functioning, though better than for autism. The treatment is similar.

Schizophrenia in older children and adolescents closely resembles that of adults. The disease is rare in preschoolers. Unlike autism, there is frequently a positive family history. The major features are disorders of thinking such as delusions and hallucinations, and a deterioration of function, which in children is often related to school performance. The key to diagnosis is the nature of the

Table 17-5. Diagnostic Criteria for Infantile Autism

A. Onset before 30 months of age.

B. Pervasive lack of responsiveness to other people (autism).

C. Gross deficits in language development.

D. If speech is present, peculiar speech patterns such as immediate and delayed echolalia, meta-phorical language, pronominal reversal.

E. Bizarre responses to various aspects of the environment, e.g., resistance to change, peculiar interest in or attachments to animate or inanimate objects.

F. Absence of delusions, hallucinations, loosening of associations, and incoherence as in schizophrenia.

(From Diagnostic and Statistical Manual of Mental Disorders, Third Edition. Washington, DC, American Psychiatric Association, copyright, 1980. Used with permission.)

delusions. The beliefs have no basis on facts or logic and are forcibly asserted. One must exclude the present or prior abuse of hallucinogenic drugs in making the diagnosis. The neurologic examination is normal and the diagnosis is usually apparent. The treatment is primarily with psychotrophic medication and psychotherapy. The prognosis is relatively good for late onset disease of short duration. The treatment of autism is unsettled. A variety of pharmacologic and behavioral therapies can be employed. The prognosis is relatively poor for achieving normal development.

CONDUCT DISORDERS

Conduct disorders are a pattern of behavior which are basically antisocial in nature. *Deliquency* is a legal term applied to children with conduct disorders and legal complications. Approximately one-third have associated learning disabilities as well as perceptual handicaps and other impairments. Conduct disorders tend to be chronic and are the best predictor of adult social behavior.

Table 17-6. Diagnostic Criteria for Pervasive Developmental Disorder

A. Gross and sustained impairment in social relationships, e.g., lack of appropriate affective responsivity, inappropriate clinging, asociality, lack of empathy.

B. At least three of the following:

1. Sudden excessive anxiety manifested by such symptoms as free-floating anxiety, catastrophic reactions to everyday occurrences, inability to be consoled when upset, unexplained panic attacks

2. Constricted or inappropriate affect, including lack of appropriate fear reactions, unexplained rage reactions, and extreme mood lability

3. Resistance to change in the environment (e.g., upset if dinner time is changed), or insistence on doing things in the same manner every time (e.g., putting on clothes always in the same order)

4. Oddities of motor movement, such as peculiar posturing, peculiar hand or finger movements, or walking on tiptoe

5. Abnormalities of speech, such as questionlike melody, monotonous voice

6. Hyper- or hypo-sensitivity to sensory stimuli, e.g., hyperacusis

7. Self-mutilation, e.g., biting or hitting self, head banging

C. Onset of the full syndrome after 30 months of age and before 12 years of age.

D. Absence of delusions, hallucinations, incoherence, or marked loosening of associations.

(From Diagnostic and Statistical Manual of Mental Disorders, Third Edition. Washington, DC, American Psychiatric Association, copyright 1980. Used with permission.)

Table 17-7. Causes for Aggressive and Violent Behavior

Medical	Systemic illness
	Hyperthyroidism
	Sydenham chorea
Neurologic	Temporal lobe epilepsy (postictal state: interictal behavior)
	Limbic encephalitis (particularly from herpes simplex)
	Hypothalamic disorder
	Migraine
Toxic	Barbiturates, including primidone (Mysoline)
	Diazepam (Valium)
	Alcohol
	Hallucinogens
	Cocaine
	Amphetamines
Psychologic	Depression
	Anxiety
	Anger
	Psychosis
Social–environmental	Lack of limit-setting
	Implicit sanction
	Culturally acceptable
	(?) Television
Genetic–constitutional	XY (normal male) karyotype
	XYY syndrome
Developmental	Sibling rivalry

(From Herskowitz J, Rossman NP: Pediatric, Neurology, and Psychiatry—Common Ground. © 1982 by Macmillan Publishing Co., New York.)

Conduct disorders are a product of both the degree of socialization and aggressiveness. The unsocialized aggressive child has the most difficulties, in that the disruptive behavior occurs in isolation. Children with social tendencies usually exhibit antisocial behavior in groups or gangs.

Neurologic assessment is occasionally requested for conduct disorders. In most instances, the purpose is to exclude the diagnosis of epilepsy. This is especially true when bouts of aggressive violence occur. In fact, it is rare for a patient who has seizures to become violent. If this does occur, the violence is usually nondirected and victims are more likely to be innocent bystanders trying to restrain the patient than a specific object of the violence. Occasionally EEG abnormalities are noted in such patients, which include slowing or spike discharges from a temporal lobe. These patients may also have seizures. Episodes of deliberate violence are rarely, if ever, associated with an ictal discharge. Treating the seizures in such patients does not necessarily improve the antisocial behavior. However, carbamazepine is often used for the treatment of episodic behavioral disturbances. Table 17-7 lists causes for aggressive and violent behavior.

CONVERSION SYMPTOMS

Conversion reactions are frequently misdiagnosed as neurologic disorders. Conversion is relatively common in older children and adolescence, but is rare in preschool children. Prior to puberty both sexes are affected equally but after

Table 17-8. Approximate Incidence of Conversion Reaction in Children

Conversion Symptom	Approximate Incidence (%)
Episodic disturbances	
Pseudoseizures	20
Syncope	10
Other	3
Motor	
Paralysis	10
Gait disturbance	7
Dystonia or posturing	2
Other	2
Sensory	
Abdominal pain	13
Headache	6
Other pain	7
Visual impairment	6
Speech and hearing	5
Other	9

(Material obtained from review of 225 children reported in the literature.)

puberty there is a 2:1 female-to-male ratio. The most common conversion symptoms are shown in Table 17-8. The child with the conversion reaction frequently has a role model such as another family member with a similar illness or is reliving a past experience in which significant secondary gain was achieved. The symptoms in the child are usually monosymptomatic and uncomplicated. Malingering can also be confused with a conversion reaction, in that a child produces symptoms to specifically avoid certain situations. It can be a sign of separation anxiety. A careful neurologic evaluation usually differentiates the conversion reaction from an organic illness. This becomes difficult, however, in patients with episodic disturbances such as pseudoseizures. In such cases the neurologic exam can be normal without any signs of physical impairment.

A conversion reaction in the simplest form is a monophasic illness and frequently susceptible to suggestive therapy by the physician. It should be remembered, however, that many diagnosed conversion reactions eventually are determined to have an organic basis. For this reason such symptoms should be taken seriously. An appropriate examination and if necessary specific tests should be performed to eliminate the possibility of an organic disease as well as to reassure the child of no significant illness. Most important in the treatment is the elimination of secondary gain.

A recently described syndrome, Munchausen's by proxy, is a disorder of the parent. In this syndrome, the parent reports a variety of complaints ascribed to the child. In fact, the child has no organic disease. Problems such as seizurelike activity, apnea, and hematemesis may be reported by the parent. The signs are produced by putting blood in the child's mouth, strangling the child, or other maneuvers. This syndrome is a subtle variety of child abuse. The parent usually actively seeks medical services and goes from hospital to hospital with the undiagnosable condition.

DISORDERS OF ELIMINATION

Elimination disorders cause considerable concern for parents and physicians, particularly encopresis. Approximately 15 percent of 5-year-olds have functional nocturnal enuresis, which diminishes to 2 percent in adolescents. About 1.5 percent of children more than 4 years old have encopresis. Neurologic causes for this disorder are rare but should be sought in each case to exclude organic, treatable diseases.

The most common neurologic cause of nocturnal enuresis is seizures and usually there is an obvious history of seizures. A common neurologic cause for daytime bowel and bladder incontinence is spinal cord disease. Signs of congenital cord lesions include discrepancy in leg growth, sacral dimple, skin marks or hair patches, and focal neurologic deficits in the legs. Almost all patients will have spina bifida occulta on plain radiographs of the spine. Acquired disorders often have symptoms of back pain and a gait disturbance as well as neurologic signs. Scoliosis or leg deformities are other important clues to spinal cord disease. Myelography is the definitive test for cord diseases (see Ch. 13).

Occasionally incontinence is associated with diffuse disease as seen in degenerative disorders, progressive hydrocephalus, and others. Personality changes, a deterioration in school performance, and diffuse neurologic signs are present and usually obvious in these patients. Hirschsprung's disease must also be considered in children with bowel incontinence.

SELECTED READINGS

Hansen CR, Jr., Cohen DJ: Multimodality approaches in the treatment of attention deficit disorders. Pediatr Clin North Am 31:499–513, 1984

Herskowitz J, Rosman NP: Pediatrics, Neurology, and Psychiatry—Common Ground. Macmillan, New York, 1982

Howell DC, Huessy HR, Hassuk B: Fifteen year follow up of a behavior history of attention deficit disorder. Pediatrics 76:185–190, 1985

Lumbroso CT, Lerman P: Breathholding spells (cyanotic and pallid infantile syncope). Pediatrics 39:563–581, 1967

McClelland CQ, Stapler WI, Weisenberg I, Bergen MF: The practitioner's role in behavioral pediatrics. J Pediatr 82:325, 1973

Ottenbacher KJ, Cooper MM: Drug treatment of hyperactivity in children. Dev Med Child Neurol 25:358–366, 1983

Schneider SS, Rice DR: Neurologic manifestations of childhood hysteria. Pediatrics 94:153–156, 1979

Shaywitz SE, Shaywitz BA: Diagnosis and management of attention deficit disorder: a pediatric perspective. Pediatr Clin North Am 31:429–458, 1984

Shaywitz SE, Hunt RD, Hatlow P et al: Psychopharmacology of attention deficit disorder. Pharmacokinetic, neuroendocrine, and behavioral measures following acute and chronic treatment with methylphenidate. Pediatrics 69:688–694, 1982

Starfield B: Behavioral pediatrics and primary health care. Pediatr Clin North Am 29:377–390, 1982

SECTION 5

Neurodegenerative and Metabolic Diseases

Progressive loss of neurologic function, episodic neurologic dysfunction, and neonatal encephalopathy characterize this diverse group of disorders. There are over 600 known degenerative diseases of both genetic and nongenetic origins. They account for a large percentage of hospitalized pediatric patients. An accurate diagnosis is important for the treatment of some disorders, genetic counseling for most, and exclusion for the treatable acquired disease of the nervous system. Most standard textbooks on pediatric neurology cover these diseases in detail.

18

OVERVIEW OF METABOLIC AND DEGENERATIVE DISEASES

Metabolic and degenerative diseases differ only insofar as our knowledge concerning the etiology: *degenerative* usually implies a lack of understanding, whereas *metabolic* refers to inborn errors of metabolism in which an enzyme defect has been determined. Classification of these disorders thus becomes confusing and changes as our knowledge expands. All such disorders are probably due to altered enzymatic function with excessive production, abnormal synthesis, or abnormal catabolism of metabolic substrates, proteins, or other cellular constituents.

As a group, the clinical course is one of progression of signs and symptoms which may lead to either death or a limited level of functioning. Alternatively, many disorders are characterized by intermittent symptoms and signs which may be superimposed upon a progressive course. The effects of the disease may be pervasive, affecting all parts of the nervous system (Tay-Sachs disease), or restricted to a particular system (familial spastic paraparesis). Furthermore, a disease may be restricted to the nervous system or involve multiple organ systems.

DIAGNOSIS

The first step in approaching these disorders is the recognition of the clinical signs suggestive of a progressive disease and the exclusion of acquired treatable conditions. This is accomplished by using the usual triad of history, physical, and neurologic examination plus selective laboratory tests. As in most childhood diseases, the history is the most important diagnostic examination (Table 18-1). The history of the present illness should document progression of symptoms, developmental arrest, or loss of previously acquired milestones. Often a change in personality, behavior, or school performance is the presenting symptom. The past medical history is important to exclude acquired illnesses of the nervous system such as chronic intoxications or infections, psychiatric illnesses, and static encephalopathies such as cerebral palsy. The family history is most important to determine inherited disease (Table 1-5). A pedigree should be diagrammed for every child suspected of having a degenerative disease to determine a mode of inheritance.

The general physical examination may reveal signs of a metabolic or de-

Table 18-1. Historical Features of Metabolic and Degenerative Diseases

Symptoms
  Change in personality or behavior
  Deterioration of school performance
  Progressive visual or hearing disturbance
  Progressive ataxia, spasticity, or movement disorder
  Uncontrolled seizures
  Idiopathic mental retardation
Clinical course
  Progressive neurologic degeneration
  Failure of development
  Developmental regression
  Recurrent neurologic dysfunction
Family history
  Similar neurologic illness in a sibling or relative
  Sibling or relative with mental retardation, cerebral palsy, or poorly controlled seizures
  Consanguinity

generative disease (see Table 3-7). Attention to dysmorphism, organomegaly, and dermatologic, hair, and ocular abnormalities (see Table 3-5) will often lead to a specific diagnosis. The neurologic exam must be complete as outlined in Chapter 4. Most degenerative and metabolic diseases involve the CNS at multiple levels and diffusely. Neurologic signs that can be explained by single lesions usually imply an acquired disease. Chronic intoxications and infections cause diffuse neurologic dysfunction and may mimic a degenerative disease. The combination of CNS, systemic, or ocular abnormalities and peripheral nervous system signs is particularly suggestive of progressive disease.

Selective screening laboratory tests that are available on a routine basis can be helpful. Blood chemistries and enzymes can often give clues to the underlying disorder (Table 18-2). Of specific usefulness are findings suggestive of a metabolic acidosis, an increased anion gap, hypoglycemia, and elevated liver enzymes. The complete blood count, especially examination of the peripheral spear, often shows characteristic signs of metabolic diseases. The urinalysis can easily evaluate for melaturia and screened for amino acids using a ferric chloride tests. Selective plain radiographs may be diagnostic. More specific tests, which may not be readily available, such as lysosomal enzyme analysis, are often necessary for the diagnosis.

CLASSIFICATION

Attempts to classify disorders are fraught with difficulty. Many classifications are based upon neuropathology, known pathogenesis, or clinical features. One classification is presented in Table 18-3. "Metabolic encephalopathies" encompasses a group of disorders with defects in the major areas of intermediary metabolism. These frequently present as an acute, intermittent, or chronic en-

Table 18-2. Routine Laboratory Abnormalities Associated with Metabolic Diseases

Acidosis, increased anion gap
- Organic acidemias
- Maple syrup urine disease
- Hereditary tyrosinemia
- Hereditary fructose intolerance
- Fructosuria
- Galactosemia

Lacticacidosis
- Pyruvate dehydrogenase deficiency
- Pyruvate carboxylase deficiency
- Organic acidurias
- Multiple carboxylase deficiency
- Mitochondrial encephalomyopathies
- Glycogen storage disease type I
- Leigh's syndrome

Renal tubular acidosis
- Fanconi's syndrome
- Hereditary tyrosinemia
- Galactosemia
- Hereditary fructose intolerance
- Lowe's syndrome
- Wilson's disease
- Primary renal tubular acidosis

Hypoglycemia
- Fructosuria
- Hereditary fructose intolerance
- Galactosemia
- Glucose-6-phosphatase deficiency
- Maple syrup urine disease
- Hereditary tyrosinemia
- Organic acidemias

Hyperammonemia
- Urea cycle disorders
- Organic acidemias

Mellituria
- Hereditary fructose intolerance
- Fructosuria
- Galactosemia
- Fanconi's syndrome

Low blood urea nitrogen
- Urea cycle disorders
- Hyperuricemia
- Lesch-Nyhan disease
- Hereditary fructose intolerance
- Glycogen storage disease type I

Hyperbilirubinemia
- Galactosemia
- Hereditary tyrosinemia
- Hereditary fructose intolerance

Elevated serum glutamic-oxaloacetic transaminase, serum glutamic-pyruvic transaminase
- Hereditary tyrosinemia
- Wilson's disease
- Galactosemia
- Hereditary fructose intolerance

Uremia
- Fabry's disease
- Mucolipidosis
- Lesch-Nyhan disease
- Anemia, thrombocytopenia
- Organic acidurias

Table 18-3. Classification and Clinical Features of Metabolic and
Degenerative Disease of the Nervous System

Metabolic encephalopathies	Fulminant neonatal metabolic encephalopathy Intermittent metabolic encephalopathy Progressive metabolic encephalopathy
Storage disorders	Visceromegaly Dysmorphic features Progressive encephalopathy
Leukodystrophies	Progressive motor disturbances Progressive special sensory deficits
Poliodystrophies	Dementia Seizures
Systems degeneration	Progressive ataxia Movement disorders Progressive weakness

cephalopathy with alterations in consciousness and other neurologic signs. Abnormal accumulation of metabolites can be measured in the blood or urine and often specific therapies, especially dietary, are available to treat or ameliorate these diseases.

Storage disorders are a heterogeneous group of inborn errors of metabolism that are characterized by abnormal accumulation of substances in neural and other tissues. Almost all of these are secondary to impaired catabolism of complex molecules. Storage material can often be visualized in a variety of tissues, such as leukocytes, skin, cutaneous nerves, liver and, of course, brain. The progression is usually slow and often organomegaly and dysmorphic features are present on physical examination.

The leukodystrophies primarily involve the white matter of the CNS. Spasticity, optic atrophy, and ataxia are prominent signs. The poliodystrophies are diseases of gray matter in which seizures and dementia are the major features. There is often considerable overlap, however, in the clinical signs between these two groups of disorders. Systems degeneration is restricted to predominantly one system of the CNS, at least initially. The spinocerebellar ataxias are an example. Unlike most of the other disorders discussed in this section, many are dominantly inherited and have unknown etiologies.

The neurocutaneous diseases are not progressive in the sense of causing diffuse degeneration of the nervous system. They are genetic diseases, usually associated with neurologic features, which may result in clinical deterioration.

The subsequent chapters will outline the clinical features, diagnosis, and therapy, when available, of these disorders. Degenerative diseases are fortunately rare. Their importance is more related to the degree of understanding of the nervous system we can acquire from their study. Although most of the degenerative diseases cannot be treated, when they are properly diagnosed, invaluable genetic counseling can be made available.

SELECTED READINGS

Brady RO, Rosenberg RN: Autosomal dominant neurologic disorders. Ann Neurol 4:548–552, 1978

Dyken P, Krawiecki N: Neurodegenerative diseases of infancy and childhood. Ann Neurol 13:351–364, 1985

Kolodny EH, Cable WJL: Inborn errors of metabolism. Ann Neurol 11:221–232, 1982

Rosenberg RN: Biochemical genetics of neurological disease. N Engl J Med 305:1181–1193, 1981

19

METABOLIC ENCEPHALOPATHIES

Metabolic encephalopathies are disturbances of CNS function caused by inborn errors of intermediary metabolism. These typically present as either acute fulminant neonatal encephalopathy with vomiting, seizures, hypotonia, and coma, or as intermittent encephalopathy with additional signs such as ataxia. Some disorders present with chronic neurologic impairment and retardation. In comm are measurable accumulations in the blood or urine of intermediary metabolites due to deficient enzyme catabolism. Secondary metabolic disturbances such as acidosis, hypoglycemia, ketosis, and hyperammonemia are common and may be the principle pathogenic mechanism of the encephalopathy.

Table 19-1 outlines the major classes of metabolic encephalopathies. These disorders are quite rare (Table 19-2). One should suspect a metabolic encephalopathy if an acquired disease has been excluded (especially intoxication), if there is a family history of a similar illnesses, or if the symptoms and signs are recurrent. Often the physical findings are nonspecific and the diagnosis must be made from laboratory tests. One physical finding that is somewhat unique for the metabolic encephalopathies is an unusal odor (Table 19-3).

AMINO ACID DISORDERS

Table 19-4 outlines the major disorders of amino acid metabolism. These include those which are due to impaired catabolism of amino acid and those that are due to abnormal membrane transport amino acids. Those defects which are thought to be benign or do not affect the nervous system have been omitted from Table 19-4. Symptoms usually occur following protein ingestion with subsequent toxic accumulation of amino acids or their intermediates. For this reason, the patients may appear normal when fasted. The pathophysiology is quite variable. Phenylketonuria (PKU) affects the developing brain to a much greater extent than the mature brain, particularly myelin formation. For this reason the disease becomes static after the first 6 years or so, although learning and behavior may be improved through continued dietary control. The fetus can be damaged because of high phenylalanine levels in the asymptomatic mother who has PKU. The metabolism of phenylalanine and that of tyrosine are closely related (Fig. 19-1). Homocystine is an important constituent of connective tissue and homocystinuria is associated with a number of connective tissue abnormalities. Most of the other disorders amino acid cause encephalopathy by overwhelming acidosis. Maple syrup urine disease (MSUD), caused by incomplete catabolism of

Table 19-1. Metabolic Encephalopathies from Inborn Errors of
Metabolism

Amino acid disorders
Organic acidurias
Disorders of carbohydrate metabolism
Urea cycles disorders
Purine and pyrimidine disorders
Porphyrias

branched-chain amino acids, is an example. The metabolism of branched-chain amino acids is also involved in the organic acidemias (see below and Fig. 19-2).

A presumptive diagnosis can be made from a variety of screening tests. Every state has a PKU screening program for neonates and many states screen for other diseases. The Guthrie test is the most widely used screening test. This is a bacterial inhibition test using bacteria sensitive to phenylalanine concentrations. Several days of protein intake may be necessary for the test to become positive. Other screening tests are listed in Table 19-5. These are far less sensitive and concentrations of amino acids must be relatively high for them to be positive. The most accurate method for diagnosis is amino acid chromotography and specific enzyme assay. Treatment is usually dietary restriction of the amino acid. Therapy

Table 19-2. Incidence of the Most Common Inborn Errors of
Intermediary Metabolism

Congenital hypothyroidism	1:4,000
Hyperphenylalaninemia	1:9,400
Phenylketonuria	1:16,000
Hereditary fructose intolerance	1:30,000
Argininosuccinicaciduria	1:70,000
Tetrahydrobiopterin deficiency (phenylketonuria variant)	1:80,000
Galactosemia	1:100,000
Hereditary tyrosinosis	1:100,000
Glycine encephalopathy	1:170,000
Maple syrup urine disease (neonatal)	1:186,000
Von Gierke's disease	1:200,000
Propionicacidemia	1:300,000
Methylmalonicacidemia	1:300,000

(Modified from Fenichel GM: Neonatal Neurology. 2nd Ed. Churchill Livingstone, New York.)

Table 19-3. Characteristic Odors of Metabolic Disease

Musty, mousy	Phenylketonuria
Rotten cabbage	Tyrosinemia
Maple syrup	Branched-chain ketoacids
Yeast	Oasthouse disease
Ketonic	Ketotic hyperglycinemias
Sweaty socks	Isovalericacidemia
	Glutaricacidemia
Tom cat	Multiple carboxylase deficiency

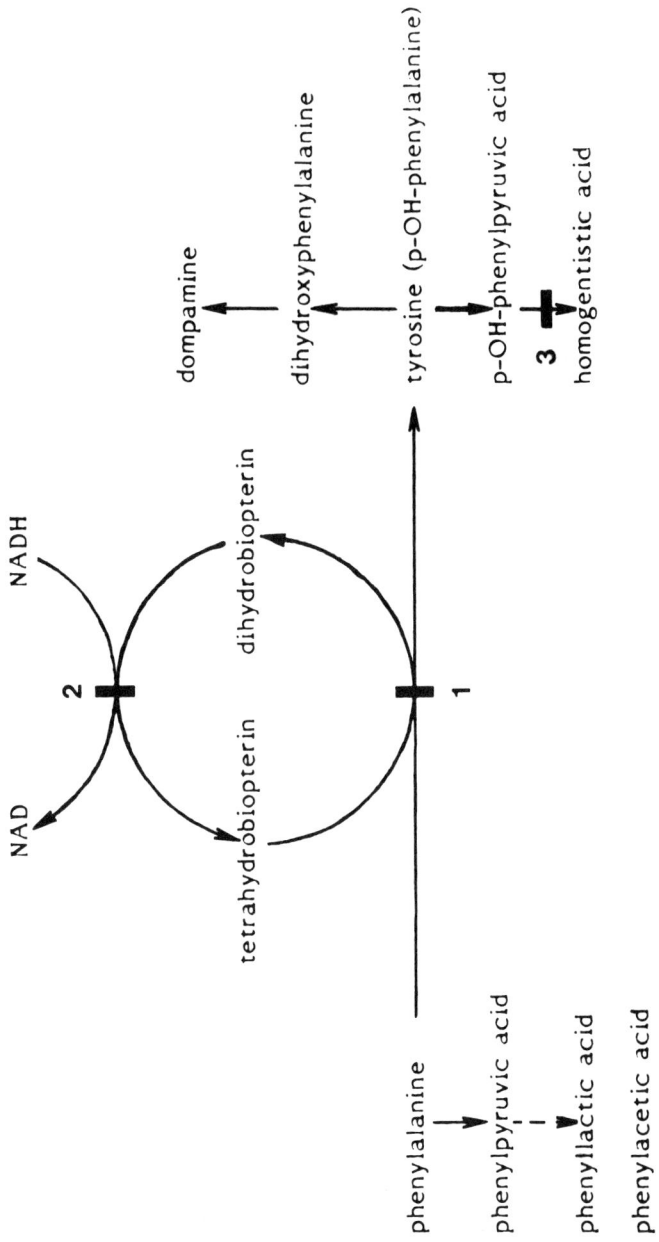

Fig. 19-1. Phenylalanine and tyrosine metabolism: (1) phenylalanine hydroxylase, classic PKU and atypical PKU, (2) dihydrobiopterin reductase, atypical PKU, (3) p-hydroxyphenylpyruvic acid oxidase, hereditary tyrosinemia and transitory neonatal hypertyrosinemia, and hyperphenylalaninemia.

Table 19-4. Disorders of Amino Acid metabolism and Transport[a]

Disorder (Enzyme)	Major Neurologic Features	Other Clinical Features	Metabolic Accumulations	Treatment
Classic PKU[b] Phenylalanine hydroxylase absent	Progressive MR[c]	Pale complexion Infantile spasms Seizures "Mousy" odor Tremor	Phenylalanine Phenyllactate Phenylpyruvate Phenylacetate	Dietary restriction (Lofenalac) to maintain blood phenyl-alanine to 3–8 mg/dl
Atypical PKU Phenylalanine hydroxylase reduced	MR		Phenylalanine Phenyllactate Phenylpyruvate Phenylacetate	Dietary restriction (Lofenalac) to maintain blood phenyl-alanine to 3–8 mg/dl
PKU variant Diphenylhydropterine reductase	MR	Bulbar Weakness Myoclonic seizures Hypotonia	Phenylalanine Phenyllactate Phenylpyruvate Phenylacetate	Dietary restriction (Lofenalac) to maintain blood phenyl-alanine to 3–8 mg/dl
Hereditary tyrosinemia para-Hydroxyphenylpyruvic acid oxidase	Hepatic encephalopathy	Hepatosplenomegaly "Rotten cabbage" odor Acidosis Rickets Progressive liver disease	Tyrosine Methionine Others	Dietary restriction of phenyl-alanine and tyrosine
Hypertyrosinemia Cytosol tyrosine transaminase	MR	Hyperkeratosis of palms and soles	Tyrosine Methionine Others	Dietary restriction of phenylalanine and tyrosine
Classic maple syrup urine (branched-chain ketoacid decarboxylase)	Fulminant neonatal encephalopathy	Maple syrup odor, severe acidosis	Leucine Isoleucine Valine Ketoacids	Dietary restriction

198

Disorder (enzyme)		Clinical features	Biochemical findings	Treatment
Maple syrup urine Intermittent disease (same, less severe)	MR	Intermittent ataxia Encephalopathy Odor	Leucine Isoleucine Valine Ketoacids	Dietary restriction
Multiple decarboxylase deficiency (thiamine-dependent decarboxylase)	Ataxia	Intermittent ataxia	Lactate Pyruvate	Thiamine, 1,000 mg/day
Nonketotic hyperglycinemia (serine hydroxymethyl-transferase)	Neonatal encephalopathy	Failure to thrive	Glycine	?
Beta-alaninemia (? beta-alanine transaminase)	Intractable seizures	Hypotonia	Beta-alanine Gamma-aminobutyric acid	Protein, pyrimidine restriction
Homocystinuria Cystathionine synthase	Recurrent strokes Mild MR	Marfanoid habitus Fair complexion Malar flush Livedo reticularis Ectopic lens Glaucoma Myopia	Homocystine	Restricted methionine diet Pyridoxine 100 mg/day
Sulfite oxidase deficiency	Severe MR	Ectopic lens	s-Sulfo-1-cysteine sulfite	?
Hartnup disease (neutral amino acids transport)	Episodic ataxia and psychiatric symptoms	Pellagralike rash	Neutral amino acid in urine	Protein supplement ? Nicotinamide, 10 mg/day
Oasthouse disease (methionine absorption)	MR	Seizures White hair "Yeast" odor	Methionine Others	Dietary restriction

[a] Benign disorders and those that do not cause neurologic complications have been omitted.
[b] PKU = phenylketonuria.
[c] MR = mental retardation.

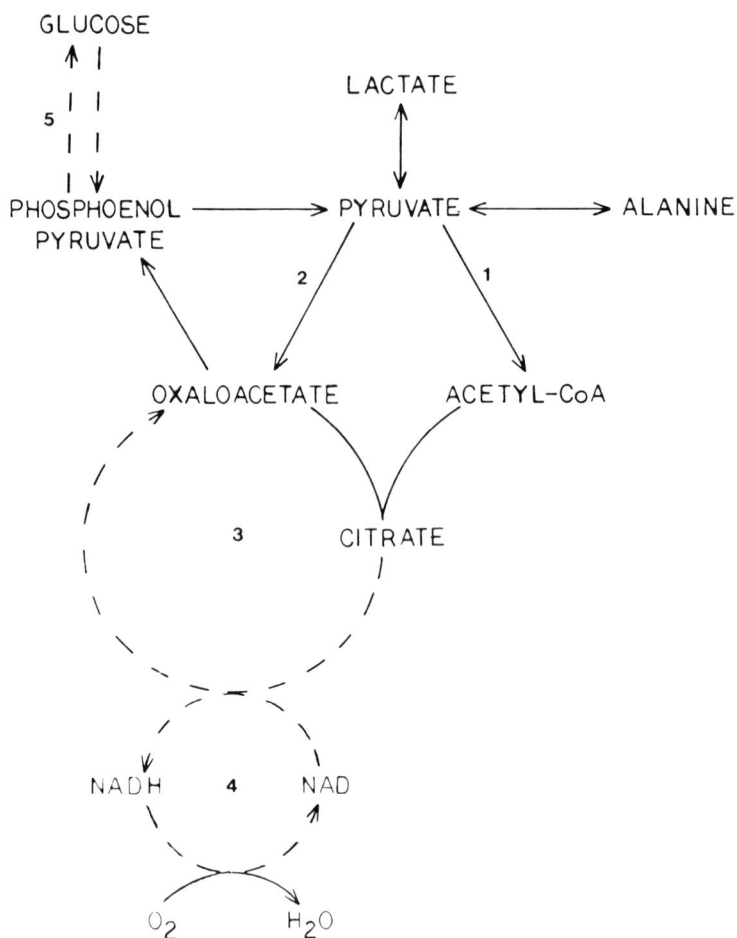

Fig. 19-2. Metabolic diseases associated with lacticacidosis: (*1*) pyruvate dehydrogenase deficiency, (*2*) pyruvate carboxylase deficiency, (*3*) tricarboxylic acid, (*4*) electron transfer system, mitochondrial encephalomyopathies, (*5*) disorders of gluconeogenesis.

should be conducted at centers experienced in metabolic diseases. Genetic counseling should be made available for families.

ORGANIC ACIDURIAS

The organic acidemias are summarized in Table 19-6. Organic acids are nonaminated intermediaries of metabolism derived principally from amino acids and pyruvate. Symptoms vary considerably, depending upon the degree of severity. The more severe the defect, the earlier the onset and more lethal the disease. Lesser degrees of deficiency cause chronic, progressive disease, often

Table 19-5. Screening Tests for Metabolic Diseases

Condition	Ferric Chloride	DNPH	Benedict's Test	Nitroprusside	Acid Albumin
Phenylketonuria	Green	+	–	–	–
Maple syrup urine disease	Occasionally navy blue	+	–	–	–
Tyrosinosis	Pale green (transient)	+	±	–	–
Histidinemia	Green brown (permanent)	±	–	–	–
Propionicacidemia	Purple	+	–	–	–
Methylmalonicaciduria	Purple	+	–	–	–
Homocystinuria	–	–	–	+	–
Glutathioninuria	–	–	–	+	–
Cystinuria	–	–	–	+	–
Mucopolysaccharidoses	–	–	–	–	+
Galactosemia	–	–	+	–	–
Fructose intolerance	–	–	+	–	–

(From Menkes JH: Textbook of Child Neurology, 3rd Ed. Lea & Febiger, Philadelphia, 1985.)

Table 19-6. Organic Acidemias

Disorder	Enzyme Deficiency	Metabolic Accumulation	Treatment
Ketotic hyperglycinemias			
α-Methyl-β hydroxybutyric acid	α-Methylacetoactyl CoA β-ketothiolase[a]	Organic acids Ammonia	Dietary protein restriction, 1.0–2.0 g/kg/day
Propionic acid	Propionyl CoA carboxylase	Glycine	Diet, biotin, 10 mg/kg/day
Methylmalonic acid	Methylmalonyl CoA mutase Methylmalonyl CoA racemase	Long-chain ketones	Diet, vitamin B_{12} 1–2 mg/day
Adenosylcobalamin synthesis		10 ng chain ketones homocystein	Diet, vitamin B_{12} 1–2 mg/d
Isovaleric acid	Isovaleryl CoA dehydrogenase		Diet
Lactic and pyruvic acidemias	Pyruvate dehydrogenase	Lactate, pyruvate alanine	Ketonic diet: thiamine, 300 mg/day; lipoic acid, 10 mg/day
	Pyruvate carboxylase	Lactate, pyruvate alanine	Ketonic diet: thiamine, 300 mg/day; lipoic acid, 10 mg/day; biotin, 10 mg/day
	Multiple carboxylase	Ketones, lactate pyruvate	Biotin, 10 mg/day
Glutaricacidemias			
Type I	Glutaryl CoA dehydrogenase	Glutaric acid, others	Dietary protein restriction
Type II	?	Glutaric acid, others	Dietary protein restriction

[a] CoA = coenzyme A.

Table 19-7. Drugs, Toxins, and Systemic Diseases Associated with Lacticacidosis

Enzymatic deficiencies
  Disorders of gluconeogenesis
    Glucose-6-phosphatase
    Fructose-1,6-diphosphatase
    Pyruvate carboxylase
    Phosphoenolpyruvate carboxykinase
  Disorders of pyruvate metabolism
    Pyruvate decarboxylase
    Lipoamide transacetylase
    Lipoamide dehydrogenase
    Pyruvate dehydrogenase phosphatase
  Other
    Multiple carboxylase
    Propionicacidemia
    Methylmalonicacidemia
    Carnitine deficiency
    Hereditary fructose intolerance
    Mitochondrial encephalomyopathies
Drug and toxins
  Biguanides: phenformin, metformin, buformin
  Antibiotics: outdated tetracycline, nalidixic acid, isoniazid
  Analgesics: salicylates, acetominophen
  Cardiovascular agents: papaverine, nitroprusside, epinephrine, paracetamol, terbutaline, salbutamol
  Tocolytics: ritodrine
  Intravenous solutions: fructose, glucose, sorbitol, xylitol
  Alcohols: ethanol, methanol, ethylene glycol, propylene glycol
  Solvents: butanone
  Other: aflatoxins, dinitrophenol, strychnine, hypoglycine, carbon monoxide, cyanide
Systemic diseases
  Hypoxia (any cause)
  Shock (any cause)
  Respiratory alkalosis (any cause)
  Liver failure (any cause)
  Renal failure (any cause)
  Diabetes mellitus
  Convulsions and other causes for excessive muscle contraction
  Neoplasms
  Reye's syndrome
  Thiamine deficiency
  Biotin deficiency

with intermittent features. Failure to thrive is a consistent feature. The two major classes are lacticacidosis and ketotic hyperglycemias.

Lacticacidosis may be associated with a number of metabolic errors, systemic diseases, and intoxication (Table 19-7). Leigh's disease is a classic pediatric neurologic disorder with perhaps many etiologies. In the typical case, growth failure and mild developmental delay begin in the first year. Ataxia, ophthalmoplegia, hypotonia, and hyporeflexia progress over the ensuing years, often associated with unusual respirations and extrapyramidal signs. There may be episodes of acute deterioration with infection or other stress. The pathology resembles that of Wernicke's encephalopathy with infarctlike lesions distributed in the midbrain and brain stem. Many children have a mild lacticacidosis which may be exacerbated by glucose challenge. Other causes of lacticacidosis include pyruvate

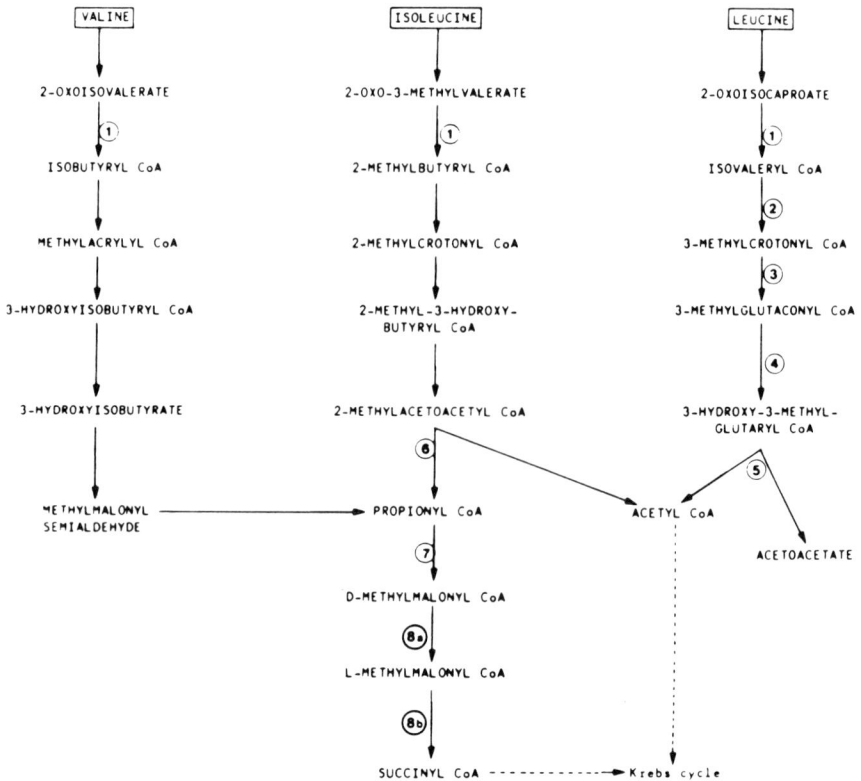

Fig. 19-3. The catabolic pathways of leucine, isoleucine, valine, and propionate: (*1*) maple syrup urine disease, (*2*) isovalericacidemia, (*3*) 3-methylcrotonylglycinuria, (*4*) 3-methylglutaconicaciduria, (*5*) 3-hydroxy-3-methylglutaryl coenzyme A lyase deficiency, (*6*) 2-oxothiolase deficiency, (*7*) propionicacidemia, (*8*) methylmalonicacidemia. (From Brett EM: Inherited disorders of the urea cycle. p. 91. In Brett EM (ed): Paediatric Neurology, Churchill Livingstone, Edinburgh, 1983.)

dehydrogenase deficiency, pyruvate carboxylase deficiency, and mitochondrial disorders. These diseases have a variable clinical course from fulminant neonatal encephalopathy to a more chronic/episodic course similar to Leigh's syndrome.

The ketotic hyperglycinemias are quite rare and are caused by defects in the branched-chain metabolite degradation pathways (Fig. 19-3). The clinical presentation is that of a fulminant neonatal encephalopathy with severe acidosis and often ketosis, hyperammonemia, and hypoglycemia. Survivors are mentally retarded and have recurrent bouts of acute encephalopathy with acidosis, hypotonia, seizures, vomiting, and stupor or coma. Glutaricacidemia type II presents similarly; type I is associated with a more chronic course of ataxia and retardation.

The diagnosis of an organic acidosis should be suspected in any child with acute neonatal metabolic acidosis and encephalopathy and in children with recurrent encephalopathy. Lactic acid can be measured in most clinical labs,

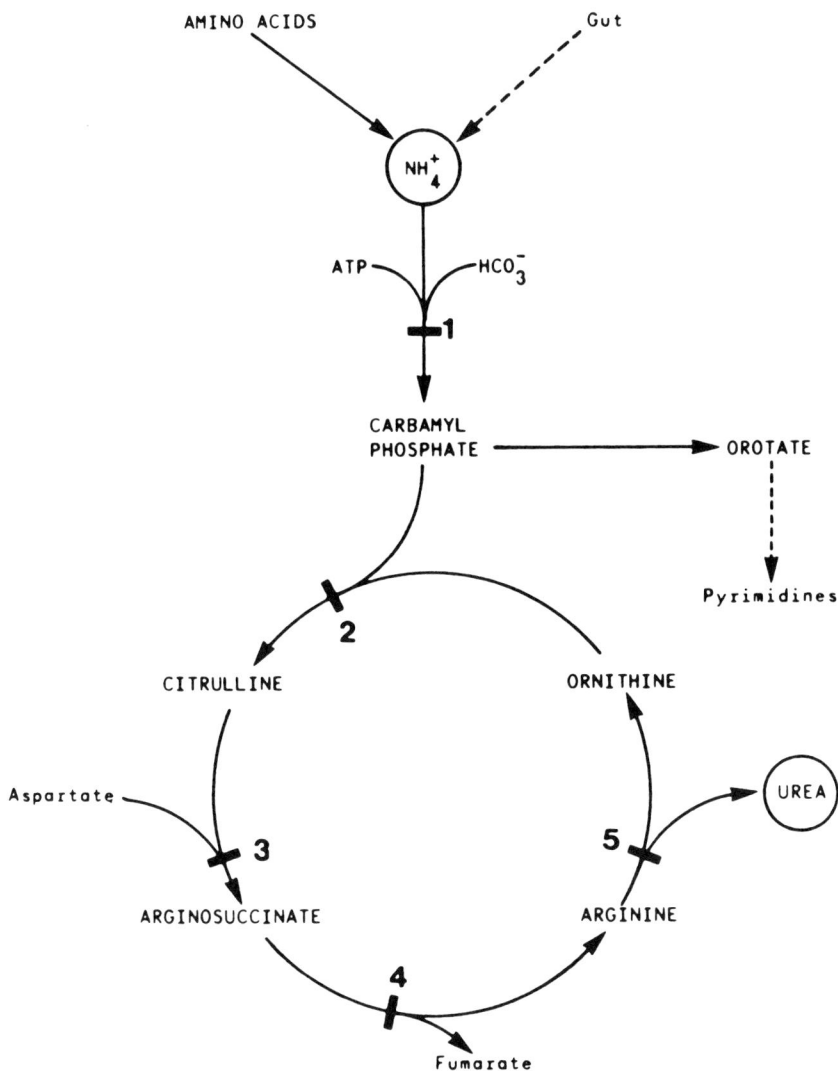

Fig. 19-4. Inherited disorders of the urea cycle: (*1*) carbamylphosphate synthetase deficiency, (*2*) ornithine carbamyltransferase deficiency, (*3*) citrullinemia, (*4*) arginosuccinicaciduria, (*5*) arginase deficiency. (From Brett EM: Inherited disorders of the urea cycle. p. 186. In Brett EM (ed): Paediatric Neurology, Churchill Livingstone, Edinburgh, 1983.)

whereas other organic acids usually require gas–liquid chromotography, which often is performed at a reference laboratory. The results may not be immediately available and, because the diagnosis may be delayed, therapy should be instituted when the diagnosis is suspected. Supportive therapy includes buffering acidosis, maintaining normal glucose concentrations if the patient is hypoglycemic, and restricting protein intake. Some of the disorders respond to vitamin therapy.

Table 19-8. Disorders of Carbohydrate Metabolism Associated with Encephalopathy

Carbohydrate	Enzyme Deficiency	Clinical Features	Treatment
Galactose	Galactose-1-phosphate uridyltransferase (classic galactosemia)	Neonatal encephalopathy Hypoglycemia, jaundice Cataracts, failure to thrive, *Escherichia coli* sepsis	Lactose-free diet
	Galactokinase	Cataracts	
Fructose	Fructose-1-phosphate aldolase (hereditary fructose intolerance)	Encephalopathy Hepatosplenomegaly Hypoglycemia, failure to thrive, seizures Fanconi's syndrome	Fructose- and sucrose-free diet
	Fructose-1,6-diphosphatase	Hypoglycemia, hepatomegaly episodic acidosis (no mellituria)	Fructose- and sucrose-free diet
Glycogen	Glycogen storage diseases (see Ch. 20) Gluconeogenesis	Hypoglycemia Myopathy Hepatomegaly	
	Fructose-1,6-diphosphatase Glucose-6-phosphatase Phosphoenolpyruvate carboxykinase Pyruvate carboxylase	Fasting hypoglycemia Seizures, lacticacidosis in some	Frequent feedings

Table 19-9. Disorders of Purine and Pyrimidine Metabolism

Disorder	Enzyme Deficiency	Clinical Features	Treatment
Purine	Hypoxanthine-guanine Phosphoribosyltransferase (Lesch-Nyahn)	Mental retardation Self-mutilation, spasticity and movement disorders Uric acid nephropathy, Gouty arthritis	Allopurinol
Pyrimidine	Oroticaciduria	Developmental delay, failure to thrive megaloblastic anemia, leukopenia	Uridine, 100 mg/kg/day
	Xeroderma pigmentosum (De Sanctis-Cacchione syndrome)	Sun sensitivity, microcephaly, ataxia Choreoathetosis, failure to thrive Progressive mental retardation	Limit sun exposure

Plasmapheresis and peritoneal dialysis may be necessary to remove lethal accumulation of toxic metabolites.

HYPERAMMONEMIAS

The urea cycle defects (Fig. 19-4) are the major causes of severe hyperammonemia in children. Other metabolic disease and some acquired diseases may also cause significant hyperammonemia (Table 18-2). The features are not unlike those of the organic acidemias with a fulminant neonatal encephalopathy occurring after protein has been introduced into the diet. Survivors experience repeated bouts of episodic encephalopathy and have severe developmental handicaps. Intermediate deficiencies may have a later onset, milder course, and episodic symptoms. One should note that ornithine transcarbamylase is an X-linked dominant disease causing a lethal condition in males and variable symptoms in females. Urea cycle defects should be suspected in the neonate with encephalopathy and elevated ammonia. Frequently the blood urea nitrogen will be unexpectedly low. Therapy is dietary protein restriction. Some of the disorders respond to supplemental dietary arginine and benzoate.

DISORDERS OF CARBOHYDRATE METABOLISM

Hypoglycemia is the major feature of this group of inborn errors of metabolism (Table 19-8). Lacticacidosis, renal tubular defects, hepatomegaly, and cataracts are additional signs. Disorders of galactose and fructose metabolism be-

Table 19-10. Porphyrias Associated with Neurologic Complications

Disorder	Enzyme Deficiency
Intermittent acute porphyria	Uroporphyrinogen I synthetase
Hereditary coproporphyria	Coproporphyrinogen oxidase
Variegate porphyria	Protoporphyrinogen oxidase

come symptomatic after dietary exposures. Disorders of gluconeogenesis become symptomatic with fasting.

The diagnosis should be suspected in the child with recurrent or severe hypoglycemia. There are many causes for hypoglycemia (see Table 18-2). Often the diagnosis may be made clinically because of distinctive clinical features of these disorders. A urine screen for reducing substances (Benedict's test) is a simple procedure and should be performed simultaneously with a glucose oxidase test to exclude glucose. Chromotography is a more quantitative method for measuring urine and blood sugars. Classic galactosemia can be diagnosed from a red cell enzyme assay. Children with defects in gluconeogenesis should be screened by carefully monitoring a fast. Blood sugar below 30 mg/dl within the first 6 hours usually indicates a primary defects in gluconeogenesis. Enzyme analysis is usually required from a liver biopsy specimen in making an exact diagnosis. Treatment is outlined in Table 19-8.

PURINE AND PYRIMIDINE DISORDERS

Table 19-9 outlines the major features of the rare purine and pyrimidine disorders. Lesch-Nyhan disease is the most common and differs from most metabolic diseases in that it is an X-linked recessive disorder. Mental retardation and self-mutilation may suggest a severe psychiatric disturbance. Although blood uric acid is usually elevated, a better screen for the disease is a urinary uric acid/creatinine ratio. Values above 0.5 are suggestive of the disease.

PORPHYRIAS

Of the many porphyrias, three have prominent neurologic symptoms and signs (Table 19-10). The major features are episodic attacks of abdominal pain with vomiting, diarrhea, and psychiatric disturbances. Motor neuropathy may also be a prominent feature and may be extensive enough to cause respiratory paralysis. The syndrome is rarely symptomatic before puberty. Interestingly, all of these disorders are dominantly inherited, which is unusual for metabolic diseases. Photosensitivity is characteristic for all the porphyrias except acute intermittent porphyria.

These disorders must be considered in patients with the recurrent symptoms described and in the child with an acute neuropathy. In acute intermittent porphyria, urine porphyrins may be elevated only during an acute attack; in the other porphyrias there are continuous elevations. Treatment is to avoid drugs which may induce an attack. Unnecessary abdominal surgery may be avoided following a correct diagnosis.

SELECTED READINGS

Barclay N: Acute intermittent porphyria in childhood. A neglected diagnosis? Arch Dis Child 49:404–406, 1974

Berry HK, Hsieh MH, Bofinger MK, et al: Diagnosis of phenylalanine hydroxylase deficiency (phenylketonuria). Am J Dis Child 136:111–115, 1982

Blass JP: Disorders of pyruvate metabolism. Neurology 29:280–286, 1979

Evans OB: Lactic acidosis in childhood. Pediatr Neurol 1:325–328, 1985

Fisher E: Developmental aspects of galactosemia from infancy to childhood. Clin Pediatr 19:38–45, 1980

Martsui SM, Mahoney MJ, Rosenberg LE: The natural history of the inherited methylmalonic acidemia. N Engl J Med 308:857–862, 1983

Menkes JH: Metabolic diseases of the nervous system. p. 1. In Menkes JH (ed): Textbook of Child Neurology. 3rd Ed. Lea & Febiger, Philadelphia, 1985

Rallison ML, Meikle AW, Zigrand WO: Hypoglycemia and lactic acidosis associated with fructose-1,6-diphosphatase deficiency. J Pediatr 94:935–939, 1979

Snyderman SE: Clinical aspects of disorders of the urea cycle. Pediatrics 68:284–289, 1981

Stanbury JB, Wyngaarden JB, Fredrickson DS (eds): The Metabolic Basics of Inherited Disease. 5th Ed. McGraw-Hill, New York, 1983

Wendel U: Maple-syrup-urine disease. N Engl J Med 308:1100–1105, 1983

Wilson JB, Young AB, Kelley WN: Hypoxanthine-guanine phospho-ribosyl transferase deficiency. The molecular basis of the clinical syndromes. N Engl J Med 309:900–904, 1983

Wolf B: Propionic acidemia: a clinical update. J Pediatr 99:835–839, 1981

20

METABOLIC STORAGE DISEASES

The metabolic storage diseases are characterized by the impaired enzyme catabolism of various complex molecules with resultant accumulation in neurons and other tissues of these substances. The major categories of storage diseases are listed in Table 20-1. The most characteristic features are progressive intellectual deterioration, blindness, and organomegaly and demonstrable storage material in tissues. The pathophysiology is variable but the accumulation of the storage material may disrupt normal cellular activity, causing cellular death. In many, a specific enzyme deficiency can be determined; however, in some the exact defect is unknown.

GLYCOGEN STORAGE DISEASES

The glycogen storage diseases have in common abnormal accumulation of glycogen in tissue. The major modes of clinical presentation are hypoglycemia, muscle weakness, and cramps on exercise. Most, but not all, are associated with hepatomegaly. An outline of the major features of the glycogen storage diseases are presented in Table 20-2 and the metabolism of glycogen is shown in Figure 20-1.

Glycogen storage disease (GSD) types I, III, and VI are associated with fasting hypoglycemia and the major neurologic features are secondary to lowered blood glucose: seizures and loss of consciousness. Pompe's disease (GSD II), debrancher deficiency (GSD type III), McArdle's disease (GSD V), and GSD type VII present with muscle disease. Infantile Pompe's disease is somewhat unique in that it is a lysosomal storage disease and affects almost all tissues. Progressive weakness, hepatosplenomegaly, cardiomegaly with heart failure, and developmental arrest from CNS involvement are the major features. The muscle pathology is distinct (Fig. 20-2) and electrocardiogram shows giant QRS complexes. The other glycogen storage diseases do not involve the CNS.

Debrancher deficiency usually presents with fasting hypoglycemia and progressive muscle weakness. The late-onset varient may have the disease restricted to muscle without hepatomegaly or hypoglycemia. McArdle's disease can present with progressive weakness, cramps on exercise, or episodic myoglobinuria. The latter is more common in childhood. A screen for this disease is an ischemic exercise test. Because of the block in glycogenolysis, lactate is not normally produced after 60 seconds of ischemic exercise. Type VII GSD is similar

Table 20-1. Metabolic Storage Diseases

Glycogen storage diseases
Lipid storage diseases
  Gangliosidoses
  Metachromatic leukodystrophy
  Globoid leukodystrophy
  Fabry's disease
  Gaucher's disease
  Niemann-Pick disease
Neuronal ceroid lipofuscinoses
Mucopolysaccharidoses
Mucolipidoses

both clinically and biochemically. Chapter 28 discusses the metabolic myopathies in more detail.

LIPID STORAGE DISEASES

Neurolipids are extremely complex macromolecules that are constructed from basic blocks of fatty acids, sugars, and other molecules (Fig. 20-3). The metabolism of neurolipids is outlined in Figure 20-4. Neural lipids are major components of cell membranes and myelin. Accumulation of the catabolic product gives rise to syndromes characterized by motor and intellectual deterioration and frequently associated with a macular cherry-red spot. Many of these disorders also cause storage in the liver, spleen, bone marrow, and other tissue. The clinical features of the lipid storage diseases are outlined in Table 20-3. Confusing are the many conditions with a similar phenotype but different genotype. Recently, phenotypic variation has been demonstrated in a single enzyme defect.

Table 20-2. Glycogen Storage Disease

Type	Enzyme Deficiency	Affected Tissue	Clinical Features
I	Glucose-6-phosphalase (von Gierke's disease)	Liver, kidney, intestines	Hypoglycemia, failure to thrive, acidosis
II	Acid maltase (Pompe's disease)	Generalized	Weakness, heart failure
III	Amylo-1,6-glucosidase (debracher, Cori's disease)	Liver, muscle	Hypoglycemia, weakness
IV	Amylo-1,4-1,6 glucosylase (brancher, Andersen's disease)	Generalized	Weakness, acidosis, liver failure
V	Muscle phosphorylase (McArdle's disease)	Muscle	Weakness, cramps on exercise
VI	Liver phosphorylase (Hers' disease)	Liver	Hypoglycemia
VII	Phosphorfuctokinase	Muscle	Cramps on exercise

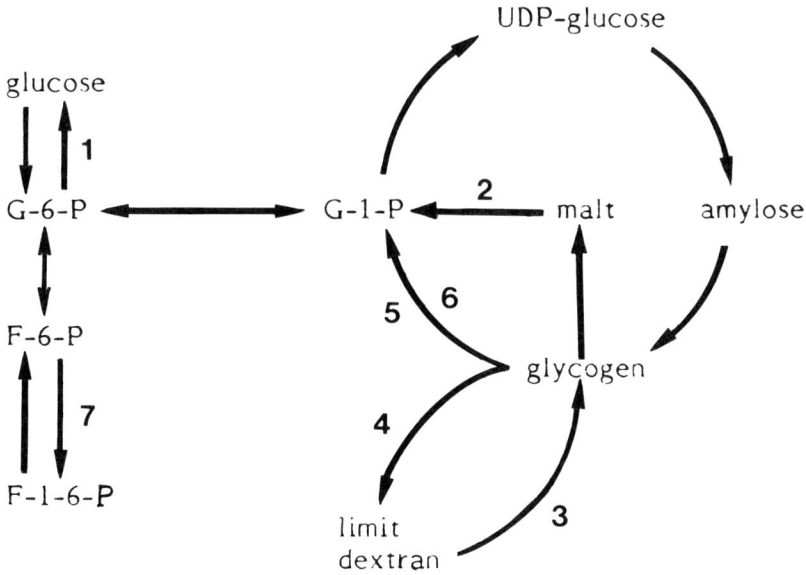

Fig. 20-1. Glycogen metabolism and associated diseases: (*1*) glucose-6-phosphatase, GSD I (von Gierke's); (*2*) acid maltase, GSD II (Pompe's); (*3*) amylo-1,6-glucosidase, GSD III (debrancher); (*4*) amylo-1,4-1,6-transglucosylase, GSD IV (brancher); (*5*) muscle phosphorylase, GSD V (McArdle's); (*6*) liver phosphorylase, GSD VI; (*7*) phosphofructokinase, GSD VII.

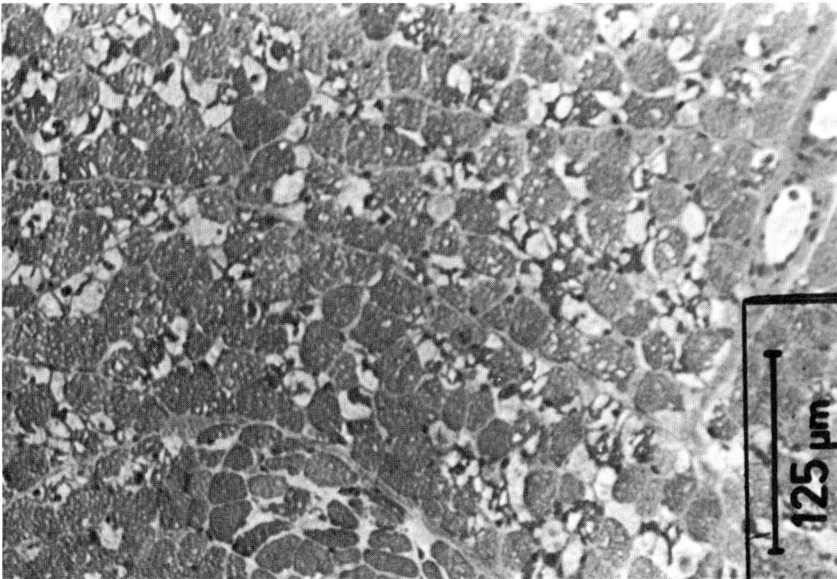

Fig. 20-2. Photomicrograph of muscle from a patient with Pompe's disease.

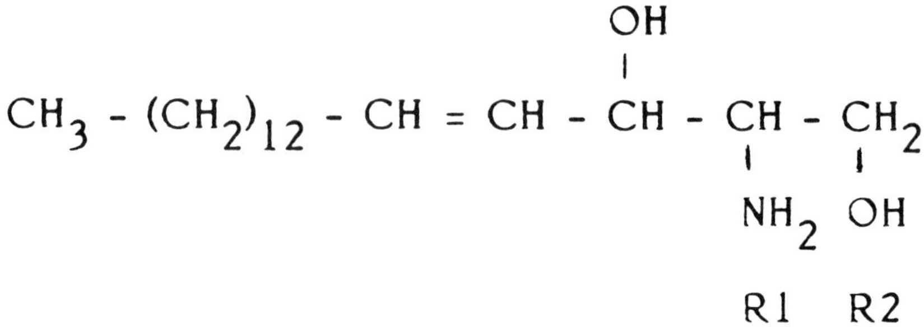

$$OH$$
$$CH_3 - (CH_2)_{12} - CH = CH - CH - CH - CH_2$$
$$NH_2 \quad OH$$
$$R1 \quad R2$$

Fig. 20-3. Neural lipids. The basis structure of sphingosine is shown. Additions at the R1 and R2 sites give the following: R1 = fatty acid (FA), ceremide; R1 = FA + R2 = phosphatidylcholine, sphingomyelin; R1 = FA + R2 = hexose, cerebroside; R1 = FA + R2 = hexoses, hexosamines, and neuramic acids, ganglioside; R1 = FA + R2 = galactosyl-3-sulfate, sulfatide.

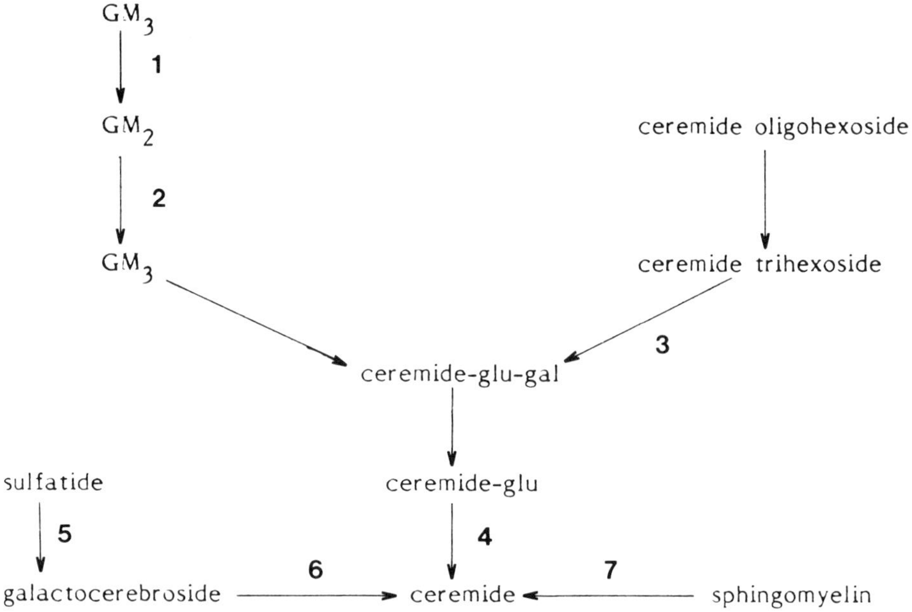

```
GM₃
 │ 1
 ▼
GM₂                                    ceremide oligohexoside
 │ 2                                          │
 ▼                                            ▼
GM₃                                    ceremide trihexoside
     ╲                                       ╱
      ╲                                     ╱  3
       ▼        ceremide-glu-gal  ◄────────
                      │
                      ▼
sulfatide        ceremide-glu
 │ 5                  │ 4
 ▼          6         ▼          7
galactocerebroside ──────► ceremide ◄────── sphingomyelin
```

Fig. 20-4. Lipid metabolism and associated defects: (*1*) β galactosidase, generalized GM₁ gangliosidosis; (*2*) hexosaminidase, Tay-Sachs and Sandhoff's disease; (*3*) α-galactosidase (trihexosidase), Fabry disease; (*4*) glucocerebrosidase, Gaucher's disease; (*5*) arylsulfatase A, metachromatic leukodystrophy; (*6*) galactocerebrosidase, Krabbe's disease; (*7*) sphingomyelinase, Nieman–Pick disease.

Table 20-3. Lipid Storage Disease

Disorder	Enzyme Defect	Visceromegaly	Age of Onset	Clinical Features
GM₂ gangliosidosis				
Type I (Tay-Sachs)	Hexosaminidase A	–	<6 months	Cherry-red spot, hyperacusis, hypotonia, spasticity, mental retardation macrocephaly, blindness
Type II (Sandhoff's)	Hexosaminidase A and B activator	+	<6 months	Cherry-red spot, hyperacusis, hypotonia, spasticity, mental retardation, macrocephaly, blindness
Type III (juvenile)	Hexosaminidase A (partial)	–	2–6 years	Ataxia, spasticity, seizures, blindness
GM₁ gangliosidosis	β-Galactosidase	+	1–2 months	Cherry-red spot in 50%, edema, hypotonia, spasticity, failure to thrive, seizures, blindness
Juvenile	β-Galactosidase (partial)	–	6 months to 2 years	Slowly progressive mental retardation, spasticity
Late onset	β-Galactosidase (partial)	–	>10 years	Cherry-red spot, ataxia, Hunter phenotype, seizures, spasticity
Niemann-Pick disease				
Type A (infantile)	Sphingomyelinase	+	<6 months	Cherry-red spot in 50%, seizures, progressive mental retardation
Type B (nonneuropathic)	Sphingomyelinase	+	<6 months	Nonneurologic
Type C (chronic)	Sphingomyelinase	+/–	>2 years	Ataxia, seizures, dystonia, mental retardation
Type D (Nova Scotia)	?	+	>2 years	Ataxia, seizures dystonia, mental retardation
Gaucher's disease				
Type I (adult)	Glucocerebrosidase	+	>10 years	Anemia, cirrhosis, fractures
Type II (infantile)	Glucocerebrosidase	+	<6 months	Spasticity, opisthotonous, seizures, stridor
Type III (juvenile)	Glucocerebrosidase	+	>10 years	Spasticity, myoclonus, mental retardation, fractures, cirrhosis
Fabry's disease	Trihexosidase	–	>5 years	Intermittent pain, angiokeratoma, corneal opacities, cerebrovascular accident, renal disease, neuropathy

(Continued)

Table 20-3. Lipid Storage Disease (*Continued*)

Disorder	Enzyme Defect	Visceromegaly	Age of Onset	Clinical Features
Farber's lipogranulomatosis	Ceramidase	—	<6 months	Arthritis, vomiting, subcutaneous, nodules, mental retardation
Krabbe's disease (globoid cell leukodystrophy)	Galactosylcerebrosidase	—	<6 months	Spasticity, seizures, mental retardation, blindness, deafness
Metachromatic leukodystrophy	Arylsulfatase A	—	12–18 months	Hypotonia, areflexia, weakness, mental retardation, spasticity, seizures, blindness, cherry-red spot
Juvenile	Arylsulfatase	—	5–10 years	Dementia, ataxia, spasticity
Late onset	Arylsulfatase	—	>10 years	Dementia
Multiple sulfatase deficiency	Arylsulfatase A, B, and C and others	—	1–2 years	Similar to juvenile metachromatic leukodystrophy

Table 20-4. Disorders of Lipid Metabolism

Disorder	Enzyme Defect	Age of Onset	Clinical Features
Wolman's disease	Acid cholesterol ester hydrolase	<3 months	Hepatosplenomegaly, vomiting, abnormal calcifications, failure to thrive
Refsum's disease	Phytanic acid α-hydroxylase	>2 years	Ataxia, polyneuropathy, retinitis pigmentosa, deafness
Cerebrotendinous xanthomatosis	? (Cholesterol accumulation)	>5 years	Ataxia, spasticity, cataracts, tendon xanthomas
Abetalipoprotinemia (Bassen-Kornzweig)	? (Causes vitamin E deficiency)	Birth	Steatorrhea, retinitis, neuropathy, ataxia, joint deformities, anemia
Hypobetalipoprotinemia	? (Causes vitamin E deficiency)	Birth	Same as above, but much milder
Tangier disease	?	>3 years	Orange tonsils, episodic weakness, corneal opacities, paresthesias, hepatosplenomegaly
Carnitine deficiency generalized muscle	? ?	Birth Birth	Reye syndrome-like episodes, myopathy Cardiomyopathy, myopathy
Carnitine palmityltransferase deficiency	Carnitine palmityltransferase	?	Muscle cramps and weakness with prolonged exercise

The gangliosidoses are caused by abnormal accumulation of gangliosides. Tay-Sachs disease is perhaps the most common and representative of this group. Most children with this disease are of Eastern European Jewish extraction. In the classic form, development is normal for the first several months of life and then irritability, hyperacusis, and excessive startle develop. Progressive intellectual decline, hypotonia, and visual loss are the intermediate stage before blindness, spasticity, seizures, and macrocephaly develop. Terminally, a vegetative

Table 20-5. The Neuronal Ceroid Lipofuscinoses

Disorder	Age of Onset	Clinical Features
Infantile (Santavuori)	<2 years	Early blindness, ataxia, seizures
Late infantile (Batten-Bielschowsky)	2–4 years	Late blindness, marked ataxia, photoconvulsive response, typical occasional retinal pigmentation
Variant (Batten)	5–7 years	Early blindness, ataxia, seizures
Juvenile (Spielmeyer-Vogt)	4–7 years	Early blindness, mild and late ataxia, retinal pigmentation
Late onset (Kufs)	>20 years	Dementia, psychosis

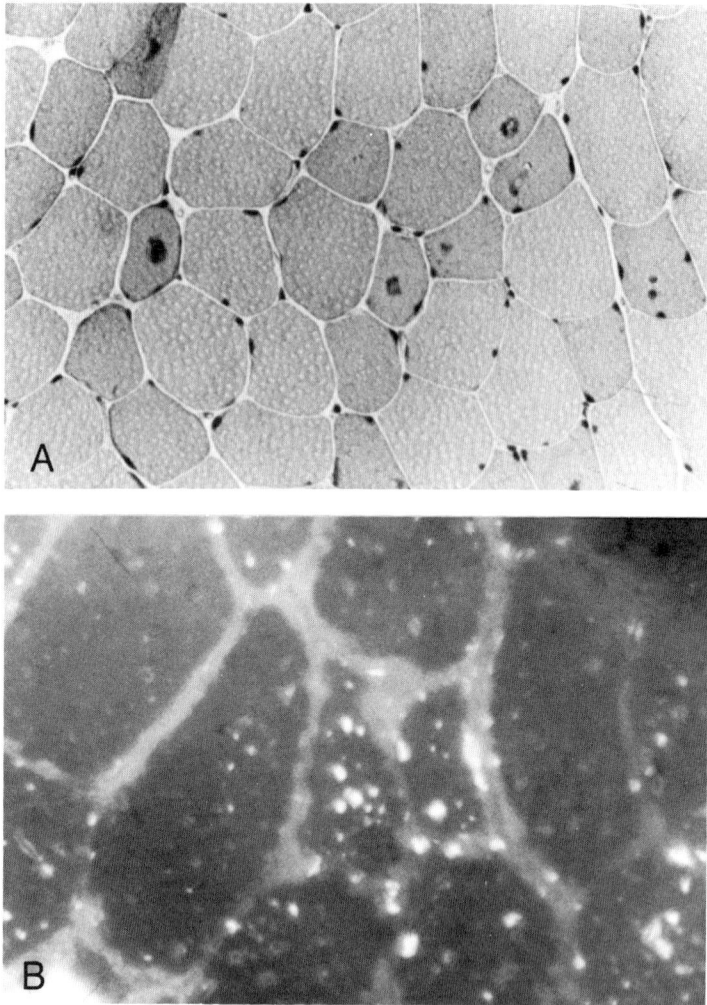

Fig. 20-5. Neuronal ceroid lipofuscinosis. (A) Photomicrograph of muscle biopsy stained with hematoxylin–eosin. (B) Fluorescent photomicrograph of same specimen.

existence persists until death at 2 to 3 years. A macular cherry-red spot is a constant finding and there is no visceromegaly.

Gaucher's disease and Nieman–Pick disease are characterized primarily by splenomegaly and intellectual deterioration. A number of variants exist, some of which are relatively benign. Metachromatic leukodystrophy and Krabbe's disease are often discussed with leukodystrophies because of the abnormal formation of myelin. These two diseases involve the peripheral nervous system, causing a polyneuropathy, and the cerebrospinal fluid protein is usually elevated.

Disorders of oxidation, transport, and absorption of lipids are very rare and

Table 20-6. Major Features of the Mucopolysaccharidoses

Type	Enzyme Defect	Corneal Clouding	Dwarfism	Mental Retardation	Urinary Mucopolysaccharides[a]
IH (Hurler's)	α-L-Iduronidase	+	+	+	DS, HS
IS (Scheie's)	α-L-Iduronidase	+	+/−	−	DS, HS
II (Hunter's)	L-Iduronosulfate sulfatase	−	+/−	−	HS
III A (Sanfilippo's)	Heparan sulfate sulfatase	−	+/−	+	HS
B	N-Acetyl-glucosaminidase	−	+/−	+	HS
C	Acetyl coenzyme A-glucosaminide N-acetyltransferase	−	+/−	+	HS
D	N-Acetyl-α-glucosaminide-6-sulfatase	−	+/−	+	HS
IV A (Morquio's)	N-Acetylgalactosamine-6-sulfatase	+/−	+	+	KS
B	β-Galactosidase				
V (Scheie's)	(see MPS type 1 S)				
VI (Maroteaux-Lamy)	N-Acetylgalactosaminase-4-sulfatase	+	+	−	DS
VII	β-Glucuronidase	+/−	+	+/−	HS, DS

[a] HS = heparan sulfate, DS, dermatan sulfate, KS = keratan sulfate.

Table 20-7. Differential Diagnosis of Hurler's
Phenotype

MPS I (Hurler's disease)
MPS II (Hunter's disease)
MPS III (Sanfilippo's disease)
MPS IV (Morquio's disease)
MPS VI (Maroteaux-Lamy syndrome)
MPS VII
GM_1 gangliosidosis (pseudo-Hunter's disease)
Sialidosis
I-Cell disease
Mucolipidosis type III
Mannosidosis
Fucosidosis
Aspartylglucosaminuria
Cretinism

are summarized in Table 20-4. Ataxia and polyneuropathy are common features. Two disorders deserve special comment, since they are treatable: Refsum's disease, by dietary restriction of phytanic acid (green vegetables), and abetalipoproteinemia, by vitamin E supplementation.

NEURONAL CEROID LIPOFUSCINOSIS

A discussion of neuronal ceroid lipofuscinosis is difficult because of the unknown etiology and the complicated eponyms ascribed to the various subtypes. The major features are progressive loss of vision, motor and intellectual

Table 20-8. Mucolipidoses and Disorders of Glycoprotein Metabolism

Disorder	Enzyme Defect	Age of Onset	Clinical Features
Mucolipidoses			
Type IA (sialdosis)	Neuraminidase	<5 years	Hurler phenotype, cherry-red spot, myoclonus, increase urine sialic acid
Type IB (I-cell disease)	Neuraminidase	Puberty	Cherry-red spot, myoclonus, ataxia, angiokeratoma corporis diffusum
Type III	?	2–4 years	Mild Hurler phenotype, normal mentation
Type IV	?	Birth	Corneal clouding, microcephaly, mild mental retardation
Glycoproteins			
Mannosidosis	α-Mannosidase	<1 year	Mild Hurler phenotype
Fucosidosis A	α-Fucosidase	<1 year	Hurler phenotype
Fucosidosis B	α-Fucosidase	<1 year	Angiokeratoma corporis diffusum, mild neurologic features
Aspartylglucosaminuria	Aspartylglucosamine amidohydrolase	<5 years	Hurler phenotype
Familial myoclonic epilepsy	?	Puberty	Myoclonic, generalized motor seizures, dementia, spasticity

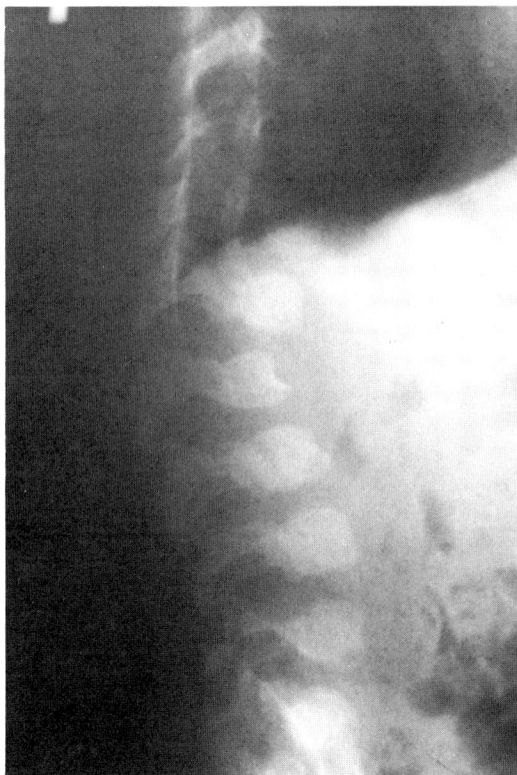

Fig. 20-6. Dysostosis multiplex.

deterioration, and seizures. The diseases share similar features with some of the juvenile lipid storage diseases and together form the "amaurotic idiocy" group. A "salt and pepper" retinitis may be present rather than a cherry-red spot. The EEG may show a characteristic photoconvulsive response in some children and the electroretinogram is abolished. The major characteristics are the neuronal ceroid lipofuscinosis subtypes are outlined in Table 20-5. Diagnosis can be made only by electron microscopy of tissue to visualize the storage material. The major storage material is a dolichol which accumulates in almost all tissues. The substance has autofluorescence and characteristic features on electron microscopy. Biopsy of apocrine skin or muscle shows the pathogenic features most consistently (Fig. 20-5).

MUCOPOLYSACCHARIDOSES AND RELATED DISORDERS

The "gargoyle" habitus together with corneal clouding, organomegaly, and mental retardation characterize the mucopolysaccharidosis (MPS) disorders. The dysmorphic features include short stature, megencephaly, coarse facial features

Table 20-9. Tissue Analysis for Metabolic Storage Disease

Disease	Tissue	Pathologic Features
Glycogen storage disease		
Type I	Liver	Cytoplasmic glycogen
Type II	Liver, muscle	Lysosomal glycogen
Type III	Liver, muscle	Cytoplasmic glycogen
Types V and VI	Muscle	Subsarcolemma glycogen
Gangliosidosis		
GM_1	Bone marrow	Foamy histiocytes
Tay-Sachs disease	Brain	Cytoplasmic lamellar inclusions
Sandhoff's disease	Bone marrow	Foamy histiocytes
Niemann-Pick disease	Bone marrow	Foamy histiocytes
Gaucher's disease	Bone marrow	Lipid-laden histiocytes
Metochromatic leukodystrophy	Nerve	Metachromasia
	Cerebrospinal fluid	Increased protein
Krabbe's disease	Nerve	Demyelinization
	Cerebrospinal fluid	Increased protein
	Brain	Globoid cells
Fabry's disease	Bone marrow	Foamy macrophages
Wolman's disease	Bone marrow	Foamy macrophages
Refsum's disease	Nerve	Hypertrophic neuropathy
	Cerebrospinal fluid	Increased protein
Bassen-Kornzweig	Red blood cells	Acanthocytes
Hypobetalipoproteinemia	Red blood cells	Acanthocytes
Tangier disease	Bone marrow	Lipid-laden histiocytes
Farber's disease	Nodule	para-Aminosalicylic acid-positive material
	Cerebrospinal fluid	Increased protein
Mucopolysaccharidoses	Urine	Mucopolysaccharide
	Bone marrow	Vacuolated cells with mucopolysaccharide
	Others	
Neuronal ceroid lipofuscinosis	Lymphocytes, apocrine skin, muscle	Electron microscopy: curvilinear bodies, fingerprint bodies, osmophilic granules
Mucolipidosis type I	Urine	Sialic acid
	Bone marrow	Foamy macrophages
I-cell disease and mucolipidosis type II	Fibroblasts	Mucopolysaccharide and membrane lysosomal inclusions
Familial myoclonic epilepsy	Liver, muscle	Lafora bodies
Fucosidosis	Liver	Vacuoles containing polysaccharides
Aspartylglycosaminuria	Lymphocytes	Vacuolated cells
Chédiak-Higashi	Neutrophils	Giant peroxidose-positive granules

with hypertelorism and thick lips, a protuberant abdomen (often with a large umbilical hernia), and short, spadelike hands and feet. The many types of MPS vary according to the predominance of one of the clinical features and the type of mucopolysaccharides excreted in the urine (Table 20-6). Hurler's disease is by far the most common, and its phenotype is seen in a number of other disorders (Table 20-7). Hunter's MPS is an X-linked recessive disease. The diagnosis can be suspected if the patient has suggestive clinical features and a screening test (acid albumin test) performed. A definitive diagnosis requires enzyme assay of fibroblasts or leukocytes.

The mucolipidoses have biochemical and clinical features similar to those of the mucopolysaccharidoses except that mucopolysaccharide is not excreted in the upine (Table 20-8). Familial myoclonic epilepsy, or Unverricht's dementia, usually presents in later childhood with the onset of myoclonic seizures and progressive motor and mental deterioration. The etiology is unknown; however, the characteristic storage material can be found from muscle, skin, and liver.

DIAGNOSIS

A presumptive diagnosis of a metabolic storage disease is made from the clinical features, especially visceromegaly, blindness with mental retardation, muscle weakness, and a Hurler-like clinical appearance. The ophthalmologic examination is particularly helpful, with corneal clouding and opacities, cataracts, retinitis, optic atrophy, and a cherry-red spot often present. Radiographs of the spine may reveal dysostosis multiplex which is present in the Hurler syndrome (Fig. 20-6). Urine screening tests are only available for the MPS disorders. Examination of the cerebrospinal fluid may show elevated protein in some disorders (Table 20-9). The EEG is not particularly helpful, except for the photoconvulsive response of the neuronal ceroid lipofuscinoses. Electromyograms and nerve conduction velocities show characteristic abnormalities in diseases which cause myopathy (glycogen storage disease) and in some of the lipid storage diseases. Although a definitive diagnosis can be made only by enzyme assay of fibroblast of biopsied tissue, most of the metabolic storage diseases demonstrate characteristic pathology from easily accessible biopsied tissues (Table 20-9).

SELECTED READINGS

Arsanio-Nunes ML, Coutires F, Aicardi J: An ultramicroscopic study of skin and conjunctival biopsies in chronic neurological disorders of childhood. Ann Neurol 9:163–169, 1981

Engel HG, Gomez MR, Marjorie E, et al: The spectrum and diagnosis of acid maltase deficiency. Neurology 23:95–106, 1973

Farrell DF, Sumi SM: Skin punch biopsy in the diagnosis of juvenile neuronal ceroid-lipofuscinosis. Arch Neurol 34:39–43, 1977

Johnson WG: The clinical spectrum of hexosaminidase deficiency disease. Neurology 31:1453–1456, 1981

Menkes JH (ed): Textbook of Child Neurology. 3rd Ed. Lea & Febiger, Philadelphia, 1985

Mueller DPR, Lloyd JK, Bird AC: The long term management of abetalipoproteinemia, a possible role for vitamin E. Arch Dis Child 52:209–212, 1977

Stanburgy JB, Wyngaarden JB, Fredrickson DS: The Metabolic Basis of Inherited Disease. 5th Ed. McGraw-Hill, New York, 1983

Werlin SL, Grand RJ, Perman JA, et al: Diagnostic dilemmas of Wilson's disease: diagnosis and treatment. Pediatrics 62:47–51, 1978

Young ID, Harper PS: The natural history of the severe form of Hunter's syndrome: a study on 52 cases. Dev Med Child Neurol 25:481–490, 1983

Zeman W, Dyken P: Neuronal ceroid-lipofuscinosis. Pediatrics 44:570–583, 1969

21

LEUKODYSTROPHIES AND DISEASES OF GRAY MATTER

Degenerative diseases are often approached based upon whether the features are caused by neuronal disease (gray matter disease) or demyelinization (white matter disease) (Table 21-1). There is considerable overlap in the neurologic signs and clinical course, however. This chapter discusses those diseases which typify these disorders, many of which have no known etiology.

LEUKODYSTROPHIES

Progressive spasticity, intellectual deterioration, and optic atrophy characterize the leukodystrophies. Movement disorders, ataxia, and muscle weakness frequently develop during the course of the illness. Seizures may occur but are rarely a prominent sign. The pathologic features are abnormal myelinization (dysmyelinization) or loss of myelinization (demyelinization). Attenuation of the white matter is a common finding on computed tomographic (CT) scan and electrophysiologic studies show delayed evoked responses. Table 21-2 lists the major degenerative diseases of myelin. Leukodystrophy traditionally refers to a degenerative disease of CNS white matter caused by a known or suspected enzyme defect. Multiple sclerosis and related acquired demyelinating diseases are probably immunologically mediated. Chronic viral infections, acute disseminated leukoencephalitis, and related conditions which cause demyelination are discussed in separate chapters.

Metabolic Leukodystrophies

Metachromatic leukodystrophy (MLD) is the characteristic disease of the metabolic leukodystrophies. There are several forms of MLD, including infantile, juvenile, and late onset. A distinct feature of MLD is that it involves both central and peripheral nervous system myelin. Metachromatic leukodystrophy is caused by arylsulfatase A deficiency (see Fig. 20-4). This causes storage of metachromatic material in central and peripheral myelin and diffuse demyelination. The clinical features vary with the age of onset. Infantile MLD often presents with hypotonia and areflexia. Spasticity and CNS signs progress rapidly. Juvenile MLD onset, on the other hand, presents with ataxia and movement disorders which progress to spasticity. Later hypotonia and areflexia develop as the pe-

Table 21-1. Clinical Features of Gray and White Matter
Diseases

	Clinical Features	
Disorder	Early	Late
Leuokodystrophies	Spasticity	Retardation
	Ataxia	Seizures
	Weakness	
	Vision loss	
Gray matter diseases	Dementia	Spasticity
	Seizures	Vegetative state
	Vision loss	

ripheral nervous system becomes increasingly involved. The late-onset variant presents primarily as a dementia in adults. All of the MLD variants are inherited in an autosomal recessive manner. The diagnosis is suggested by demonstrating slowed peripheral nerve conduction velocities, delayed evoked responses, and elevated cerebrospinal fluid (CSF) protein. Metachromatic inclusions are found on the sural nerve biopsy. Measurement of arylsulfatase A activity in leukocytes or fibroblasts confirms the diagnosis.

Krabbe's disease, or globoid cell leukodystrophy, shares many characteristics with MLD. The principle differences are an earlier onset and greater involvement of the CNS. Spasticity is a major feature early in the course of the disease. Seizures are more frequent in this disorder than in MLD. Pathologically there is extensive demyelination and multinucleated giant cells (globoid cells) in the brain. The diseases is caused by β-galactosylcerebrosidase deficiency (see Fig. 20-4). The electrodiagnostic abnormalities are similar to those of MLD, and the CSF protein is elevated. An enzymatic assay on fiberblasts is the definitive test.

Adrenoleukodystrophy is an X-linked recessive disorder which can present at any age in childhood. The major features are progressive spasticity, extrapyramidal signs, vision loss, and seizures. Some of the patients develop a pseudobulbar palsy with emotional instability and difficulty with swallowing. Central

Table 21-2. Diseases of Central Nervous
System Myelin

Metabolic
    Metachromatic leukodystrophy
    Krabbe's disease
    Adrenoleukodystrophy
Degenerative
    Pelizaeus-Merzbacher disease
    Canavan's disease
    Alexander's disease
Acquired
    Multiple sclerosis
    Neuromyelitis optica (Devic's)
    Schilder's disease
    Progressive multifocal leukoencephalitis
    Acute disseminated leukoencephalitis

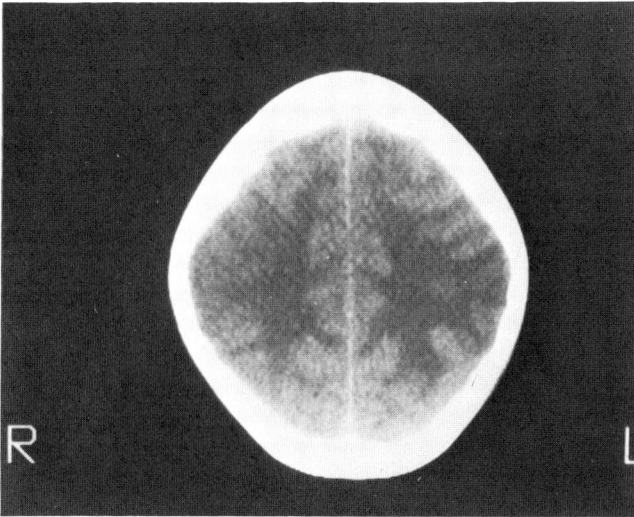

Fig. 21-1. CT scan showing extensive demyelinization in a patient with leukodystrophy.

nervous system demyelinization is often striking on CT scan (Fig. 21-1). The peripheral nervous system is not involved and intellectual deterioration is less severe than in other leukodystrophies. The majority of patients also show adrenal insufficiency which may be either severe or quite subtle. Cutaneous manifestations of Addison's disease may be present.

Pathologically, lipid material is found in macrophages throughout the white matter and adrenal glands. Demyelinization is extensive, though often sparing the subcortical fibers. The etiology is thought to be secondary to impaired catabolism of long-chain fatty acids (C22 through C30). Diagnosis should be suspected in a child with progressive white matter symptoms, optic atrophy, and electrophysiologic evidence of delayed auditory and visual evoked responses. Adrenal insufficiency can be demonstrated by failure to respond to adrenocorticotropic hormone stimulation. There is no enzyme marker for the disease; however, an increased ratio of C26 to C21 fatty acids is typically found in the plasma. Older literature often refers to sudanophilic cerebrosclerosis, which is probably the same disorder as adrenoleukodystrophy.

Pelizaeus-Merzbacher Disease

The original description attributed X-linked recessive inheritance to Pelizaeus-Merzbacher disease. Similar cases, however, have shown other types of inheritance. The major features are progressive spasticity and a somewhat slower clinical course than for the other disorders discussed above. The onset is usually within the first year, with coarse nystagmus and roving eye movements. Later ataxia, optic atrophy, and involuntary movements progress to spasticity in later

Table 21-3. Presenting Symptoms in Children
with Multiple Sclerosis

Symptom	Percentage of Cases
Ataxia	55
Visual disturbances	34
Sensory disturbances	23
Dizziness, headache, vomiting	18
Vertigo	11
Incontinence	4
Other	5

Modified from Menkes JH (ed): Textbook of Child Neurology, 3rd Ed. Lea & Febiger, Philadelphia, 1985, p. 449.

life. There are no specific diagnostic tests short of a brain biopsy. The pathology shows a dysmyelinating condition rather than one of demyelination.

Cockayne's Syndrome

Dysmorphic features, growth failure, decreased subcutaneous fat, developmental regression, and retinal degenerations are the major features of Cockayne's syndrome. The children are sensitive to sunlight and there is evidence for defective DNA and RNA repair similar to that of ataxia telangiectasia.

Canavan's and Alexander's Diseases

Canavan's and Alexander's diseases affect infants and are best characterized by progressive spasticity and marked developmental regression. Progressive macrocephaly is also a characteristic feature. The two diseases differ pathologically in that Canavan's shows a spongy degeneration in the subcortical white matter while Alexander's disease is characterized by the presence of Rosenthal fibers which have accumulations of eosinophilic material and demyelinization. There is no specific diagnostic test for these diseases short of a brain biopsy. In Canavan's disease the CT scan is said to show a characteristic spongy appearance. The CT scan in Alexander's disease is similar to that of other diseases of the white matter.

Multiple Sclerosis and Related Disorders

Multiple sclerosis is rare prior to adolescence. The major feature is a remitting course involving multiple areas of the CNS; ataxia and visual disturbances are the most common presenting symptoms (Table 21-3). The attacks usually progress over days to weeks and remissions take place over similar periods of time. The remissions may not be complete and rarely the disease is slowly progressive rather than remitting.

There are two related syndromes. Devic's disease, or neuromyelitis optica, is characterized by the acute onset of optic neuritis and transverse myelitis. Children who present with this syndrome have a high incidence of developing more characteristic features of multiple sclerosis at a later age. Schilder's disease, or diffuse sclerosis, is a fulminant demyelinating disease with progressive intellectual, motor, and visual failure.

Pathologically, patients with multiple sclerosis have islands of demyelinization. In Schilder's disease there are large areas of diffuse demyelinization which frequently spare the arcuate fibers. Cerebral edema may occur in some children secondary to the rapid destruction of white matter throughout the CNS. Baló's disease is a pathologic variant of Schilder's diffuse sclerosis and is often termed *encephalitis periaxialis concentrica* because of the concentric bands of demyelinization within the white matter.

Diagnostic Evaluation of Leukodystrophies

In children presenting with predominantly motor signs and optic atrophy, a disorder of white matter should be considered. Age of onset, inheritance (if known), and certain clinical features such as macrocephaly may lead to a specific diagnosis. Electrodiagnostic features of delayed evoked responses are consistent with a diagnosis of white matter disease. Measurement of nerve conduction velocities will separate those entities which involve both peripheral and central myelin, particularly MLD and Krabbe's disease. Biopsy of the sural nerve may be diagnostic for these disorders as well. Many diseases of white matter have increased CSF protein. The CSF protein in multiple sclerosis often shows an increase in gammaglobulin and the presence of myelin basic protein. The CT scan shows white matter attenuation in most of the leukodystrophies. In multiple sclerosis, magnetic resonance imaging often shows very distinct plaques.

DISEASES OF GRAY MATTER

It is more difficult to determine which disorders to exclude than to include in diseases of gray matter. Most metabolic and degenerative diseases of the nervous system affect cortical neurons either primarily or secondarily. The metabolic storage diseases are an excellent example and are discussed in Chapter 20. Included in the present chapter are other disorders which primarily affect neuronal activity of the cerebral cortex and some disorders which are difficult to classify elsewhere (Table 21-4).

The major clinical features of gray matter diseases are dementia and seizures. *Dementia* is a term frequently used in adult neurology to describe progressive loss of previously acquired higher cortical functions such as memory, language, reasoning, and abstraction. In children, dementia may present initially as a halt in development. A child may plateau at a given level of development and then begin to regress. Documenting this pattern is important for the diagnosis of any degenerative disease. Seizures in gray matter diseases tend to occur early in the course of the disease and are often severe and unresponsive to therapy. The

Table 21-4. Diseases of Gray Matter

Metabolic storage diseases (Ch. 20)
Alper's syndrome
Zellweger's syndrome
Mitcohondrial encephalomyopathies
Menkes' kinky hair syndrome
Rett's syndrome
Epileptic encephalopathies
Chronic viral infection (Ch. 32)

epilepsy is a mixed type with generalized tonic–clonic, myoclonic, and other seizures. In some cases, the seizures themselves are the major feature and obscure the other clinical aspects of the diseases.

Alper's Syndrome

The eponym Alper's syndrome is best used to describe those children with progressive gray matter disease of unknown cause. The onset is usually in the second or third year with a mixed seizure disorder. Progression occurs over 2 to 3 years, with dementia and later spasticity. A CT scan may show progressive cortical atrophy as a result of a marked loss of cortical neurons (Fig. 21-2). The prognosis is uniformly poor, with the child eventually becoming vegetative.

Zellweger's Syndrome

This disorder is also called the cerebrohepatorenal syndrome because of its multiorgan involvement. The major clinical features are minor dysmorphic features, severe hypotonia, and hepatosplenomegaly shortly after birth. Renal cysts,

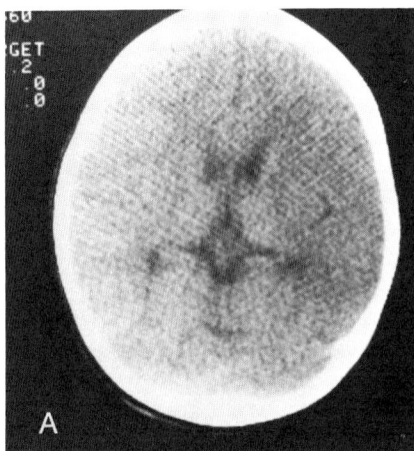

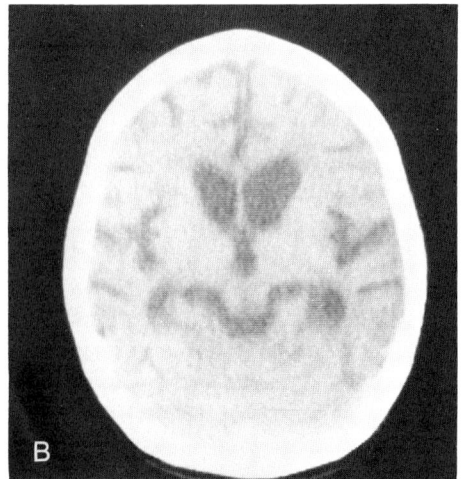

Fig. 21-2. Two CT scans showing progressive cortical atrophy of unknown etiology: (A) at $2\frac{1}{2}$ years and (B) at 4 years.

Table 21-5. Encephalomyopathies

Cytochrome complex deficiencies
  Infantile muscle weakness and encephalopathy
  Subacute necrotizing encephalomyelopathy (Leigh's)
  Progressive sclerosis poliodystrophy (Alper's)
  Trichopoliodystrophy (Menkes')
Ophthalmoplegia, retinal degenerations
  Heart block, ataxia, dementia (Kearns-Sayer syndrome)
Myoclonus epilepsy with ragged red fibers
Mitochondrial encephalopathy, myopathy, lacticacidosis, and stroke like episodes

liver failure, seizures, and severe developmental delay complete the syndrome. Recently, increased serum pipecolic acid in these patients have been reported. On pathologic examination, there is neuronal loss and microgyria.

Mitochondrial Encephalomyopathies

Although many of the mitochondrial myopathies present with hypotonia and weakness, some also have prominent CNS features (encephalomyopathy). This group of disorders, also called poliodystrophies, is thought to be caused by abnormalities of mitochondrial function resulting in deranged energy metabolism. Those disorders with known defects are listed in Table 21-5. The major clinical features are failure to thrive, dementia, seizures, and ophthalmoplegia. Strokelike episodes occur in some children. Cardiomyopathy, renal tubular disease, and lacticacidosis are systemic manifestations. Ragged red fibers on Gomori trichrome stain of a muscle biopsy and spongiform degeneration of the brain are found in many patients. Electron microscopy shows abnormal mitochondrial morphology frequently associated with lipid storage (Fig. 21-3). Because mitochondrial DNA is derived from the cytoplasm of the ovum, most of these disorders have a sex-linked inheritence.

Menkes' Kinky Hair Syndrome

A disorder of copper metabolism, Menkes' kinky hair syndrome, presents with the early onset of seizures, hypotonia, and developmental arrest. The hair is "kinky," colorless, and brittle. Microscopic examination of the hair shows pili torti (twisted hair) and trichorrhexis nodosa (fractured hair). Serum copper and ceruloplasmin concentrations are reduced. Copper is a component of several metalloenzymes and this disorder may be related to the mitochondrial encephlomyopathies. Dietary copper supplementation does not appear to reverse the disease progression.

Rett's Syndrome

This recently described disorder occurs only in females, with onset in the first few years of life. After a period of normal development there is developmental arrest followed by the onset of autistic features, seizures, acquired mi-

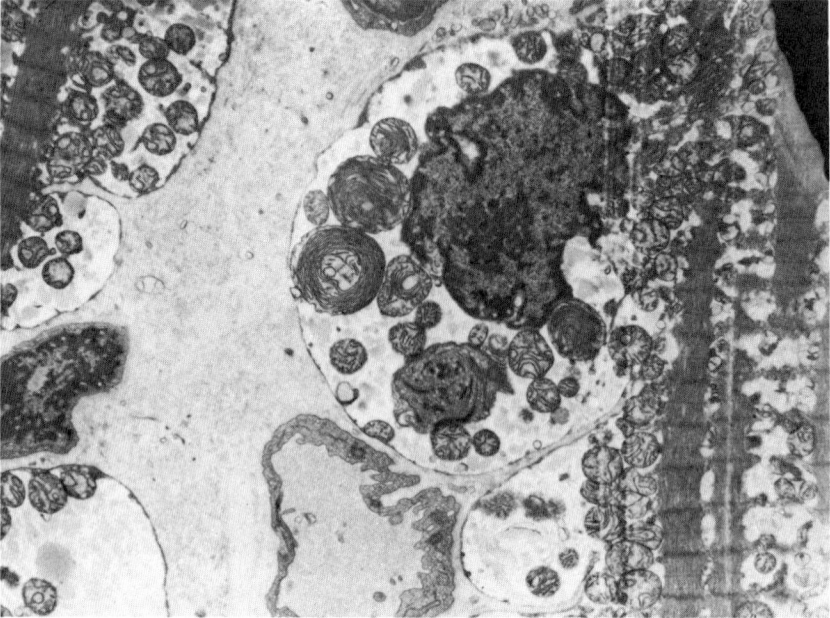

Fig. 21-3. Electron photomicrograph of a patient with mitochondrial encephalomyopathy.

crocephaly, and loss of hand use and ambulation. Handwringing activity is characteristic. The disease progresses and then plateaus at a low level of function for years. The etiology is unknown, as is its exact mode of inheritence. There is no diagnostic test for Rett's syndrome.

Epileptic Encephalopathies

Some of the epileptic syndromes closely resemble the disorders discussed in this chapter and will be briefly mentioned here. A more detailed review is found in Chapter 36. Cryptogenic infantile spasms occur in the setting of developmental arrest and a hypsarrhythmic EEG (West's syndrome) in the otherwise normal child. Other types of seizures may be present. The prognosis is poor, in that 50 percent will develop retardation and most will have continued epilepsy. Although the prognosis is better than for those children whose infantile spasms are associated with an underlying disease (e.g., tuberous sclerosis and congenital infections), it is clear that many children with West's syndrome have a severe gray matter disease.

The Lennox-Gastaut syndrome is similar to West's syndrome but occurs in older children. It is associated with a mixed seizure disorder, including generalized tonic–clonic and atonic, and atypical absence and slow spike wave discharge on EEG. As with infantile spasms, many of these cases have an unknown etiology. The prognosis is similarly poor.

SELECTED READINGS

Buknell WE, Haslam RH, Holtzman NA: Kinky-hair syndrome: response to copper therapy. Pediatrics 52:653–656, 1973

Dimauro S, Bonilla E, Zivieni M et al: Mitochondrial myopathies. Ann Neurol 17:521–528, 1985

Farrell DF, Swedberg K: Clinical and biochemical heterogeneity of globoid cell leukodystrophy. Ann Neurol 10:365–370, 1981

Hagberg B, Aicardi J, Dias K, et al: A progressive syndrome of autism dementia, ataxia, and loss of purposeful hand use in girls: Rett's syndrome—report of 35 cases. Ann Neurol 14:471–478, 1983

Hauser SL, Bresnan MJ, Reinherz EL, et al: Childhood multiple sclerosis: clinical features and demonstration of changes in T cell subsets with disease activity. Ann Neurol 11:463–468, 1982

Kurokawa T, Goya N, Fuckuyama Y et al: West syndrome and Lennox-Gastaut syndrome: a survey of the natural history. Pediatrics 65:81–88, 1980

MacFaul R, Cavanagh N, Lake BD, et al: Metachromtic leukodystrophy: review of 38 cases. Arch Dis Child 57:168–175, 1982

Moser HW, Moser AE, Trojak JE, et al: Identification of female carriers of adrenoleukodystrophy. J Pediatr 103:54–58, 1983

22

SYSTEM DEGENERATIONS

The system degenerations are progressive disorders predominantly involving one neurologic system. Rarely is there a pure system degeneration, in that most of the disorders affect more than one system of the brain. This chapter divides the system degenerations into the ataxias, basal ganglia/movement disorders, and the motor neuron diseases (Table 22-1). Other disorders that enter into the differential diagnosis but which are not truly progressive will be discussed for convenience.

PROGRESSIVE ATAXIAS

Ataxia is one of the most common presenting signs of progressive neurologic disease. Many disorders can cause ataxia at some point in their course (Table 22-2). Interruption of the sensory or motor afferent tracts, the cerebellar efferent tracts, or disease within the cerebellum itself causes ataxia. Although many disorders cause ataxia, this discussion will focus on childhood diseases which are primarily degenerative with an unknown cause.

Friedreich's ataxia is the most common cause of progressive ataxia in childhood. It is a recessively inherited spinocerebellar disease with onset before puberty. The most common presenting complaint is gait disturbance. A rare patient may present with cardiomyopathy or scoliosis. At the time of diagnosis, all patients will have lower limb areflexia, ataxia, and limb dysmetria. Eventually, all patients have scoliosis, pes cavus deformities of the feet, muscle weakness, posterior column signs, and dysarthria. The majority of patients develop cardiomyopathy and some have optic atrophy and hearing loss. The disease is relentlessly progressive and most patients are nonambulatory by the end of the second decade. Pulmonary or cardiac complications result in death during the third or fourth decade.

The diagnosis is usually not difficult in the typical case. Characteristic patterns of electrodiagnostic abnormalities are found in Friedreich's ataxia which separate these patients from those with hereditary neuropathies. Motor conduction velocities are slow to normal and the sensory evoked amplitudes and sensory nerve conduction velocities are absent or markedly reduced. Patients with Friedreich's ataxia have a higher incidence of diabetes than the general population. A defect in oxidative metabolism has been suspected and a patient with similar clinical findings has been shown to have hexosaminidase A deficiency.

Table 22-1. Systems Degenerations

Progressive ataxia
  Spinocerebellar degenerations
  Ataxia-telangiectasia
  Ataxia associated with metabolic diseases
Movement disorders and diseases of basal ganglia
  Huntington's disease
  Hallervorden-Spatz disease
  Wilson's disease
  Fahr's disease
  Dystonia musculorum deformans
  Tremor
  Parkinson's disease
  Tourette's syndrome
  Spasmus nutans
Motor neuron disease
  Familial spastic paraparesis
  Sjögren-Larssen syndrome
  Amyotrophic lateral sclerosis
  Spinal muscular atrophies

Ataxia-telangiectasia is also considered with the neurocutaneous syndromes. It is a recessively inherited disease of children. Oculomotor apraxia is the initial sign. Ataxia presents at the time of walking, with telangiectasia of the conjunctiva, malar cheeks, and ear lobes at 3 to 5 years. Approximately two-thirds of patients have deficient immunoglobulins and show an increase susceptibility to recurrent infections. Neoplasms are common. The disease is progressive and during the latter stages of the disease there is variable mental retardation, choreoathetoid movements, and dystonia. Electrodiagnostic studies may show similar abnormalities to that of Friedreich's ataxia but usually at a much later age. Serum α-fetoprotein is elevated to greater than 30 µg/dl in all cases, making it a marker for the disease. Death usually occurs after the first decade from infection or cancer. The defect is thought to be one of faulty DNA repair.

Leigh's disease, or subacute necrotizing encephalomyelitis, presents in early childhood with hypotonia. As the child matures, ataxia, dysmetria, ophthalmoplegia, and weakness become apparent. Children also have growth failure, abnormal respiration, and developmental delay. Most are not severely retarded. Other findings include dysarthria, dystonia, and seizures. Children with Leigh's disease are prone to episodic attacks of severe ataxia and weakness with intercurrent infections or other stresses. Many have lacticacidosis with attacks, which can be provoked by a glucose challenge. Electrodiagnostic studies show evidence of polyneuropathy. Some have specific defects in oxidative metabolism, particularly pyruvate oxidation, while others have a defect in thiamine metabolism, which is a cofactor for pyruvate dehydrogenase enzyme. The neuropathology is similar to that of Wernicke's encephalopathy.

A number of other syndromes present with a wide variety of signs and symptoms, including progressive ataxia. Table 22-2 summarizes these by age of onset. A recessive ataxia, often associated with spasticity in the lower extremities,

Table 22-2. Familial Degenerative Ataxias

Onset of Disease	Metabolic Error	Distinguishing Signs	Inheritance[a]	Screening Test
0–6 months				
Marinesco-Sjögren	?	Dementia, cataracts	R	CT scan: cerebral atrophy
Gillespie syndrome	?	Aniridia, dementia	R	CT scan: cerebral atrophy
Joubert syndrome	?	Hyperpnea, dementia	R	CT scan: cerebral atrophy
6 months to 6 years				
Ataxia-telangiectasia	Faulty DNA repair	Recurrent infections, oculomotor apraxia	R	α-Fetoprotein
Spastic ataxias (several)	?	Spastic paraplegia, dementia, other	R	
Tay-Sachs variant	Hexosaminidase A	None	R	Skin, rectal, conjunctiva biopsy
Juvenile GM₁	β-D-Galactosidase	Cherry-red spot, dementia, seizures	R	Skin, rectal, conjunctiva biopsy
Neuronal lipofuscinosis	?	Optic atrophy, dementia, spasticity	R	Skin, rectal muscle biopsy
Chédiak-Higashi	?	Recurrent infections	R	Leukocyte inclusions
Subacute necrotizing encephalomyelitis	Pyruvate oxidation	Ophthalmoplegia, neuropathy	R	Blood lactate, pyruvate, urine TPP inhibition
Sandhoff's	Hexosaminidase A and B	Dementia	R	Rectal, skin, conjunctiva biopsy
Cerebrotendinous xanthomatosis	?	Dementia, xanthoma, spasticity	R	Tendon biopsy
6–16 years				
Friedreich's ataxia		Joint deformities, neuropathy	R	
Adrenoleukodystrophy		Seizures, adrenal insufficiency	X	Adrenocorticotropic hormone stimulation test, long-chain fatty acids
Metachromatic leukodystrophy		Dementia, rigidity, neuropathy	R	urine arylsulfatase A, nerve biopsy
Refsum's disease	Phytanic acid hydroxylase	Retinitis, deafness, neuropathy	R	Serum phytanic acid
Bassen-Kornzweig	Abetalipoproteinemia	Retinitis, acanthocytosis	R	Blood lipoproteins, cholesterol, vitamin E
Sjögren-Larssen		Retinitis, spasticity, icthyosis	R	
Pelizaeus-Merzbacher		Dementia, seizures	X	
Neuroaxonal dystrophy		Dementia, myoclonic epilepsy	R	Nerve biopsy
Ramsay Hunt		Myoclonic epilepsy	? R	
Lafora body disease		Myoclonic epilepsy	R	Liver biopsy
Hypobetalipoproteinemia		None		Blood lipoproteins
Roussy-Lévy		Tremor, neuropathy	D	
Machado-Joseph		Dystonia, movement disorders	D	(Portuguese ancestry)

[a] R = recessive, D = dominant, X = X linked.

is perhaps most common. Optic atrophy may be an additional feature. This syndrome resembles some of the olivopontocerebellar atrophies, which generally have a later onset and are normally dominantly inherited. The Ramsa Hunt syndrome (dentorubral atrophy) is the combination of myoclonic epilepsy and ataxia. This syndrome is probably nonspecific and there are a number of conditions with similar features but different etiologies. The early-onset ataxias have been included in Table 22-2, although they may not be clearly progressive in nature.

Diagnosis

It is essential whether the course is chronic and nonprogressive or progressive. The chronic nonprogressive ataxias are the result of either malformations or injury to the cerebellum and comprise the ataxic cerebral palsy syndromes. A computed tomographic (CT) scan may show agenesis of the cerebellar vermis or other abnormalities in the posterior fossa. The subacutely progressive ataxias are caused by posterior fossa tumors until proven otherwise. The CT scan should be the first test performed; if negative, then other causes such as chronic intoxications, infections, or other diseases can be considered. Occasionally anatomic defects of the upper spine or cranium, such as platybasia and the Klippel-Feil anomaly, can cause progressive signs. Diagnosis of a progressive ataxia syndrome is frequently based upon the family history, major features or the neurologic exam, and a few selected tests, as outlined in Table 22-2.

MOVEMENT DISORDERS AND DISEASES OF THE BASAL GANGLIA

Movement disorders are generally involuntary and result from disease of the basal ganglia. The signs include chorea, athetosis, dystonia, and tics. As with ataxia, involuntary movements may accompany a number of metabolic and degenerative diseases of the brain, as listed in Table 22-2. This discussion will focus on those disorders in which a movement disorder is the prominent feature. In the absence of a positive family history, a clinical diagnosis of a specific disorder may be difficult.

Huntington's disease is a dominantly inherited disorder characterized by involuntary movements and dementia. Seizures and dystonia are much more common in the child than in the adult. The most common presentation is dementia between the ages of 5 and 10 years. A Parkinson-like syndrome follows with muscle rigidity and hypokinesia. Seizures and choreoathetosis develop in the majority of cases. The disease is relentlessly progressive and death occurs within 10 years. There are no specific tests for the disease, although caudate atrophy on the CT scan is highly suggestive. A DNA marker for the disease has recently been determined. The disease affects primarily the caudate nucleus and the frontal lobes. The exact cause is unknown.

Hallervorden-Spatz disease is a recessively inherited disorder of iron metabolism. There is pigmentation of the basal ganglia with storage of iron-containing material. The clinical features are progressive rigidity, hypokinesia, and dementia. Some patients develop choreoathetosis. The etiology is unknown and there is no specific diagnostic test or treatment.

Wilson's disease (hepatolenticular degeneration) is a recessively inherited disease of copper metabolism. Approximately one-third present with heptic disease, usually as an acute hepatitis. One-third will present with cerebral symptoms of progressive dystonia and a gait disturbance and another third have both hepatic and neurologic symptoms. Mid-childhood is the usual time of onset; the disease is rare in the preschool child. Untreated, the disease has a tendency to progress, although the course may wax and wane. Extraparamedial symptoms include dystonia, tremor, choreoathetosis, and rigidity. Hepatic cirrhosis and renal tubular disease can complicate the course.

The disease is caused by an abnormal accumulation of copper in tissue. There is an absent or low serum ceruloplasmin in 95 percent of the patients and increased excretion of copper in the urine in all patients. The most important physical finding is the presence of a Kayser-Fleischer ring. This is present in all patients with neurologic findings and in 75 percent of those with liver disease. It is characterized by ring-shaped pigmentation around the iris in the cornea which may only be visualized on slit-lamp examination.

Wilson's disease disorder can be treated by dietary restriction of copper and administering a chelating agent (penicillamine, 0.5 to 1.0 g/day). Therapy should be started prior to the onset of neurologic symptoms by identifying children at risk within the family. After neurologic symptoms develop, less than one-half of patients will have complete recovery with therapy.

Familial calcification of the basal ganglia goes by the eponym of Fahr's disease. This is probably a syndrome rather than a specific entity. Dominantly inherited calcification of the basal ganglia can be asymptomatic. There are also a number of calcium and phosphate disorders such as hypoparathyroidism and hyperparathyroidism which cause calcification of the basal ganglia. The symptomatic childhood cases present with early mental retardation, dystonia, and choreoatheosis. The diagnosis is made by demonstrating the characteristic calcifications on CT scan.

Dystonia musculorum deformans is a disorder of marked increase in muscle tone. The initial manifestation may be torticollis or abnormal positioning of the foot when walking. As the disease progresses, the limbs and trunk constantly become distorted during the waking hours. During sleep the spasms are absent. The earlier the onset, the more rapidly progressive the disease. There is usually no intellectual impairment or seizures. There is no distinct neuropathology. While the inheritance is variable, the majority have Eastern European background and recessive inheritance.

Localized forms of dystonias are encountered as writers' cramp, torticollis, and others which may remain localized or progress to generalized disease. Dystonia may occur in conjunction with other acquired diseases of the brain and may coexist with other diseases of the basal ganglia.

Table 22-3. Clinical Features of Tourette Syndrome

Defining criteria
  Onset during childhood
  Multiple motor tics
  Vocal tics
  Changing symptoms, pattern
  Changing severity, independent of treatment
Variable features
  Complex sterotyped movements
  Compulsive behavior (touching, smelling, biting, rubbing, etc.)
  Coprolalia
  Copropraxia
  Echolalia
  Echopraxia
  Palilalia
  Obsessive thinking
  Family history of tics
  Learning disability

(From Golden CS: Tics in childhood. Pediatr Ann, 12:821–824, 1983.)

Familial tremor is a dominantly inherited disease characterized by a fine rhythmic tremor which is worse with activity and absent with rest. There are no other neurologic symptoms and it usually does not significantly interfere with activities. Tremor without a family history is essential tremor but has similar clinical features.

The clinical picture of Parkinson's disease is more often found in Huntington's disease than in other diseases. Muscle rigidity, resting tremor, and hypokinesia are the major features. Dementia is not a common symptom early in the disease. Because of its rarity in childhood, other diseases of the basal ganglia and the spinocerebellar degenerations should be considered first.

Tics are very common in childhood, particularly in the early school years. Simple tics are characterized by a single repetitive movement and rarely last longer than 6 months. The movements are quick, stereotyped activities most frequently affecting the face or neck. These are called habit spasms. They differ from myoclonus and chorea, which are random movements. Tics are under partial voluntary control in that with great effort the child can refrain from the activity for a short period of time. Clinically they may appear to be involuntary.

Complex tics involve multiple portions of the body and have a ritualistic character. The tics may be multiple and complex tics tend to persist throughout childhood. The most severe form of a tic disorder is the Tourette syndrome, which is associated with complex tics, vocal utterances and coprolalia (Table 22-3). Approximately one-third have learning disabilities and attention deficit disorder. It is possible for treatment of an attention problem with stimulant medications to precipitate Tourett's syndrome.

Spasmus nutans is a curious condition that is nonprogressive and presents in infants at 3 to 6 months of age. It is characterized by a disassociated nystagmus (one eye shows greater nystagmus than the other), head nodding, and a head tilt. This does not cause developmental impairment and in most children the disease resolves over 2 to 3 years. Rarely, patients with spasmus nutans have

Table 22-4. Pharmacologic Management of Common Movement Disorders

Disorder	Drug	Total Daily Dose (mg)	Schedule
Tics	Haloperidol	2.0–5.0	bid
	Clonidine	0.05–0.15	bid
	Pimozide	0.1–0.3/kg	bid
Essential tremor	Propranolol	0.5–2.0/kg	tid
Dystonia	Diazepam	0.1–0.3/kg	tid
	Benztropine	.05–0.1/kg	hs
	Trihexyphenidyl HCl	0.1–0.3/kg	tid
	Carbidopa/levodopa	10–20/kg	tid
Myoclonus	Clonazepam	0.1–0.2/kg	tid
	Valproic acid	30–50/kg	tid

been shown to have optic gliomas. The "bobble-headed doll" syndrome occurs in small children with hydrocephalus or other midline disease and involves involuntary head nodding.

EVALUATION AND TREATMENT OF MOVEMENT DISORDERS

The evaluation of movement disorders depends upon the family history and clinical course of the movement problem. Nonprogressive disorders are more likely to be caused by acquired injury such as perinatal asphyxia or hypoxia. Progressive movement disorders can be caused by infections (subacute sclerosing panencephalitis) intoxications (lead), and tumors of the diencephalon. Rarely vasculitis (lupus) on anti-immune disease (multiple sclerosis) enters the differential diagnosis. The evaluation includes a CT scan, examination of the cerebrospinal fluid slit-lamp examination, quantitation of urine copper excretion and serum ceruloplasmin, and measurement of ANA, anti-DNA, and antistreptolysin O titers.

Treatment of movement disorders can be difficult (Table 22-4). Chorea and tics will often respond to a phenothiazine, notably haloperidol, starting at a low dose and increasing gradually until there is a clinical response. Dystonia and related disorders are often treated with a combination of benzodiazepines and anticholinergic medication. Propranolol is useful in the treatment of essential or familial tremors. Anti-Parkinson drugs, particularly carbidopa/levodopa, may be useful in any disorder in which akinesis is present. Stereotaxic surgery should be considered a treatment of last resort for severe dystonias and rarely for other movement disorders.

MOTOR NEURON DISEASE

The most common motor neuron disease in children is spinal muscular atrophy. This is a disease of lower motor neurons which causes progressive weakness (see Ch. 25). Motor neuron diseases which involve the upper motor

Table 22-5. Classification of Motor Neuron
Diseases

Upper motor neuron
  Familial spastic paraparesis
  Primary lateral sclerosis
  Sjögren-Larssen syndrome
Upper and lower motor neuron
  Amyotrophic lateral sclerosis
  Familial amyotrophic lateral sclerosis
Lower motor neuron
  Spinal muscular atrophy
    Infantile (Werdnig-Hoffmann disease)
    Late Infantile
    Juvenile (Kugelberg-Welander disease)
    Progressive bulbar palsy
    Fazio-Londe disease
    Focal spinal muscular atrophy
    Reactivated poliomyelitis

neurons are discussed here. A classification of the motor neuron diseases is presented in Table 22-5.

Familial spastic paraparesis is a disease of unknown etiology that is usually inherited as a dominant trait, although recessive and X-linked inheritance can rarely be encountered. The clinical expression is quite variable. Both early and late onset can occur within the same family and the severity can be mild to incapacitating. The typical features are progressive spasticity and weakness of the lower extremities. occasionally cerebellar and other signs may be present. Sjögren-Larssen syndrome consists of spastic paraparesis, mental retardation, retinitis, and icthyosis. Primary lateral sclerosis occurs in adults as an amyotrophic lateral sclerosis variant.

Amyotrophic lateral sclerosis rarely occurs in children. The clinical features are those of both upper and lower motor neuron signs. Fasciculations and muscle wasting coexist with hyperreflexia and spasticity. The etiology is unknown and there is no known therapy. The major differential is compressive myelopathy, and a myelogram should be considered for patients with progressive spasticity. Hydrocephalus and midline brain tumors can also present with progressive spasticity.

SELECTED READING

Goebel HH, Heipertz R, Scholz W, et al: Juvenile Huntington's chorea: clinical ultra-structural and biochemical studies. Neurology 28:23–30, 1978

Golden GS, Hood OJ: Tics and tremors. Pediatr Clin North Am 29:95–103, 1982

Hogan GR, Bauman MC: Familial spastic ataxia: occurrence in childhood. Neurology 27:520–525, 1967

Martin WE, Resch JA, Baker JB: Juvenile Parkinsonism. Arch Neurol 25:494–497, 1981

Menkes JH (ed): Textbook of Child Neurology. 3rd Ed. Lea & Febiger, Philadelphia

Nelson JS, Prenksky AL: Sporadic juvenile amyotrophic lateral sclerosis. Arch Neurol 27:300–306, 1972

Stumpf DA: The inherited ataxias. Pediatr Neurol 1:85–95, 1985

23

NEUROCUTANEOUS DISEASES

The association of characteristic skin lesions and neurologic signs and symptoms constitute the heterogeneous neurocutaneous syndromes, also called the phakomatoses. The cutaneous manifestations are usually distinctive enough to make a specific diagnosis without requiring further tests. The family history may also provide important clues to the diagnosis. The major neurocutaneous syndromes are summarized in Table 23-1. Von Hippel-Lindau disease and ataxia-telangiectasia are included, although they are not strictly neurocutaneous syndromes. Other neurologic diseases which are occasionally associated with skin manifestations are not included (see Table 3-9).

NEUROFIBROMATOSIS

Neurofibromatosis (von Recklinghausen's disease) is a dominantly inherited disease with the characteristic skin lesion being a café au lait spot 0.5 cm in diameter or greater (Fig. 23-1). A minimum of five such lesions strongly suggest the diagnosis. Axillary freckling is another prominent skin manifestation. Subcutaneous nodules resulting from growth of neurofibromas on cutaneous nerves may cause a cobblestone texture of the skin when they are extensive. Giant plexiform neurofibromas cause overgrowth of limbs and occasionally of the trunk and face (elephantiasis). The major neurologic manifestations are the result of neurofibromas growing on peripheral nerves and tumors arising in the CNS. Acoustic neuromas and meningiomas are frequent CNS manifestations of the disease in adults but are rare in children. Optic gliomas, however, do occur in childhood. Neurofibromas can cause dysfunction in almost any cranial or spinal nerve and result in neurologic symptoms. Gliomas of the spinal cord and "dumbbell" neurofibromas arising in the spinal region cause scoliosis. Other neurologic manifestations include seizures, retardation, and macrocephaly. The causes for these are symptoms and signs are often unknown.

The pressing neurologic symptoms, characteristic skin lesions, and family history determine the diagnosis. As in many dominantly inherited diseases, the parents may be asymptomatic and unaware of their own disease; however, careful examination of the parent may demonstrate the lesions. The McCune-Albright syndrome consists of café au lait lesions, fibrous dysplasia of bone, mild retardation, and precocious puberty in females and can cause confusion in the diagnosis.

Table 23-1. The Major Neurocutaneous Syndromes

Disorder	Skin Manifestations	Neurologic Manifestations	Inheritance
Neurofibromatosis	Café au lait spots Axillary freckling Subcutaneous neurofibromas Plexiform neuromas	Compressive neuropathy Compressive myelopathy Scoliosis Intracranial tumors Mental retardation Seizures	Dominant
Tuberous sclerosis	Ash-leaf spot Shagreen patch Adenoma sebaceum Subungual, retinal tubers	Mental retardation Infantile spasms Seizures Brain tumors	5/6 sporadic 1/6 dominant
Sturge-Weber	Port-wine stain of the face	Hemiparesis Seizures	sporadic
Von Hippel-Lindau	Retinal hemangioblastomas	Cerebellar and spinal cord hemangioblastoma	Dominant
Ataxia-telangiectasia	Conjunctival, facial, ear telangiectasia	Oculomotor apraxia Ataxia Mental retardation	Recessive
Albrights' syndrome	Café au lait spots	Mental retardation	Sporadic
Klippel-Trenaunay	Port-wine stain	Mental retardation, limb hypertrophy	Sporadic
Incontinentia pigmenti	Vesicular eruptions as infant	Seizures Mental retardation	X-Linked dominant
Linear sebaceous nervus	Midline, facial epidermal nevus	Seizures Mental retardation	Sporadic
Progressive hemifacial atrophy	Bone and soft tissue atrophy of face	Seizures	Sporadic
Hypomelanosis of Ito	Pastterns of hypopigmentation of the skin	Mental retardation Seizures	Sporadic

TUBEROUS SCLEROSIS

Tuberous sclerosis (Bourneville's disease, epiloia) usually presents in early childhood. The characteristic skin lesion is the amelanotic nevi ("ash-leaf" spot; see Fig. 23-2), which can occur on any part of the body. In children of fair complexion the lesions are best visualized by using a Wood's lamp and they are variable in size and multiple number. Another characteristic lesion is adenoma sebaceum, which occurs primarily over the bridge of the nose and in a butterfly distribution on the face. These appear as small reddish nodules similar to acne (Fig. 23-3) and are rarely present before the age of 2 to 3 years. Other cutaneous manifestations include the shagreen patch, which is a large, leathery patch of skin found most often on the back subungual fibromas, and café au lait spots (5 percent). On funduscopic examination retinal tubers may be seen.

The neurologic signs of the disease are more severe than those of neuro-

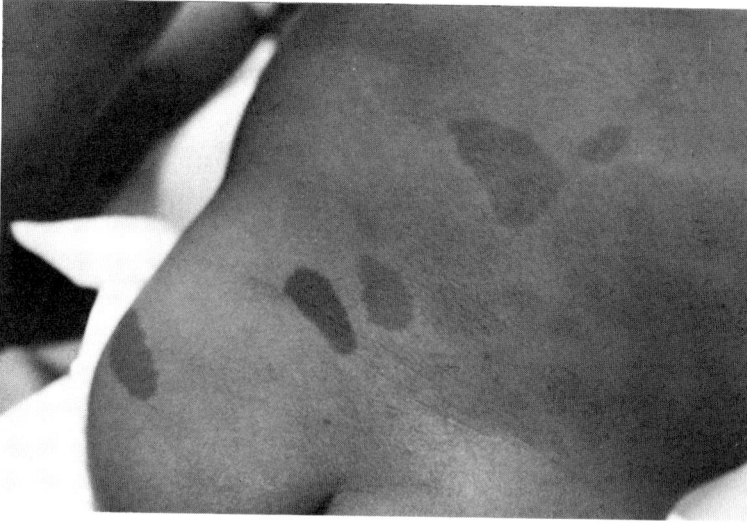

Fig. 23-1. Café au lait spots in a child with neurofibromatosis.

fibromatosis. The earliest manifestation is frequently developmental delay. Many children will develop normally only to experience infantile spasms at approximately 6 months of age. Frequently associated with this are developmental arrest and hypsarrhythmic pattern on EEG (West's syndrome). Mixed seizures frequently follow. The majority of children with tuberous sclerosis will develop some degree of mental retardation. Other neurologic manifestations of the disease are related to intracranial tumors. These tumors vary widely in size and have a tendency to calcify. "Brain stones" (Fig. 23-4) are large calcified tumors located in the brain parenchyma. The descriptive term *candle guttering* is often used to describe the periventricular calcifications and tumors lining the ventricular wall, when seen on pneumoencephalogram. Occasionally these tumors undergo malignant degeneration. Systemic manifestation of tuberous sclerosis includes sarcomas of the heart and kidneys and cystic lesions in the lungs.

The diagnosis of this disease is usually not difficult. Genetic counseling may be difficult, with one one-sixth of the cases having a positive family history and the remainder being sporadic occurrences. To exclude the disease in the asymptomatic parent, a careful examination of the skin with a Wood's lamp, a computed tomographic (CT) scan, and possibly heart and renal scans may be necessary.

STURGE-WEBER SYNDROME

The Sturge-Weber syndrome is characterized by the clinical triad of a facial port-wine nevus, hemiplegia, and seizures. The skin lesion is a flat, reddish capillary hemangioma located in the ophthalmic division of the trigeminal nerve.

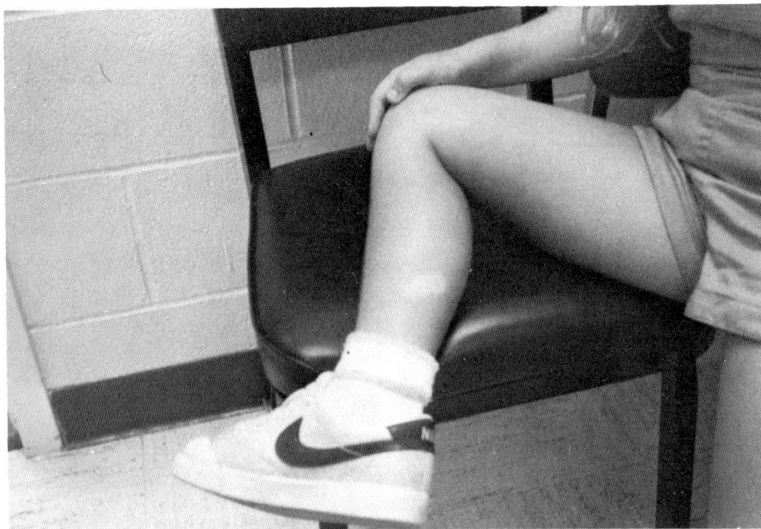

Fig. 23-2. Ash-leaf spot in a child with tuberous sclerosis.

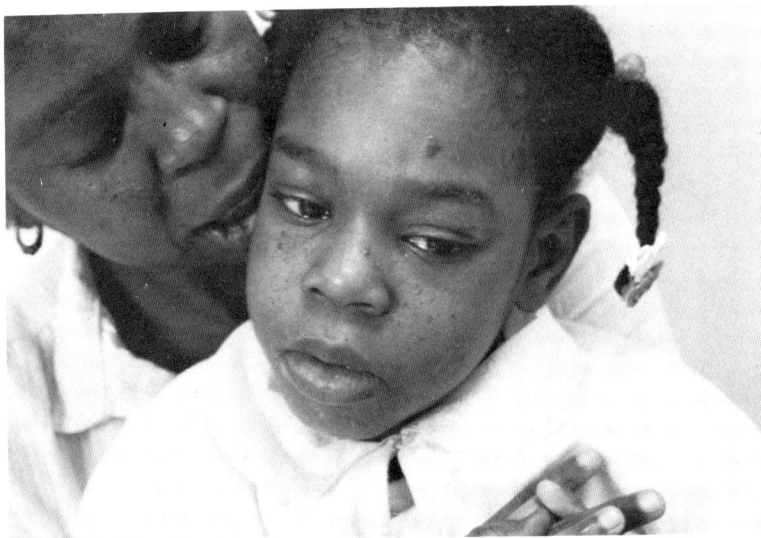

Fig. 23-3. Adenoma sebaceum in a child with tuberous sclerosis. Note the small shagreen patch on the forehead.

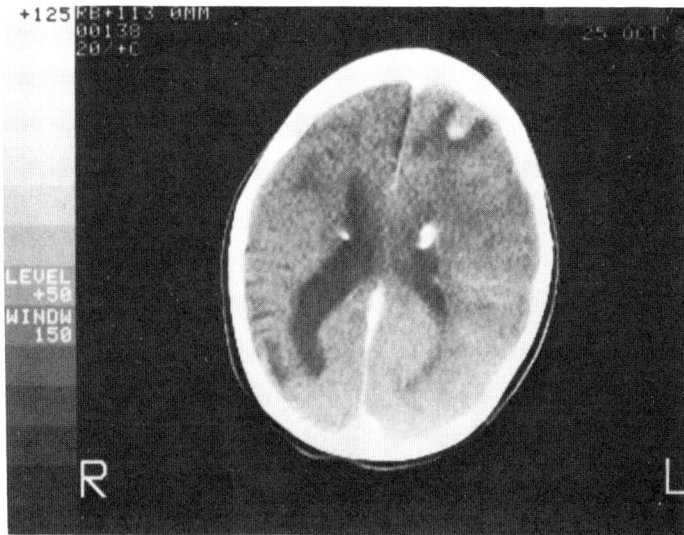

Fig. 23-4. Large calcified tuber ("brain stone") in a child with tuberous sclerosis.

It may involve the entire distribution of the trigeminal nerve and is bilateral in approximately one-fourth of the patients. There are no other skin manifestations. The neurologic manifestations result from angiomatous malformations involving the leptomeninges of the ipsilateral cerebral cortex. Occipital and parietal areas are most often involved. In a minority of cases, the cortex is involved bilaterally.

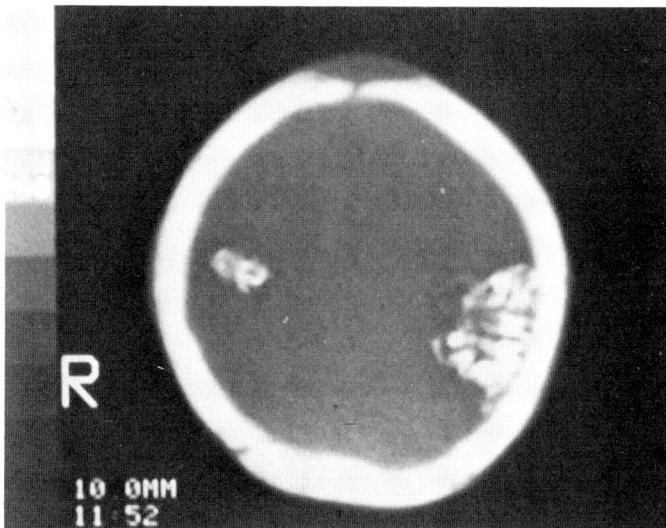

Fig. 23-5. Angiomatous calcifications in a CT scan in a child with Sturge-Weber syndrome.

The angiomatous malformation has a tendency to calcify, resulting in the "tram track" pattern seen on both skull radiographs and CT scans (Fig. 23-5). Rarely the cerebral and radiographic manifestations are seen in the absence of a port-wine nevus.

The neurologic manifestations are progressive hemiplegia and seizures, usually beginning in the first year of life. These seizures may become increasingly difficult if not impossible to control. The majority of children show a progressive intellectual decline with resultant mental retardation. Glaucoma is another complication of this disease.

VON HIPPEL-LINDAU DISEASE

Von Hippel-Lindau disease, or multiple hemangioblastomas, occurs as a dominantly inherited disorder and may present in children with a variety of neurologic signs and symptoms. There are no real cutaneous manifestations, although the hemangiomas may be seen in the retina. The most common CNS manifestations are due to a cerebellar hemangioblastoma and include ataxia, long track signs, and other signs typical of a posterior fossa tumor. Hemangioblastomas may also be found in the spinal cord and may be associated with syringomyelia. Cystic tumors can occur in the kidney, pancreas, and epididymis.

ATAXIA-TELANGIECTASIA

Ataxia-telangiectasia (Louis-Bar syndrome) is a progressive disease of children characterized primarily by ataxia, telangiectasias of the conjunctiva, and recurrent infections. The earliest manifestation is ocular motor apraxia. This is the inability to voluntarily direct gaze. Breaking fixation is difficult and patients have to blink or turn their head and drag their eyes away to refixate on another object. Ataxia is present as soon as the child starts walking. Truncal and gait ataxia are early manifestations, with limb ataxia and ataxic dysarthria developing later. A progressive decline in intellectual abilities occurs in the majority of patients.

The skin manifestations do not usually occur until 3 to 5 years of age. Telangiectasias of the conjunctiva are the characteristic feature (Fig. 23-6); however, similar lesions can occur over the ears and chest or on the face. Systemic manifestations of the disease cause the major morbidity and mortality. Approximately two-thirds of the patients have recurrent upper and lower respiratory infections leading to chronic otitis media and bronchiectasis. A more serious complication is the tendency to develop malignancies such as leukemia and lymphoma.

The diagnosis is usually not difficult on clinical grounds. Immunoglobins are decreased in the majority of patients, but not all. Serum α-fetoprotein is elevated (more than 30 mg/ml) in all children with the disease and serves as a diagnostic marker. In older children, there may be evidence of peripheral neuropathy.

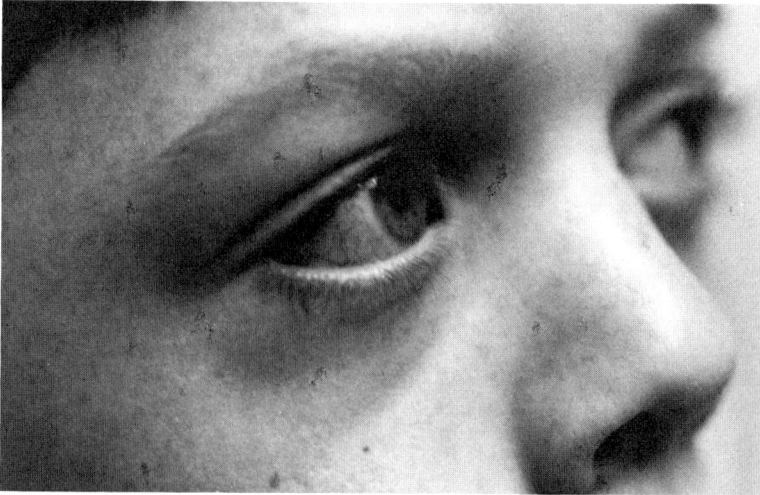

Fig. 23-6. Telangiectasia of the conjunctiva in a patient with ataxia-telangiectasia.

The Osler-Weber-Rendu syndrome presents with similar skin and mucosal telangiectasias which are prone to rupture, causing recurrent ataxia. Vascular anomalies may be found in other organs and brain.

KLIPPEL-TRENAUNAY SYNDROME

This disorder has skin features similar to those of the Sturge-Weber syndrome. The skin manifestations are port-wine nevi located over any part of the body, but characteristically on the extremities. In the distribution of the port-wine stain, there is hypertrophy of the underlying bones and soft tissue which causes progressive growth and enlargement. Neurologic manifestations are relatively uncommon, with mild mental retardation often being the only abnormality.

INCONTINENTIA PIGMENTI

Incontinentia pigmenti is an X-linked dominant disorder and is thought to be lethal for males. It is a rare condition characterized by the eruption of bullae and other lesions in infancy. These tend to resolve with time and may not be present in the adult. Seizures and retardation occur in a minority of patients.

LINEAR SEBACEOUS NEVUS

The linear sebaceous nevus is usually a midline nodular lesion over the forehead and scalp. This is also a rare disorder without an inheritance pattern. The associated neurologic signs are mental retardation and seizures.

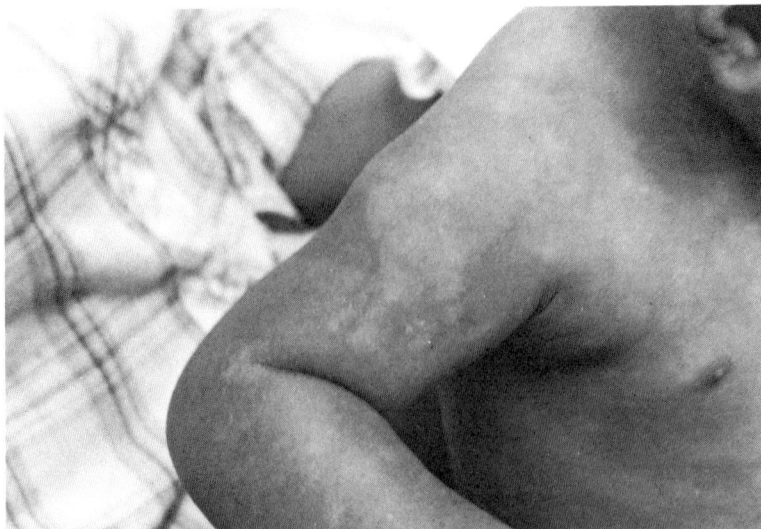

Fig. 23-7. Skin features of hypomelanosis of Ito.

PROGRESSIVE HEMIFACIAL ATROPHY

Progressive atrophy of the soft tissues and underlying bone of one-half of the face constitutes the major feature progressive hemifacial atrophy. A small percentage of cases will have associated seizures and mental retardation. The inheritance is unknown.

HYPOMELANOSIS OF ITO

Mental retardation, seizures, and abnormal pigmentation of the skin constitute the major features of hypomelanosis of Ito. The skin manifestations consist of alternating linear streaks of hyper- and hypopigmentation (Fig. 23-7). These lesions often end abruptly at the midline. Macrocephaly and mild mental retardation may also be associated with this disorder.

NEUROCUTANEOUS MELANOSIS

Neurocutaneous melanosis is the association of a giant hairy nevus and leptomeningeal carcinomatosis with a malignant melanoma. The disorder is quite rare and is not inherited.

SELECTED READINGS

Chalhub EG: Neurocutaneous syndromes in children. Pediatr Clin North Am 23:499–516, 1976

Fienman NL, Yakovac WC: Neurofibromatosis in childhood. J Pediatr 76:339–346, 1970

Gomez MR: Tuberous Sclerosis. Raven Press, New York, 1979

Ricardi VM: Von Recklinghausen's neurofibromatosis. N Engl J Med 305:1617, 1981

Riopelle RJ, Riccardi VM, Faulkner S, et al: Serum neuronal growth factor levels in von Recklinghausen's neurofibromatosis. Ann Neurol 16:54, 1984

Whitehouse D: Diagnostic value of the café-au-lait spot in children. Arch Dis Child 41:316–319, 1966

SECTION 6

Neuromuscular Diseases

The neuromuscular diseases represent the largest group of inheritable diseases. Weakness is a major symptom and sign of a variety of handicapping conditions in children. With the modern approach to diagnosis, including muscle histochemistry and electromyography, a diagnosis can be made in the majority of cases. This is important, because some disorders are treatable, most allow genetic counseling, and a prognosis is important for most parents. This section discusses the major neuromuscular diseases in children.

24

WEAKNESS

Movement is one of the major expressions of the nervous system and is dependent upon muscle strength, tone, and coordination. Many parts of both the central and peripheral nervous systems are involved in the complex movements of human behavior, so that a child who presents with weakness has a relatively large differential diagnosis. The purpose of this chapter is to present a general view of the various causes of weakness and a method for pursuing the diagnosis by a careful history, neurologic exam, and judicious use of laboratory tests.

PATHOPHYSIOLOGY

Movement is initiated from the cerebral cortex and brain stem and is modulated and coordinated by the extrapyramidal and cerebellar systems. Injury to the upper motor neuron of the motor cortex causes muscle weakness and hypotonia initially. Spasticity develops weeks to months after the injury. Hypotonia, but not necessarily weakness, is also a characteristic early feature of the cerebellar injury and patients who later develop choreoathetosis. Metabolic and toxic disturbances can temporarily suppress neuron function of the brain and cause hypotonia and weakness. All of the upper motor neuron and extrapyramidal influences are transmitted via the descending tracts of the spinal cord. Injury to the spinal cord causes spinal shock which lasts for days to weeks. During this period, the muscles below the injury will be flaccid and other cord functions will be inhibited. Segmental reflexes return after spinal shock resolves and spasticity develops over the ensuing weeks.

The influences of the upper motor neuron and extrapyramidal system converge on the internuncial and lower motor neurons in the anterior gray horn of the spinal cord. The lower motor neuron, or anterior horn cell, thus becomes the final common pathway for muscle contraction. The motor unit consists of the anterior horn cell, its axonal extension in the peripheral nerve and its surrounding myelin sheath, the neuromuscular junction, and the muscle fibers innervated by the motor neuron (Fig. 24-1). The motor unit is a functional unit such that injury to any part causes a similar loss of function. Flaccid paralysis and hypotonia are the consistent signs of motor unit disease.

DIAGNOSIS

One can approach weakness in the child based upon the history of progression, episodic, acute, subacute, or chronic progressive (Table 24-1). One must remember that acute weakness may be the first sign of an episodic illness

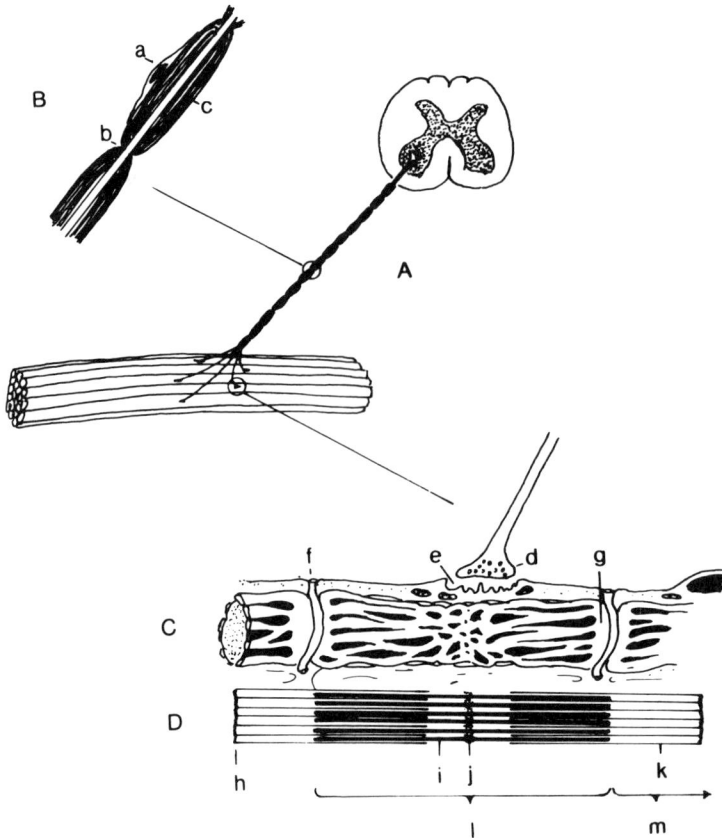

Fig. 24-1. The motor unit. (A) Diagram of the anterior horn cell, peripheral nerve fiber, neuromuscular junction, and innervated muscle fibers. (B) Myelinated nerve: (*a*) Schwann cell, (*b*) node of Ranvier, (*c*) myelin lamellae. (C) Neuromuscular junction: (*d*) Nerve terminus and synaptic vesicles, (*e*) synaptic cleft, (*f*) T-tuble, (*g*) sarcoplasmic reticulum. (D) Sarcomere: (*h*) Z line, (*i*) myosin, (*j*) M line, (*k*) actin, (*l*) A band, (*m*) I band.

and that some disorders have more than one type of presentation. Aside from the weakness, other aspects of the history are important, especially the family history. Most of the neuromuscular diseases have a familial tendency and one can often determine the diagnosis based on the history, physical findings, and family history alone. The major neuromuscular disorders and their inheritances are listed in Table 24-2. The pitfalls in obtaining an accurate family history include distinguishing X-linked recessive disease from an autosomal, recessively inherited disorder, and the sporadic case from one of recessive inheritance without affected siblings. Finally, dominantly inherited disorders can be difficult to determine if the parents are unaware of their own disease or exhibit denial of their disease.

Weakness is usually not difficult to demonstrate in the child on examination. In young children and infants, formal manual muscle testing cannot be done.

Table 24-1. Differential Diagnosis of Weakness

Progression	Brain	Spinal Cord	Anterior Born Cell	Peripheral Nerve	Neuromuscular Junction	Muscle
Acute	Vascular accident	Transverse myelitis Epidural abscess Vascular accident Multiple sclerosis	Poliomyelitis	Guillain-Barré syndrome	Botulism Toxins Myasthenia gravis	Myositis
Episodic	Migraine Multiple sclerosis Metabolic encephalopathies	Multiple sclerosis		Chronic relapsing polyneuropathies Porphyria	Toxins Myasthenia gravis	Metabolic myopathies Periodic paralysis
Subacute	Tumor Intoxications	Tumor Malformations	Infantile spinal muscular atrophy	Toxic neuropathies Chronic Guillain-Barré syndrome	Myasthenia gravis	Inflammatory myopathies
Chronic	Tumor Metabolic encephalopathies Malformation	Tumor Malformation	Spinal musculature atrophy	Familial neuropathies Metabolic neuropathies	Myasthenia gravis	Musculature dystrophies Congenital myopathies Metabolic myopathies Inflammatory myopathies

Table 24-2. Inheritance of the Major Familial Neuromuscular Disorders

	Dominant	Recessive	X Linked
Motor neuron disease	Familial spastic paraparesis	Spinal muscular atrophies	
Polyneuropathy	Charcot-Marie-Tooth	Inborn errors of metabolism with neuropathy	
Neuromuscular junction	?	Congenital myasthenias ? Infantile myasthenias	
Myopathies	Facioscapulohumeral dystrophy	Limb-girdle dystrophy	Duchenne's dystrophy
	Myotonic dystrophy	Metabolic myopathies	Becker's dystrophy Emory-Dreifus dystrophy

There are several maneuvers, however, that one can use to test the major muscle groups (see Fig. 4-5). A child should be able to suspend himself by his grip and stand on his toes and heels. These maneuvers are a test of distal strength. Similarly, a child should be able to suspend his weight by the proximal arm muscles (vertical suspension) as well as do a deep knee bend without the use of his arms. The gait may also yield information, such as the typical waddling gait of

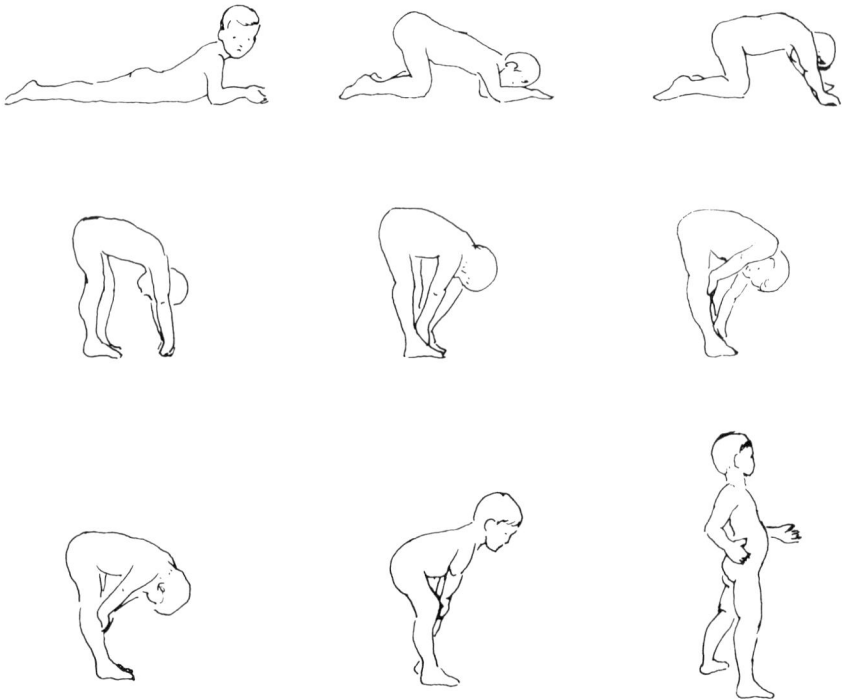

Fig. 24-2. Gowers' maneuver. (Redrawn from Chusid JG: Correlative Neuroanatomy and Functional Neurology. 14th Ed. © 1970 by Lange Medical Publications, Los Altos, CA.)

Table 24-3. Neurologic Features of Muscle Weakness by Etiology

Etiology	Weakness	Reflexes	Babinski Sign	Sensory Loss	Other
Brain	Hemiparesis, generalized	Increased	Present	Unilateral, generalized or normal	Other signs of CNS involvement
Spinal cord	Paraparesis	Increased	Present	Segmental level	Incontinence
Anterior horn cell	Proximal, generalized	Decreased	Absent	Normal	Fasciculations
Peripheral nerve	Distal	Decreased	Absent	Distal	Distal wasting
Neuromuscular junction	generalized, ocular	Present	Absent	Normal	Fatiguability, ptosis
Muscle	Proximal, generalized	Present	Absent	Normal	Proximal wasting, myotonia, pseudohyper-trophy in some

proximal weakness, the scissoring gait of spastic paraparesis, the hemiparetic gait, and the steppage gait of distal weakness. Observing the child arise from the floor will demonstrate the Gowers' maneuver in a child with proximal weakness (Fig. 24-2).

The most important part of the examination for weakness is determination of its distribution. Weakness can be generalized or focal with either the distal or proximal musculature more involved. Unilateral weakness indicates a hemiparesis which is almost always due to an upper motor neuron lesion in the brain or spinal cord. Weakness in the legs only (paraparesis) is suggestive of a spinal cord lesion but may be found in early peripheral nerve disease and midline brain disease (early hydrocephalus, tumor). Bulbar weakness can have many causes, but true ocular weakness and ptosis are almost always associated with diseases of the motor unit. Other important parts of the neurologic exam include testing of deep tendon reflexes, muscle mass and tone, Babinski sign, sensation, the presence of fasciculations, myotonia, and fatiguability, and general physical findings such as joint deformities and skin lesions. Table 24-3 summarizes the char-

Table 24-4. Laboratory Investigation for Muscle Weakness[a]

Disease	Creatine Kinase	Electrodiagnosis			Muscle Biopsy
		Nerve Conduction Velocities	Electromyography	Repetitive Stimulation	
Spinal muscular atrophy	Normal to slight increase	Normal	Diagnostic	Normal	Neuropathic
Polyneuropathy	Normal	Diagnostic	Neuropathic	Normal	Neuropathic
Myasthenia	Normal	Normal	Normal	Diagnostic	Normal
Myopathy	Normal to marked increase	Normal	Myopathic	Normal	Diagnostic

[a] The expected results are indicated with the characteristic features. Those indicated as "diagnostic" are the most specific test for that group of disorders.

acteristic features of the neurologic examination for the different causes of weakness.

LABORATORY TESTS

The history and physical examination should determine the differential diagnosis for the muscle weakness. Laboratory tests are used to confirm the diagnosis or to specify the etiology. The mainstays of laboratory investigation of muscle weakness include the measurement of muscle enzymes, electrodiagnostic studies, and muscle biopsy. Table 24-4 summarizes the laboratory findings in the diseases of the motor unit. Subsequent chapters will cover these disorders in greater detail.

Muscle enzymes generally refer to cytosol enzymes that are found in abundance in muscle fibers. Injured fibers release these enzymes into the circulation. Creatine kinase is the most reliable enzyme to measure, although aldolase, serum glutamic-oxaloacetic transaminase, lactic dehydrogenase and others can be elevated in muscle disease. Electrodiagnostic tests, including electromyography, nerve conduction velocities, and repetitive stimulation are discussed in Chapter 5. These procedures investigate the electrical properties of muscle, the electrical conduction of peripheral nerve, and neuromuscular transmission. The muscle biopsy is the most specific test for myopathies and also may confirm the presence of denervation. In general, if the electromyogram and muscles enzymes are normal, it is unlikely that the biopsy will be of benefit. In some peripheral nerve diseases, a nerve biopsy can be diagnostic.

SELECTED READINGS

Brooke MH: A Clinician's View of Neuromuscular Disease. Williams & Wilkins, Baltimore, 1977

Dubowitz V: Muscle Disorders in Childhood. WB Saunders, London, 1978

Florence JM, Brooke MH, Carroll JE: Evaluation of the child with muscle weakness. Orthop Clin North Am 9:409–430, 1978

Spiro AJ: Approach to diagnosis in the child with muscle weakness. Pediatr Ann 6:149–161, 1977

Swaiman KF, Wright FS: Pediatric neuromuscular disease. CV Mosby, St. Louis, 1979

25

SPINAL MUSCULAR ATROPHIES

The clinical spectrum of motor neuron disease in humans ranges from infantile spinal muscular atrophy to the adult disease of amyotrophic lateral sclerosis. The former is a disease of lower motor neurons, whereas the latter involves both upper and lower motor neurons. Familial spastic paraparesis, which is a purely upper motor neuron disease, is often classified in the group of motor neuron diseases as well. In children, the spinal muscular atrophies are relatively common and are the most common cause of death due to a recessive disease after cystic fibrosis. This chapter reviews the spinal muscular atrophies in childhood. Other motor neuron diseases are discussed in Chapter 22.

PATHOPHYSIOLOGY

The cause for spinal muscular atrophy is unknown. During fetal development, a greater number of lower motor neurons are formed than are needed. During the maturation of the peripheral and central nervous systems, motor neurons are lost in the spinal cord in those areas in which there is little peripheral innervation, such as the thoracic region. One hypothesis is that in spinal muscular atrophy this process of motor neuron dropout continues in all areas of the cord and does not reach the maturational arrest that normally occurs. Loss of anterior horn cells is the characteristic pathologic finding. There are few other changes. Inflammation and gliosis are notably absent. Occasionally the few surviving neurons show chromatolysis, pyknosis, and neuronophagia.

Loss of motor neurons causes the typical features of spinal muscular atrophy: marked muscle wasting and weakness, fasciculations, and the characteristic features on the muscle biopsy and electromyography. In contrast to peripheral nerve disease, the distribution of weakness in spinal muscular atrophy tends to be more proximal than distal. The cranial nerves are almost always involved in the generalized form of the disease, although ocular motility is spared. In children with little subcutaneous fat, fasciculations can be seen. The best place to observed fasciculations is in the tongue. Fasciculations can have a number of etiologies, including intoxications, metabolic abnormalities, and peripheral nerve disease. The most common cause is destruction of the anterior horn cell.

Nerve conduction velocity measurements show normal or minimally decreased motor nerve conduction velocities. Electromyography shows fibrillation potentials and other signs of denervation. Fasciculations are found in approx-

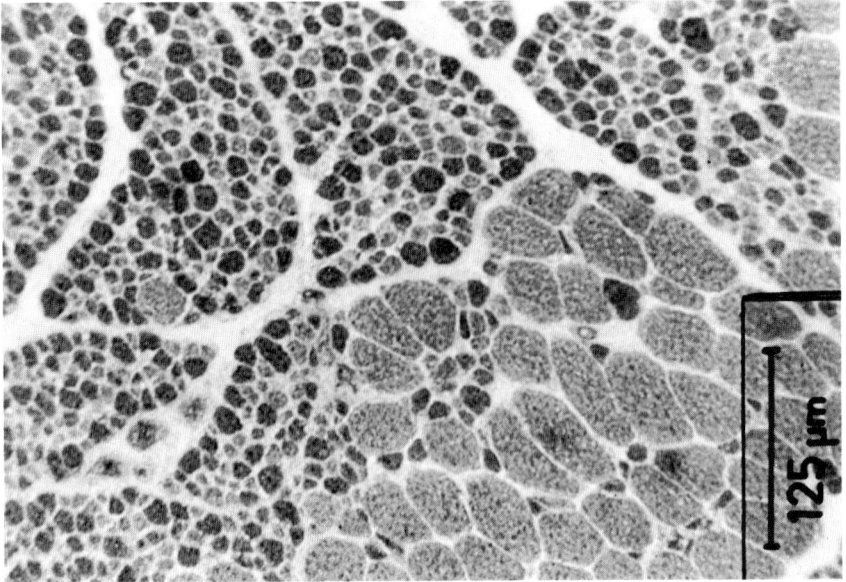

Fig. 25-1. Infantile spinal muscular atrophy. There is marked fiber atrophy and fascicular atrophy with preservation of a few hypertrophied fibers (ATPase pH 9.4). Compare with Figure 28-1.

imately one-third of patients. During voluntary contraction, there is reduced recruitment and long-duration polyphasic potentials.

The muscle biopsy in spinal muscular atrophy shows a relatively characteristic picture. In the acute form, one finds large hypertrophied fibers scattered throughout numerous small, atrophic fibers (Fig. 25-1). If the disease is slowly progressive, reinnervation occurs such that there is grouping of fiber types (Fig. 25-2). Fascicular atrophy, in which a whole muscle fascicle is composed of nothing but small rounded fibers, is characteristic of infantile spinal muscular atrophy.

CLASSIFICATION AND CLINICAL FEATURES

The classification is determined by the clinical course, distribution of weakness, and inheritance. Table 25-1 lists one such classification of the spinal muscular atrophies.

Werdnig-Hoffmann Disease

Werdnig-Hoffmann disease, or acute spinal muscular atrophy, has its onset in the first 6 months. In about one-third of cases, the onset is thought to be prenatal with a history of decreased fetal movements during the third trimester.

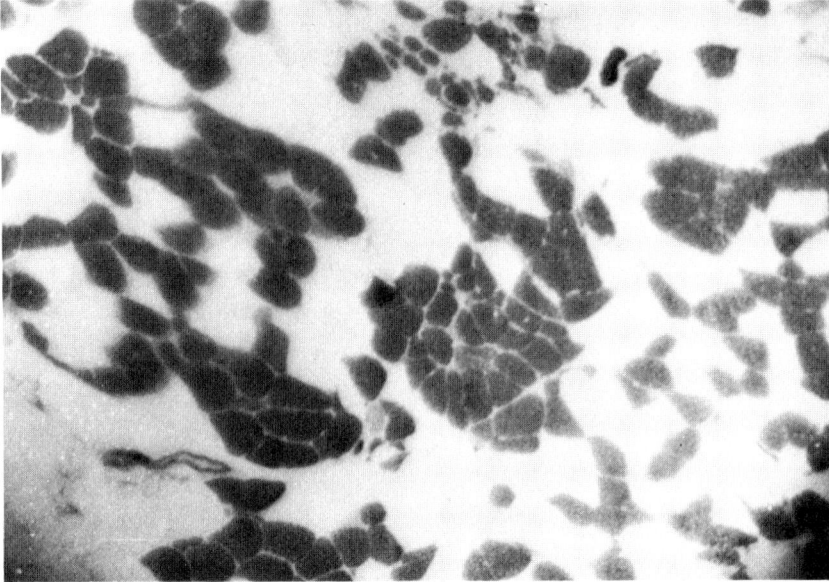

Fig. 25-2. Chronic spinal muscular atrophy. Fiber-type grouping is apparent for both type I and type II fibers (ATPase pH 4.3). Compare with Figure 28-1.

The most common presenting symptom is hypotonia or weakness, followed by decreased suck and delayed motor milestones. The examination shows marked hypotonia and generalized weakness which is more severe proximally than distally. Ocular motility is normal. Reflexes are absent and sensation is normal. Tongue fasciculations are common. The child is alert and responsive and developmentally normal except for motor skills. In the acute form of the disease, the child will not develop head control or the ability to sit. The natural course is one of progressive weakness, difficulty with feeding, and finally compromise

Table 25-1. Classification of Lower Motor Neuron Spinal Muscular Atrophies

Generalized
  Spinal muscular atrophies
    Werdnig-Hoffmann disease type I (acute infantile spinal muscular atrophy)
    Kugelberg-Welander syndrome
      Type II (chronic childhood spinal muscular atrophy)
      Type III (arrested Werdnig-Hoffmann disease)
  Neurogenic arthrogryposis
Focal
  Distal spinal muscular atrophy
  Neurogenic scapuloperoneal spinal muscular atrophy
  Neurogenic facioscapulohumoral spinal muscular atrophy
  Progressive juvenile bulbar palsy (Fazio-Londe disease)
  Möbius syndrome
  Late activation of poliomyelitis

of respiratory function. These patients usually succumb secondary to an inter-current respiratory illness and the median time of death is 7 months. The later the onset, the better the prognosis. Occasionally, death is sudden. It is rare for a child to live beyond the third year with this disorder. The diagnosis is made by the typical clinical features, a consistent electromyogram, and muscle biopsy. This diagnosis should only be made in the absence of other congenital abnor-malities of the CNS. At present, there is no known treatment. Because recessive inheritance is common, genetic counseling is indicated. Type II spinal muscular atrophy has a later onset and a slower course.

Kugelberg-Welander Syndrome

The onset of this disease can occur at any time after the second year. The earlier the onset, the worse the prognosis. Most children with late onset spinal muscular atrophy learn to sit, many learn to walk, and they have a prognosis in terms of years. Clinical features are similar to those of the acute infantile disease, but less rapidly progressive. The weakness tends to be greater in the proximal muscles and the ocular muscles are spared. Fasciculations are more easily seen and swallowing and respiratory difficulties occur only late in the course. Areflexia or marked hyporeflexia is characteristic. In some patients, pseu-dohypertrophy of the calves can be found. The creatine kinase is mildly elevated in some conditions, although never more than two to three times normal. The electromyographic changes are similar to those seen in infantile spinal muscular atrophy; however, one usually finds giant polyphasic potentials indicating ex-tensive reinnervation. The muscle biopsy also shows evidence of reinnervation and extensive fiber-type grouping.

There is no specific therapy to arrest or treat the underlying disease; how-ever, many of these children need rehabilitative therapy and physical therapy to help prevent joint contractures and scoliosis. Early management of scoliosis with a jacket or, rarely, an operative procedure, may prevent pulmonary com-promise and improve longevity.

Other Spinal Muscular Atrophies

Distal spinal muscular atrophy has its onset in infancy and is characterized by distal rather than proximal weakness. Patients usually have a normal life span, although they have increasing weakness of the hands, feet, and lower legs and usually require ambulatory aids by the second or third decade. The physical findings are diffuse hyporeflexia and distal wasting. Electromyography shows typical features of denervation in the distal muscles. This disorder resembles that of the neuronal form of Charcot-Marie-Tooth disease; however, there is no sensory involvement and the inheritance is probably recessive rather than dominant.

Scapuloperoneal spinal muscular atrophy is a rare disorder, with onset in the second or third decade, and is characterized by proximal weakness in the upper extremities and distal weakness in the lower extremities. Weakness may be distributed throughout other muscles but is not as severe. It resembles scapuloperoneal dystrophy, but the biopsy shows the typical features of a neuropathic disorder as opposed to a myopathic disease.

Fazio-Londe disease, or progressive juvenile bulbar palsy, is a disease which affects the muscles innervated by the cranial nerves. There is marked facial and tongue weakness which begins toward the end of the first decade or early in the second decade. This is a progressive disorder that later involves the spinal cord. Death usually ensues within 5 to 10 years.

The Möbius syndrome is a congenital absence of cranial nerve nuclei. The lower cranial nerves, along with the fourth cranial nerve, are most involved. The children are born with a marked internal strabismus, flattened facial expression, difficulty swallowing, and atrophy of the tongue. Occasionally there is evidence of dysfunction of other parts of the CNS. These children do not have a progressive disease; however, their bulbar weakness is relatively severe.

Neurogenic arthrogryposis multiplex congenita is a congenital disease of multiple joint deformities caused by a neuropathic process. Anterior horn cell disease, radiculopathy, and peripheral nerve disease have all been implicated. There are many other causes of arthrogryposis (see Table 11-2).

Poliomyelitis is seldom encountered since the advent of widespread immunization. Years following paralytic poliomyelitis, patients may experience further progression of muscle weakness. The signs are similar to amyotrophic lateral sclerosis. The cause of the late activation is unknown.

SELECTED READINGS

Byers BK, Banker BQ: Infantile muscular atrophy. Arch Neurol 5:140–164, 1961

Low NL: Spinal muscular atrophy syndromes. Pediatr Ann 6:162–168, 1977

Pearn JH: Classification of spinal muscular atrophies. Lancet Apr, 919–921, 1980

Pearn JH, Wilson J: Acute Werdnig-Hoffmann disease. Arch Dis Child 48:425–430, 1973

Pearn JH, Gardner–Medwin D, Wilson J, et al: A genetic study of subacute and chronic SMA in childhood. J Neurol Sci 227:37–42, 1978

26

NEUROPATHY

Polyneuropathy is a generalized disease of peripheral nerves characterized by muscle weakness, sensory loss, hyporeflexia, and autonomic dysfunction. The severity of one or more of these signs varies with the underlying cause and the type of peripheral nerve involved. Mononeuropathy is a disorder of a single peripheral nerve, and mononeuropathy multiplex is a disorder of multiple single nerves. Radiculopathy is a disease of spinal nerve roots. This chapter reviews the pathophysiology, etiologies, and evaluation of peripheral nerve diseases.

PATHOPHYSIOLOGY

The peripheral nerve is composed of the axonal extension of the neuron and its surrounding myelin sheath. The axon diameter and the degree of myelination varies according to the nerve's specific function (Table 26-1). In general, motor fibers and position and vibratory sensory fibers are the largest and most heavily myelinated peripheral nerves. Autonomic fibers and other sensory fibers are smaller and less myelinated. A peripheral nerve is composed of many nerve fiber types. Myelin is formed from the Schwann cells and enables the nerve fiber to propagate an electrical potential by saltatory conduction, which is much faster than propagation by spreading deplorization. As a result, large myelinated fibers conduct an electrical impulse much more quickly than smaller fibers. The electrodiagnostic hallmark of demyelinating neuropathies is slowed nerve conduction velocities.

As an extension of the neuron, the axon has an excitable membrane and, when depolarized, will propagate an action potential. Special sensory receptors and motor neurons initiate action potentials. The axon transports from the motor neuron metabolic products that are essential for axonal function and "trophic" factors necessary for normal maintenance of muscle function. Without innervation muscle atrophies. After several weeks of denervation the muscle develops denervation hypersensitivity. This causes the major neuropathic features on electromyograph: fibrillations, positive sharp waves, and increased insertional irritability.

The clinical signs of neuropathy reflect the function of the peripheral nerves: weakness, sensory loss, loss of deep tendon reflexes, and autonomic dysfunction. The severity of these findings varies, depending upon the cause, the extent of the disease, and the peripheral nerve's primary function. In many patients, particularly young children, a gait disturbance is an early feature. The high steppage

Table 26-1. Peripheral Nerve Fibers

Type	Diameter (mm)	Conduction Velocity (m/sec)	Function
Motor			
α	12–20	70–120	Skeletal muscle innervation
γ	2–8	10–50	Muscle spindle innervation
Sensory			
Muscle			
Ia	12–20	70–120	Muscle spindle (annulospiral)
Ib	12–20	70–120	Golgi tendon organs
II	6–12	30–70	Muscle spindle (flower spray)
Cutaneous			
A	6–20	30–120	Joint receptors, deep tendon, proprioception
AS	2–6	4–30	Touch, temperature, pain
C	<2	0.5–2	Pain
Autonomic			
Motor			
B	<3	3–30	Preganglionic efferents
C	<1	0.5–2	Postganglionic efferents
Sensory			
A	2–12	4–70	Variable, visceral receptors
C	<2	0.5–2	Visceral receptors

or foot-drop gait is frequently seen in motor neuropathies. In neuropathies principally involving sensory nerves, an ataxic gait and a positive Romberg test may be found. Objective sensory testing is difficult at any age, but particularly in the young child. Patients with chronic neuropathies often have other physical findings as well. Skeletal deformities, such as pes cavus foot deformities, "hammer" toes, and scoliosis may be the presenting complaint, particularly in those with familial neuropathies. Skin ulcerations can occur in the rare hereditary sensory neuropathies.

CLASSIFICATION

There are many methods for classifying neuropathies, including by age of onset, etiology, and clinical progression. Perhaps the best classification is that separating peripheral nerve disease pathophysiologically into either myelinopathic or neuronopathic disorders. Myelinopathies are caused by lack of myelin formation, abnormal myelin synthesis or catabolism, acute inflammatory destruction, and hereditary disorders of chronic myelin destruction (Table 26-2). Myelinopathic disorders affect the large myelinated nerves preferentially so that weakness, position and vibratory sensory loss, and hyporeflexia are the most common findings. Slowed motor nerve conduction velocities are characteristic.

The neuronopathies or axonopathies have many causes (Table 26-3). The majority are associated with acquired metabolic disorders, intoxications, or other systemic disease, although some are inherited. Because the axon is primarily involved, many patients will have decreased pain and temperature sensation and some will have dysesthesias. Many of the conditions listed in Table 26-3

Table 26-2. Myelinopathic Neuropathies

Failure of myelin formation
 Congenital hypomyelinating polyneuropathy
Abnormal myelin synthesis or catabolism
 Metachromatic leukodystrophy
 Krabbe's disease
 Refsum's disease
 Abetalipoproteinemia (vitamin E deficiency)
 Tangier disease
 Fabry's disease
Inflammatory, demyelinating neuropathies
 Guillain-Barré syndrome
 Chronic progressive polyneuropathy
 Chronic relapsing polyneuropathy
 Diphtheric neuropathy
Hereditary demyelinating neuropathies
 Hereditary sensorimotor neuropathies
  Type I: Charcot-Marie-Tooth disease
  Type III: Dejerine-Sottas disease

(Modified from Hobson AK: Peripheral neuropathy in childhood. Pediatr Ann 12:814–820, 1983.)

Table 26-3. Neuronopathic Neuropathies

Metabolic neuropathies
 Vitamin deficiencies: thiamine, niacin, pantothenic acid, vitamin B_{12}, folate
 Systemic disease: uremia, diabetes, multiple myeloma, malignancy
 Inborn errors of metabolism: porphyrias, adrenoleukodystrophy, pyruvate dysmetabolisms
Toxic neuropathies
 Drugs: vincristine, nitrofurantoin, phenytoin, isoniazid, tricyclics
 Chemicals: N-hexane, triorthocresylphosphate, carbon monoxide, acrylamide, hexachlorophene, heavy metals
 Biologic: buckthorn, tic paralysis
Vasculitic neuropathies
 Polyarteritis nodosa
 Lupus erythematosis
 Rheumatoid arthritis
 Sjögren's syndrome
 Hypersensitivity angiitis
Hereditary neuropathies
 Hereditary amyloid neuropathy
 Hereditary sensorimotor neuropathies
 Hereditary sensory neuropathies
 Familial dysautonomia
 Ataxia-telangiectasia
 Friedreich's ataxia
 Giant axonal neuropathy
Infectious neuropathies
 Herpes zoster
 Leprosy

(Modified from Hobson AK: Peripheral neuropathy in childhood. Pediatr Ann 12:814–820, 1983.)

Table 26-4. Electrodiagnostic Abnormalities in Neuropathies

Conduction Studies	Myelinopathies	Neuronopathies
Conduction velocity	Marked decrease	Normal to mild decrease
Latency	Marked delay	Minimal delay
Amplitude	Marked reduction	Dispersion
Electromyography		
Denervation hypersensitivity	Variable[a]	Marked increase
Recruitment	Variable[a]	Decreased
Motor units	Variable[a]	Polyphasic

[a] Depends upon concomitant axonal involvement.

are actually quite rare in children. Neuropathy of diabetes, carcinoma, multiple myeloma, and the porphyrias are mainly adult diseases. The most common toxic polyneuropathy in childhood is from vincristine, because of its widespread use in chemotherapy. Electrodiagnostic studies, electromyography and nerve conduction velocities, are essential for separating the two types of disorders (Table 26-4).

CLINICAL SYNDROMES

It is impossible to cover every cause of neuropathy in detail; however, there are some that are encountered more frequently and should be discussed specifically.

Mononeuropathies

Mononeuropathies can be divided into inflammatory, entrapment, traumatic, and vasculitic neuropathies (Table 26-5). The most common inflammatory mononeuropathy is Bell's palsy. This may occur at any time during childhood and usually has an abrupt onset. The exact etiology is unknown, but it is thought to be a postinfectious event. The physical findings depend upon the completeness of the seventh cranial nerve injury. It is important to document that the facial paralysis involves both the upper and lower portions of the face, differentiating this disease from upper motor neuron facial hemiparesis. The condition lasts from weeks to months, and recovery can generally be anticipated. The role of steroids and transcutaneous stimulation in the treatment of this disorder is somewhat controversial.

There are many entrapment neuropathies. The most common is the carpal tunnel syndrome, caused by entrapment of the median nerve. Pain and weakness in the hand are the usual symptoms, and electrodiagnostic studies show conduction block at the wrist. Carpal tunnel syndrome may be associated with rheumatoid arthritis and other systemic diseases, as well as with certain occupations or activities. It is caused by hypertrophy of the synovial sheaths and muscle fibers which accompany the nerve in the carpal tunnel. Relief may be obtained by splinting the wrist, although surgical release is often necessary. Other

Table 26-5. Mononeuropathy and Mononeuropathy Multiplex

Inflammatory mononeuropathies
  Facial nerve: Bell's palsy
  Brachial plexitis
  Lumbar plexitis
Entrapment mononeuropathies
  Median nerve: carpal tunnel syndrome
  Ulnar nerve: medial epicondyle, Guyon's canal
  Radial nerve: "Saturday night palsy"
  Lateral femoral cutaneous nerve: meralgia paresthetica
  Sciatic nerve: sciatica
  Peroneal nerve: fibular head
  Posterior tibial: tarsal tunnel syndrome
  Spinal roots: radiculopathy
  Brachial nerves: thoracic outlet syndrome, brachial plexus syndrome
  Lumbar, sacral nerves: cauda equina syndrome
  Cranial nerves: skeletal dysplasias
Vascular mononeuropathies
  Acute, chronic meningitis
  Vasculitides: lupus, rheumatoid arthritis, etc.
  Systemic diseases: amyloidosis, diabetes
Traumatic neuropathies
  Mononeuropathy
  Plexus neuropathies
  Reflex autonomic dystrophy
Hereditary, recurrent mononeuropathies: tomaculus neuropathy

entrapment syndromes involving virtually all peripheral nerves have been described.

Traumatic mononeuropathies are usually obvious because of the history or physical signs of trauma. If the nerve has been completely severed (neurotmesis), then recovery will be slow and usually incomplete. If the nerve sheath has been preserved but the axon damaged (axonotmesis), then recovery depends upon regrowth of the axon, which usually occurs at a rate of 1 to 3 mm/day and may be complete. Recovery from compression of the peripheral nerve without axonal damage (neuropraxia) usually is a matter of days to weeks.

Occasionally a vasculitis will cause a mononeuropathy. In the pediatric setting the most common vasculitic mononeuropathies are those associated with meningitis, in which one or more cranial nerves may be involved. These are most frequently the sixth, seventh, and eighth cranial nerves. Recovery of facial and ocular motility weakness is usually complete; however, eighth nerve dysfunction may not recover.

Mononeuropathy multiplex is rare in children. In adults, periarteritis nodosa is particularly common, and it can be seen in other vasculitic disorders. Multiple cranial nerve neuropathies are very common in chronic infectious meningitis, carcinomatous meningitis, and in those rare conditions such as mucopolysaccharidoses which cause an abnormal growth of the skull with entrapment of the cranial nerves at their cranial foramina.

Brachial plexitis presents with peripheral nerve dysfunction in the upper extremities which, on careful neurologic exam, can be traced to the proximal cervical roots and brachial plexus. This condition often begins with pain in the shoulder or arm followed by weakness, particularly in the muscles supplied by the upper portion of the brachial plexus and the C5 and C6 roots. In approximately one-third of cases the condition will be bilateral. Recovery takes place over several months.

Polyneuropathy

The syndrome of polyneuropathy is usually easily diagnosed and can be divided into acute and chronic disorders. The prototype of acute polyneuropathy is the Guillain-Barré syndrome, which is an inflammatory neuropathy, probably of immune origin. This affects all children of both sexes, with an incidence of about 2 to 3 per 100,000 per year. There may be some sensory complaints of pain or discomfort in the extremities at the beginning of this syndrome. Weakness then ensues quickly in an ascending fashion, from the lower extremities to the upper extremities. In some cases the upper extremities or the cranial nerves are involved first. Progression reaches a maximum deficit over several weeks to a month. This is followed by a plateau phase and gradual recovery over several months. The weakness may be quite severe, requiring ventilatory support in 10 to 30 percent of cases; 30 to 40 percent have cranial nerve weakness. Autonomic dysfunction, particularly tachyarrhythmias, can occur and can be life threatening. In some children, the sensory component is more prominent than the motor component, such that in the early stages the child may be ataxic.

Diagnosis of the Guillain-Barré syndrome is based upon the clinical presentation and laboratory studies. An elevated cerebrospinal fluid protein is found in almost every case but may not be present until 5 to 7 days into the disease. Electrodiagnostic studies are usually abnormal as well, but again may take several weeks before being definitive. There is no evidence that steroids improve the course of the disease. Plasmapheresis has been shown to improve the short-

Table 26-6. Differential Diagnosis of Acute Polyneuropathy

Encephalopathy
  Acute cerebellar ataxia
Myelopathy
  Cord compression
  Transverse myelitis
  Poliomyelitis
Polyneuropathy
  Guillain-Barré syndrome
  Diphtheria
  Porphyria
  Tic paralysis
Myasthenic disorders
  Botulism, other toxins
  Myasthenia gravis
Myopathies
  Acute polymyositis
  Acute rhabdomyolysis
  Periodic paralysis

Table 26-7. Differential Diagnosis of Chronic Neuropathy

Myelopathy
   Cord compression
   Tethered cord

Anterior horn cell
   Spinal muscular atrophy

Polyneuropathy
   Disimmune polyneuropathies
      Chronic progressive
      Chronic relapsing
   Hereditary polyneuropathies
      Hereditary sensorimotor neuropathies
         Type I Charcot-Marie-Tooth disease (demyelinating)
         Type II (Charcot-Marie-Tooth disease (neuronal)
         Type III Dejerine-Sottas disease
         Type IV Refsum's disease
      Hereditary sensory neuropathies
   Toxic neuropathies (see Table 26-3)
   Vasculitic neuropathies (see Table 26-3
   Acquired metabolic neuropathies
      Vitamin deficiencies
      Uremia
      Diabetes
   Inborn errors of metabolism (see Tables 26-2 and 26-3)
   Infectious neuropathies
      Herpes zoster
   Leprosy

Myasthenic disorders
   Myasthenia gravis
   Congenital myasthenias
Myopathies
   Muscular dystrophies
   Inflammatory myopathies
   Metabolic myopathies

term prognosis. In general, recovery is complete. A variant of the Guillain-Barré syndrome called the Fisher syndrome, is associated with ophthalmoplegia and ataxia. The differential diagnosis of acute polyneuropathy is listed in Table 26-6.

Chronic relapsing polyneuropathy and chronic progressive neuropathy show laboratory and clinical findings similar to those of acute Guillain-Barré syndrome. These disorders may respond to steroid therapy.

Charcot-Marie-Tooth disease is the most common chronic progressive neuropathy seen in childhood. The onset of clumsiness along with foot deformities or scoliosis occurs in the first decade. Diagnosis is usually made between 10 and 16 years of age, frequently because of the foot deformities. These patients have distal weakness, areflexia, and sensory loss. A positive family history is usually present, since this is a dominantly inherited disease in the majority of patients. The parents may be asymptomatic, however, and electrodiagnostic testing may be necessary to diagnose their disease. In the myelinopathic form (type I) of the disease, the conduction velocity is markedly slowed. In the neuronopathic form (type II) the conduction velocity is minimally slowed but there are marked

Table 26-8. Evaluation of Polyneuropathy in Children

History and Evaluation	Diagnosis
Acute	
Cerebrospinal protein increased	Guillain-Barré syndrome
If cerebrospinal fluid normal, consider	
Antinuclear bodies, erythrocyte sedimentation rate, etc.	Vasculitides
Urine porphyrins[a]	Porphyria
Immunization history	Diphtheria
Chronic	
Dominant family history	
EDS,[b] myelinopathic	Hereditary sensorimotor neuropathy I (Charcot-Marie-Tooth)
EDS, neuronopathic	Hereditary sensorimotor neuropathy II
Recessive or X-linked family history	
EDS, myelinopathic	
Acanthocytes, serum	Abetalipoproteinemia, Tangier disease
Lipoproteins, serum phytanic acid	Refsum's disease
Nerve biopsy	
Hypertrophic	Hereditary sensorimotor neuropathy III (Dejerine-Sottas), Refsum's disease
Hypomyelinating	Congenital neuropathy
Storage	Metachromatic leukodystrophy, Krabbe's disease
Demyelinization	Fabry's disease, abetalipoproteinemia, Tangier disease
Lysosomal enzymes	
Arylsulfatase A	Metachromatic leukodystrophy
Galactocerebrosidase	Krabbe's disease
Ceremide trihexosidase	Fabry's disease
EDS, neuronopathic	Hereditary sensory neuropathy
Sporadic (consider chronic and recessive or X-linked family history)	
EDS, myelinopathic	Chronic disimmune neuropathy
	Chronic progressive
	Chronic relapsing
EDS, neuronopathic	
Heavy metals, toxin screen	Toxic neuropathy
Antinuclear bodies, erythrocyte sedimentation rate, etc.[a]	Vasculitic neuropathy
Vitamin levels	Nutritional neuropathy
Chemistries	Uremia, diabetes
Immunoelectrophoresis[a]	Multiple myeloma

[a] Rare before puberty.
[b] EDS = electrodiagnostic studies.

electromyographic findings of denervation. The other hereditary sensorimotor neuropathies include Dejerine-Sottas disease (type III), which is similar to Charcot-Marie-Tooth disease but presents at a much earlier age, and Refsum's disease (type IV), discussed in Chapter 20.

The Riley-Day syndrome, or familial dysautonomia, is a hereditary sensory neuropathy which presents in young children of Jewish background with failure to thrive, frequent fevers, abnormal sweating, and absent fungiform papillae of the tongue. Intradermal injection of histamine (0.1 ml of a 1:1,000 dilution) causes a wheal to form, but no surrounding flair. In normal persons the flair develops because of reflex vasodilatation. The hereditary sensory neuropathies are quite rare. These children present with complete insensitivity to pain, Charcot joints, and other evidence of neglected trauma. The differential diagnosis of chronic neuropathy is listed in Table 26-7.

EVALUATION

The evaluation begins with a history to determine whether the disorder is acute or chronic to establish the differential diagnosis. The family history is important for sorting out hereditary from acquired disorders. The physical examination differentiates other disorders of the motor unit and CNS from peripheral nerve disease. Excluding a compressive myelopathy is the most important part of the examination. A careful search for ticks in any child who presents with neuropathy (tick paralysis) during the spring and summer months should be part of the physical examination. Electrodiagnostic studies are almost always indicated to differentiate neuronopathic from myelinopathic disorders. In acute neuropathies a lumbar puncture is needed for measurement of the spinal fluid protein. Other laboratory studies are contingent upon the above findings. In rare cases a diagnostic peripheral nerve biopsy may be necessary. This is most useful in myelinopathic disorders and rarely in neuronopathic disorders, and it should be performed at a center familiar with peripheral nerve pathology. Table 26-8 outlines a general approach to the evaluation.

TREATMENT

There are limited therapies for the treatment of neuropathies. Removal of offending toxins, treatment of systemic disease, and supporting vital signs with acute disease are the mainstays of therapy. Patients who have chronic relapsing or chronic progressing neuropathy associated with increased spinal fluid protein and patients with vasculitides frequently respond to prednisone, 1 to 2 mg/kg/day. Alternate-day therapy should be instituted when a clinical response occurs. The dose should be slowly tapered to about 0.5 mg/kg every other day and continued for about 6 months after recovery. In rare nutritional causes of neuropathies, the replacement of appropriate vitamins will reverse the syndrome. The only treatable metabolic disease is Refsum's disease, in which the restriction of dietary chlorophyll improves the prognosis. Plasmapheresis for the treatment of the Guillain-Barré syndrome in children has not been studied extensively but it does appear to be effective in adults.

SELECTED READINGS

Axelrod FB, Pearson J: Congenital sensory neuropathies. Am J Dis Child 138:947–954, 1984

Byers RK, Taft LT: Chronic peripheral neuropathy in childhood. Pediatrics 20:517–537, 1957

Evans OB: Polyneuropathy in childhood. Pediatrics 64:96–105, 1979

Gamstorp I: Polyneuropathy in childhood. Acta Pediatr Scand 57:230–238, 1968

Hobson AK: Peripheral neuropathy in childhood: an update in diagnosis and management. Pediatr Ann 12:814–820, 1983

Tucker WG, Chutorian AM: Chronic polyneuritis of childhood. J Pediatr 74:699–708, 1969

27

MYASTHENIC DISORDERS

The myasthenic disorders are a group of diseases which are characterized by a dysfunction of the neuromuscular junction. Prevalence in the general population is approximately 5 per 100,000, and 20 percent have the onset before adulthood. More is known about the myasthenic disorders than any other neuromuscular disease. The results of intensive research have led to specific therapies which usually ameliorate the symptoms and frequently eradicate the disease.

PATHOPHYSIOLOGY

The neuromuscular junction consists of the terminal portion of the motor nerve and the endplate region of the muscle separated by the synaptic cleft (see Fig. 24-1). The action potential originates in the anterior horn cell and is propagated down the axon of the motor nerve. Depolarization of the nerve terminus opens calcium channels, which causes the release of acetylcholine into the synaptic cleft. Acetylcholine is synthesized in the nerve terminal from acetyl coenzyme A and choline and then packaged in small vesicles. Release of acetylcholine into the synaptic cleft allows the acetylcholine molecules to interact with the acetylcholine receptor on the muscle endplate. The receptor is a specialized protein located in the plasma membrane of the muscle fiber. This interaction alters the permeability to ions in the region of the acetylcholine receptor, causing localized depolarization of the endplate. If a sufficient number of interactions occur, then the summation of the depolarization reaches the threshold potential for the excitable muscle membrane. Once this threshold potential has been achieved, a muscle action potential is generated which is propagated along the muscle plasma membrane and into the interior of the muscle fiber by the T tubules. This initiates the muscle contraction by causing the release of calcium from the sarcoplasmic reticulum which in turn causes the interaction of actin and myosin. This process is called an excitation contraction coupling. Depolarization ceases with hydrolysis of the acetylcholine molecule by the enzyme acetylcholinesterase, which is located in the synaptic cleft. Neuromuscular transmission can fail if insufficient acetylcholine is released or if there are insufficient numbers of acetylcholine receptors to interact with the acetylcholine. Neuromuscular transmission failure can also be due to depolarization block caused by inhibition of acetylcholinesterase.

Myasthenic disorders disrupt one or more of these processes. The most common form of myasthenia, myasthenia gravis, is an autoimmune disease in which an immune globulin interferes with the number and function of the acetylcholine receptors. These antibodies not only cause destruction and increased turnover of the acetylcholine receptors but also may block the interaction between acetylcholine and the receptor. The origin of antibody production is not entirely known, although the thymus gland plays a role. The thymus may stimulate antibody production by sensitizing specific lymphocytes to produce the antibody against the acetylcholine receptor. A high percentage of patients with myasthenia gravis will show thymic hyperplasia, and myasthenia gravis is relatively common in patients who have thymic tumors.

Botulinum toxin causes botulism by inhibiting the release of acetylcholine from the nerve terminals. The Eaton-Lambert syndrome, a paraneoplastic syndrome, also causes a dysfunction in acetylcholine release. This condition has been reported only rarely in children. The congenital myasthenias are a group of disorders which are recessively inherited and represent an inborn error of metabolism in the synthesis, release, or interaction of acetylcholine with the acetylcholine receptor or the specific ion channels they regulate.

Defects in neuromuscular transmission can be shown electrophysiologically. The repetitive stimulation test usually shows a decrement in the amplitude of the muscle action potential when the motor nerve is repetitively stimulated, indicating transmission failure. These changes can be augmented by having the patient first perform ischemic exercise. The classic finding in myasthenia gravis is at least a 10 percent decrease in subsequent action potentials with repetitive stimulation (decremental response).

CLASSIFICATION AND CLINICAL FEATURES

The myasthenic disorders can be classified based on their clinical presentation and underlying pathophysiology (Table 27-1).

Juvenile Myasthenia Gravis

Juvenile myasthenia gravis is essentially the same disease as that of adults and is caused by autoimmune injury. The onset is never before the first year and is after 10 years in the majority of cases. More females are affected than males. The most common presentation is ptosis or diplopia, but rarely the disease presents with sparing of the ocular muscles. Very rarely a child will present with an acute fulminating disease progressing to respiratory paralysis over 24 hours. In children in which the disease does begin with the ocular musculature, most will develop generalized disease. Ocular myasthenia describes the group with the symptoms and signs restricted to the ocular muscles. Regardless of the distribution of weakness, the key features are susceptibility to fatigue and a waxing and waning quality. Persistent or repetitive movements are particularly affected. The patient may claim a worsening of symptoms at particular times of the day. This differs from other neuromuscular disorders, in which the symptoms are relatively constant.

Table 27-1. Myasthenic Syndromes

Immune-mediated myasthenias
  Juvenile myasthenia gravis
    Ocular myasthenia
    Acute fulminating myasthenia
    Generalized myasthenia
  Transitory neonatal myasthenia
Familial myasthenias
  Congenital myasthenia
  Familial infantile myasthenia
  Limb-girdle myasthenia
Myasthenia syndromes associated with systemic disease
  Paraneoplastic syndrome (Eaton-Lambert syndrome)
  Hyperthyroidism, hypothyroidism
  Connective tissue disease
    Lupus
    Rheumatoid arthritis
  Drug-induced
    Trimethadione
    Penicillamine

Examination shows evidence of generalized weakness in the majority of patients. Also, most patients will show some defect in extraocular motility or ptosis. Having the patient look upward is the easiest method to demonstrate fatiguability of the ocular muscles. Holding the arms outstretched or walking up stairs will also demonstrate easy fatiguability. After a brief rest the patient may be able to resume that activity for a short period of time. Reflexes are spared.

The remainder of the neurologic examination is normal. The diagnosis of myasthenia gravis is best made by performing a Tensilon test. Tensilon (edrophonium) is a short-acting and potent acetylcholinesterase inhibitor. By inhibiting acetylcholinesterase one increases the availability of acetylcholine, thus improving the chance for an interaction of acetylcholine with its receptor and the possibility of a successful neuromuscular transmission. The drug is given at a dose of 0.2 mg/kg intravenously, or 10 mg maximum. A test dose of 1/10 the total dose is given initially and the patient is monitored for heart rate and blood pressure. Some patients will be sensitive to the drug, and cardiac arrest can occur. If there are no complications with the test dose, then the full dose is given. Rapid improvement usually follows within 10 minutes and is sustained for several minutes thereafter. In questionable cases it is often useful to do this as a double-blind test.

Repetitive stimulation demonstrates the definitive electrophysiologic abnormality. A skilled examiner can make the diagnosis in the majority of patients, particularly if ischemic exercise is used and more than one muscle tested. The characteristic decremental response and post-tetanic fasciculation are diagnostic. These abnormalities can be reversed by the administration of Tensilon. In 80 to 90 percent of patients who have generalized symptoms, circulating anti-acetylcholine receptor antibodies can be detected. The antibody titer has a loose correlation with the severity of the symptoms.

Treatment of myasthenia gravis is directed toward immunologic suppression

Table 27-2. Commonly Used Drugs in the Treatment of Myasthenic Disorders

Drug	Available Dose	Dosage	Frequency
Edrophonium chloride (Tensilon)	10 mg/ml	0.2 mg/kg iv	
Neostigmine bromide (Prostigmin)	15-mg tablet	7.5–15 mg/dose po	3–4 hours
Neostigmine methylsulfate (Protstigmin)	0.25, 0.5, 1.0 mg/ml	0.04 mg/kg im	3–4 hours
		0.02 mg/kg iv	
Pyridostigmine bromide (Mestinon)	60-mg tablet	30–60 mg/dose po	4–6 hours
Prednisone	1-, 2.5-, 5-, 20-, 20-, 50-mg tablets	2–3 mg/kg/day	alternate day

and improving neuromuscular transmission (Table 27-2). In the rare fulminating disease, acetylcholinesterase inhibitors can be life saving. Neostigmine, 7.5 to 15 mg tid, or pyridostigmine, 30 to 60 mg every 4 to 6 hours, is recommended. At higher doses, one may get muscarinic effects and atropine may be needed. Definitive therapy, however, is a combination of thymectomy and immunosuppression. Thymectomy should be performed as soon as the patient is clinically stable and followed by a high dose of prednisone, 2 to 3 mg/kg/day. After approximately 1 week this can be changed to alternate day therapy and gradually tapered as the symptoms improve. Maintenance therapy, usually between 5 and 15 mg of prednisone every other day, may be required for several years. In some patients, however, symptoms persist and there is a need for the addition of either acetylcholinesterase inhibitors or other forms of immunosuppression, including plasmapheresis and chemotherapy. Myasthenias that complicate systemic disease usually respond to acetylcholinesterase inhibitors and treatment of the underlying disease.

The prognosis is relatively good. Twenty percent of patients with myasthenia gravis undergo a spontaneous remission within 2 years of the onset of their disease. Almost all, however, have pure ocular myasthenia. With generalized myasthenia gravis the combination of thymectomy and immunosuppression results in permanent remission in 60 to 70 percent of patients.

Transitory Neonatal Myasthenia

Transitory neonatal myasthenia presents at birth in infants born to mothers with myasthenia gravis. Approximately 12 percent of pregnant mothers with myasthenia gravis will have children with this syndrome. This is caused by the transplacental passage of the IgG antireceptor antibodies. The severity of the mother's illness is not necessarily correlated with that of the infant's. In the great majority, the weakness presents in the first day of life, with difficulty in sucking, generalized weakness and hypotonia, and respiratory insufficiency. Ptosis or ocular motility problems occur in only 15 percent. The mean duration of symptoms averages approximately 2 weeks but may persist for several months.

Tensilon is given subcutaneously for diagnosis and there is usually a dramatic improvement of symptoms within several minutes. With severe disease, anticholinesterase therapy may be indicated until the disease naturally abates with time. Administration of 0.1 mg of neostigmine methylsulfate 15 to 20 minutes before feeding usually ensures sufficient strength for eating purposes. In very severe cases plasmapharesis has been used successfully to treat the disease. The prognosis is excellent for recovery and subsequent normal development.

Congenital Myasthenic Syndromes

The key features of congenital myasthenia are the onset of symptoms shortly after birth, evidence for recessive inheritance without the mother having myasthenia, and prominent involvement of the extraocular muscles. In other cases there is generalized weakness, compromised respiration or feeding, as well as severe impairment of ocular motility. These conditions tend to be chronic without spontaneous remission and resistant to a variety of therapies, although patients may improve with anti-acetylcholinesterase therapy.

Familial infantile myasthenia is similar to congenital myasthenia except that ocular motility is usually spared and there is generalized muscle weakness and respiratory distress. These patients do have a tendency to spontaneous remission, although late recurrence of apnea and sudden death may occur with infection. Infants with this disorder improve an anti-acetylcholinesterase therapy.

Limb-girdle myasthenia is an unusal disorder with onset in adolescence in which there is rapidly progressive symmetric proximal weakness with ocular sparing. The distribution of the weakness and clinical progression suggest a myopathic process, and, indeed, occasional electromyographic studies have suggested a myopathy. However, repetitive stimulation shows a decremental response and there is a positive response to Tensilon. A familial incidence of this disease suggests genetic transmission. These patients do respond to the usual therapies for myasthenia gravis. The etiology is not known.

Eaton-Lambert Syndrome

The Eaton-Lambert syndrome has been reported rarely in children. It differs from myasthenia gravis in that the ocular muscles are usually spared, and it is caused by impaired release of acetylcholine from the nerve terminal. Electrophysiologic studies show an incremental response rather than a decremental response to repetitive stimulation. Patients may respond to guanidine, which facilitates acetylcholine release, rather than to acetylcholinesterase inhibitors. The syndrome also remits with removal of the tumor.

Botulism

Botulinum toxin is produced by *Clostridium botulinum* and is one of the most potent toxins known. The toxin disrupts acetylcholine synaptic transmission, causing both severe weakness and autonomic dysfunction. The parasympathetic system is involved more than the sympathetic because both pre- and postganglionic transmissions are cholinergic. Signs of sympathetic overflow include tachycardia, constipation, and urinary retention. The weakness can be severe and persist for weeks.

Infantile botulism differs from the adult disease in that the organism proliferates in the intestines and releases the toxin. In adults, the toxin is a contamination of ingested foods. The diagnosis can be made by demonstrating the toxin in the blood or culturing the organism from the stool in infants. There is no specific treatment, although guanidine has been reported to improve muscle strength.

Neuromuscular Toxins

A number of pharmacologic agents interfere with neuromuscular transmission. These can cause an acute toxic illness and confuse or compound existing disorders such as myasthenia or botulism by increasing the degree of neuromuscular transmission failure (Table 27-3). There are also a number of synthetic and naturally occurring substances that cause irreversible neuromuscular block or inhibition of acetylcholinesterase. The former group includes toxins such as curare and bungarotoxin and synthetic drugs, such as pancuronium and succinylcholine, that are frequently used in general anesthesia. The acetylcholinesterase inhibitors used in the treatment of myasthenias were discussed earlier. In higher dosages, autonomic toxicity can occur. Of greater importance are the organophosphates, such as parathion, which cause prominent autonomic signs as well as muscle paralysis.

Table 27-3. Drugs and Toxins That Interfere with Neuromuscular Transmission

Antibiotics
  Aminoglycosides
    Amikacin
    Gentamicin
    Kanamycin
    Neomycin
    Streptomycin
    Tobramycin
  Polymyxin
  Colistin
Procainamide
Quinidine
Quinine
Chlorpromazine
Propranalol
Diphenylhydantoin
Cholinesterase inhibitors
Orangophosphate insecticides

SELECTED READINGS

Fenichel GM: Clinical syndromes of myasthenia in infancy and childhood. Arch Neurol 35:97–101, 1978

Greer M, Schotland M: Myasthenia gravis in the newborn. Pediatrics 26:101–105, 1960

Rodriguez M, Gomez MR, Howard FM, et al: Myasthenia gravis in children. Long-term follow-up. Ann Neurol 13:504–508, 1983

Sarnat MB, McGarry JD, Lewis JE: Effective treatment of infantile myasthenia gravis by combined prednisone and thymectomy. Neurology 27:550–555, 1977

Snead OC et al: Juvenile myasthenia gravis. Neurology 30:732–736, 1980

28

MYOPATHIES

The muscular dystrophies and related disorders represent some of the most commonly inherited diseases of humans. Despite their high incidence, very little is known of their pathogenesis. This chapter concentrates on those conditions which are common in childhood.

PATHOLOGY

Because the diagnosis of many myopathies is made by the characteristic pathologic features on a muscle biopsy specimen, a brief discussion of muscle histopathology is warranted. An anatomic muscle is surrounded by connective tissue called the epimysium. The muscle is divided into muscle fascicles which are enclosed by the connective tissue of the perimysium. The endomysium is a network of collagen surrounding each muscle fiber. Many myopathies, especially the dystrophies, show connective tissue proliferation and often replacement by fat.

The muscle fiber is a polygonal syncytial cell of about 25 to 75 μm in diameter and up to 50 cm in length. The muscle fiber is enclosed in a cell membrane, or sarcolemma, and the nuclei are normally in the subsarcolemma position. Pathologic features of myopathy include internal nuclei, fiber atrophy, hypertrophy, fiber phagocytosis, basophilic or regenerating fibers, fiber splitting, ring fibers, and connective tissue proliferation and inflammation. Denervation causes marked fiber atrophy.

The muscle fibers have certain physiologic and metabolic properties. Type I fibers are resistant to fatigue but have slow contraction times. They are high in oxidative enzymes. Type II fibers are sensitive to fatigue, have fast contraction properties, and have a primarily glycolytic metabolism. Histochemistry can demonstrate the differences in the muscle fiber types by staining for oxidative and glycolytic enzymes and myosin adenosinetriphosphatase (ATPase) activity (Fig. 28-1). Table 28-1 summarizes the difference in the muscle fiber types.

DIAGNOSIS

The diagnosis of a myopathy is usually made based upon a complaint of weakness. There are many other symptoms which can precede actual muscle weakness and occasionally muscle disease can be diagnosed from seemingly

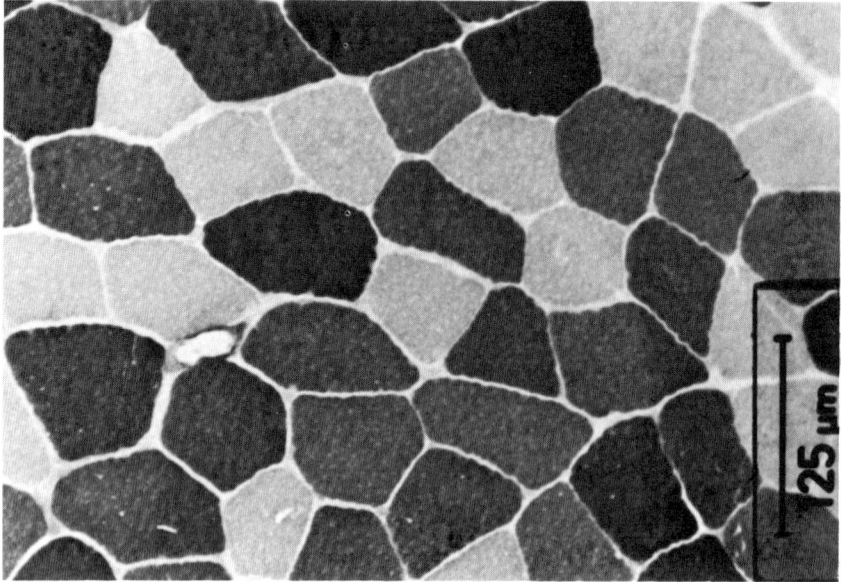

Fig. 28-1. Photomicrograph of normal muscle ATPase histochemical reaction at ph 4.6: type I, dark; type IIa, light; type IIb, intermediate.

unrelated tests. Table 28-1 lists a number of signs and symptoms that are suggestive of a muscle disease.

Of equal importance is the family history. One should ask about specific members of the patient's family and whether they have evidence of muscle weakness such as the use of braces, wheelchairs, and so on. Frequently family members will have been misdiagnosed or be unaware of the exact nature of their disease. It is not uncommon at all for children with dominantly inherited muscle diseases to have parents who deny any symptoms but have the disease.

The physical findings of the myopathies vary with the specific entity. From the general physical examination, such things as heart disease, rash, joint deformities, and cataracts may often suggest a specific diagnosis. In some disorders

Table 28-1. Muscle Fiber-Type Characteristics

Characteristic	Type I	Type IIa	Type IIb
Contraction	Slow	Fast	Fast
Fatigue resistance	High	Intermediate	Low
Metabolism	Oxidative	Oxidative/glycolytic	Glycolytic
Histochemistry			
ATPase pH 9.4	Light	Dark	Dark
ATPase pH 4.6	Dark	Light	Intermediate
ATPase pH 4.3	Dark	Light	Light
NADH-transreductase	Dark	Intermediate	Light
Succinate dehydrogenase	Dark	Intermediate	Light
Phosphorylase	Light	Dark	Light
			Dark

a mild degree of retardation may be present. The most important part of the neurologic exam is the examination of the muscles. Specific findings include atrophy or hypertrophy of muscles, muscle weakness and its distribution, and evidence of myotonia. Myopathies are usually more severe in the proximal muscles. A Gowers' maneuver is usually present (see Fig. 24-2). Unless the muscle weakness is severe, reflexes are usually preserved. Ptosis and weakness in the extraocular muscles are not generally found except in the ocular dystrophies and myotonic dystrophies. Facial muscles and other bulbar muscles may be involved in some myopathies.

Laboratory tests for the evaluation of myopathy include measurement of muscle enzymes, electromyography (EMG), and muscle biopsy. Creatine kinase (CK) and other enzymes, including serum glutamic-oxaloacetic transaminase lactic dehydrogenase, and aldolase, are released from muscle when the cell is injured. Creatinine kinase is more specific for diagnosing muscle disease than the other serum enzymes, although the CK can be nonspecific when only marginally or moderately elevated. The value of the EMG is primarily to exclude other disorders of the motor unit and occasionally to make a specific diagnosis in such disorders as myotonia. The muscle biopsy can often make a specific diagnosis when other tests cannot.

CLASSIFICATION AND CLINICAL FEATURES

One can divide myopathies into the musclar dystrophies, myotonias, metabolic myopathies, and inflammatory myopathies (Table 28-2). Excluded from this discussion will be the congenital myopathies, which are covered in Chapter 11.

MUSCULAR DYSTROPHIES

X-Linked Dystrophies

Duchenne muscular dystrophy is the most common of all muscular dystrophies and occurs in approximately 30 in 100,000 live born males. The disease can be inherited as an X-linked recessive disorder, although one-third of cases are thought to be new mutants. In another one-third of cases there is an obvious family history of X-linked inheritance of the disease, and in the remaining one-third there is no family history but the mother is a carrier or a mutant carrier. Very rarely female carriers will be symptomatic.

Infants can show an elevated CK and an abnormal muscle biopsy at birth, but children are rarely symptomatic before the second to third year. Increasing gait difficulty is the most common presenting symptom. After the third or fourth year, proximal weakness is evidenced by difficulty in climbing stairs, inability to run, and the use of the Gowers' maneuver when getting up from the floor. The disease is more or less progressive but most children are in wheelchairs by

Table 28-2. Classification of the Myopathies

Congenital myopathies
  Fiber-type disproportions
    Congenital fiber-type disproportions
    Myotubular myopathy
    Central core disease
    Nemaline rod myopathy
  Congenital muscular dystrophy
  Congenital myotonic dystrophy

Muscular dystrophies
  X-Linked inherited dystrophies
    Duchenne's muscular dystrophy
    Becker's muscular dystrophy
    Emory-Dreifus
  Recessively inherited dystrophies
    Limb-girdle dystrophy
  Dominantly inherited dystrophies
    Facioscapulohumeral dystrophy
    Ocular syndromes
    Myotonic dystrophy

Myotonias
  Myotonic dystrophy
  Myotonia congenita
  Paramyotonia congenita
  Schwartz-Jampel syndrome

Metabolic myopathies
  Glycogen storage diseases
    Pompe's disease
    Debrancher deficiency
    McArdle's disease
    Other defects in glycolysis
  Carnitine and lipid disorders
    Carnitine deficiency
    Carnitine palmityltransferase deficiency
  Periodic paralysis
    Hypokalemic periodic paralysis
    Hyperkalemic periodic paralysis
    Normokalemic periodic paralysis
    Periodic paralysis associated with thyrotoxicosis
  Mitochondrial myopathies

Inflammatory myopathies
  Childhood dermatomyositis
  Polymyositis
  Inflammatory myopathies associated with connective tissue
    disease
  Infectious myositis

12 to 14 years of age and death occurs in the second or third decade. The usual cause of death is respiratory or cardiac failure.

The physical findings early in the course of the disease are proximal weakness, joint contractures, and pseudohypertrophy of the calves. Flexion contractures of the ankles, knees, and hips and the weakness progress with time. Lordosis and a waddling gait also are typical features. When tested, the majority of patients have below-average IQs but are not severely retarded. Laboratory

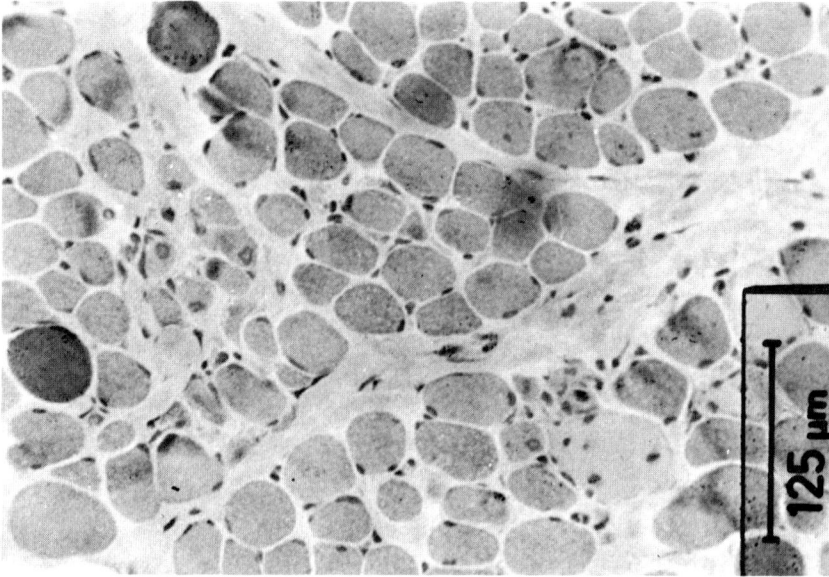

Fig. 28-2. Duchenne dystrophy. The photomicrograph demonstrates connective tissue proliferation, variation in fiber size, and opaque fibers (hematoxylin–eosin stain).

studies show a CK at least 10 times greater than normal. The EMG shows typical myopathic features and the muscle biopsy shows dystrophic changes: increased fat and connective tissue, necrosis, and opaque fibers (Fig. 28-2). The majority of patients will have some abnormalities of cardiac function with cardiac hypertrophy and heart failure, particularly toward the end of their disease. Electrocardiographic abnormalities may be seen earlier which are characterized by tall R waves in the right precordial region and deep Q waves.

A major issue in Duchenne's dystrophy is carrier detection. Until recently, measurement of serum CK in the female was the most specific method. The recommended method is three determinations performed weekly during periods of relative inactivity. Persistent elevation of serum CK is suggestive of a female carrier. This is more likely to be abnormal in younger females. Recently, however, genetic markers on the X chromosome are becoming available and will be much more specific for determining the carrier status. A female is an obligate carrier if there is another male offspring with the disease or if there are males with the disease in previous generations in the mother's pedigree. An obligate carrier is a heterozygote for the disease. Statistically, male children have a 50 percent chance of having the disease and female children a 50 percent chance of being carriers.

Becker muscular dystrophy is the other common X-linked recessive muscular dystrophy and has features similar to those of Duchenne's dystrophy. The incidence is approximately $\frac{1}{10}$ that of Duchenne's dystrophy. The major differences are later onset and slower progression. Most children with Becker mus-

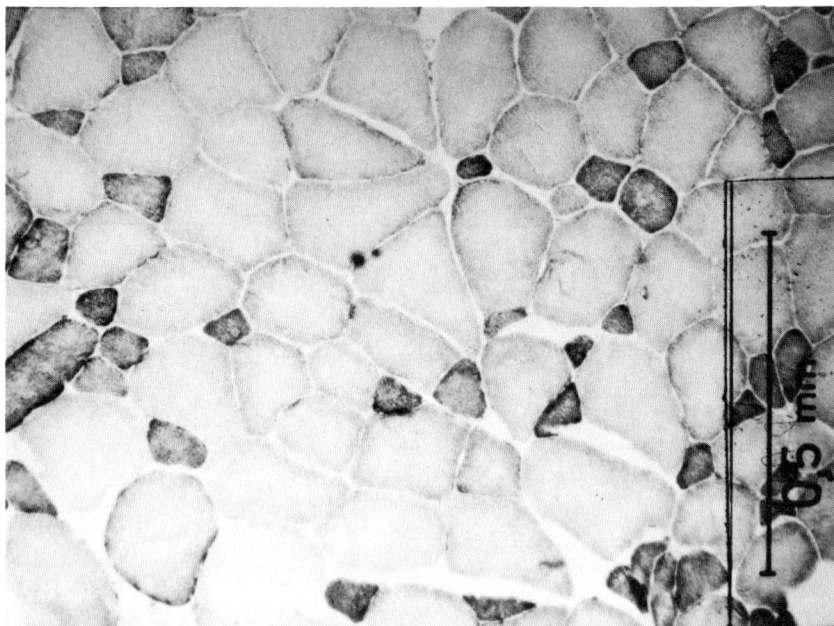

Fig. 28-3. Emery-Dreifuss dystrophy. The photomicrograph demonstrates marked type I fiber atrophy (NADH transreductase).

cular dystrophy have the onset after 6 years of age and survive for many decades. The diagnostic features are very similar to those with Duchenne's dystrophy.

The Emery-Dreifuss disease is another X-linked dystrophy that presents toward the end of the second decade or later. It is characterized by weakness, primarily in the biceps, and heart block. The muscle biopsy shows a characteristic feature of type I fiber atrophy (Fig. 28-3). These patients are at risk for sudden death and frequently require cardiac pacing.

Recessively Inherited Dystrophies

Limb-girdle muscular dystrophy is the most common recessively inherited disorder. There is some debate, however, whether or not this represents a specific entity. The onset is rare before the 10th year. Weakness in the distribution of the proximal girdle muscles is the most common presenting complaint. The course crosses many decades and most patients are able to pursue relatively normal lives. There are no distinctive clinical features on examination other than the weakness and the proximal atrophy. The laboratory studies show a moderately elevated CK, a myopathic EMG, and a muscle biopsy with a mild degree of dystrophic findings, fiber hypertrophy, and more fiber splitting than in most other dystrophies (Fig. 28-4). There is no treatment for the disease.

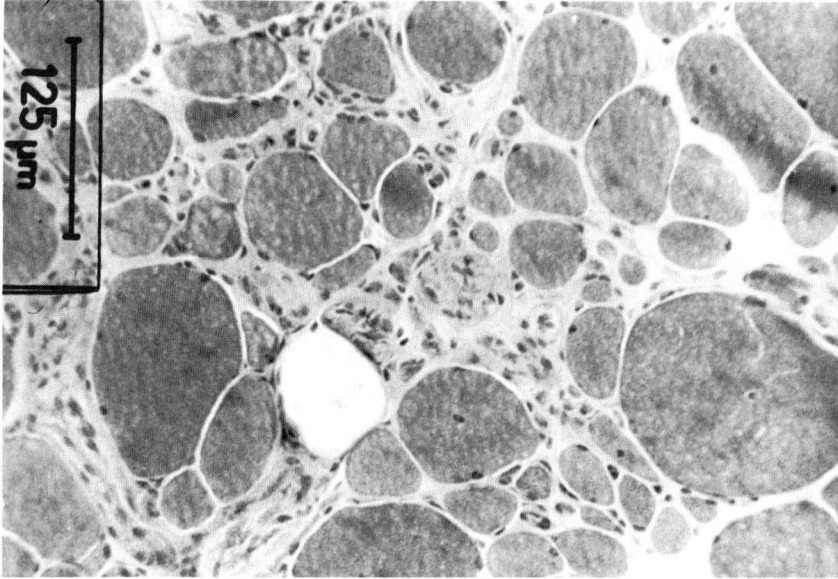

Fig. 28-4. Limb-girdle dystrophy. The photomicrograph demonstrates fiber splitting, fibrosis, and excessive variation in fiber size (hematoxylin–eosin stain).

Dominantly Inherited Muscular Dystrophies

Myotonic dystrophy is the most common dominantly inherited muscular dystrophy. The incidence is approximately 15 in 100,000. The age of onset is usually after the first decade; however it can be congenital. Neonates present with poor sucking and respiratory distress. Only infants born to mothers with myotonic dystrophy are symptomatic at birth. The symptoms with a later onset are weakness in the hands, difficulty walking, and a tendency to fall. Some patients will complain of myotonia at the initial presentation.

The physical features are somewhat distinctive. Patients almost always have ptosis and there may be some slight impairment of ocular motility. The typical facial appearance is due to wasting of the temporalis muscles, which gives a somewhat haggard or "hatchet face" appearance. The patients may have dysarthria because of weakness of the facial muscles and myotonia of the tongue. There is marked weakness and wasting in the limbs, especially distally. Myotonia is the characteristic finding and makes the clinical diagnosis in these patients. Percussion of the tongue or thenar muscles is the best way to elicit the delayed relaxation (percussion myotonia). Having the patient grip tightly and suddenly release or having the patient close his eyes tightly and then open them quickly can also demonstrate myotonia.

Myotonic dystrophy is a systemic disease and has a number of other characteristics. Ninety percent have cataracts by slit-lamp examination, frontal baldness, especially in males, and gonadal atrophy. Impaired pulmonary function, heart disease, and mental deficiency are found in the majority of patients. There

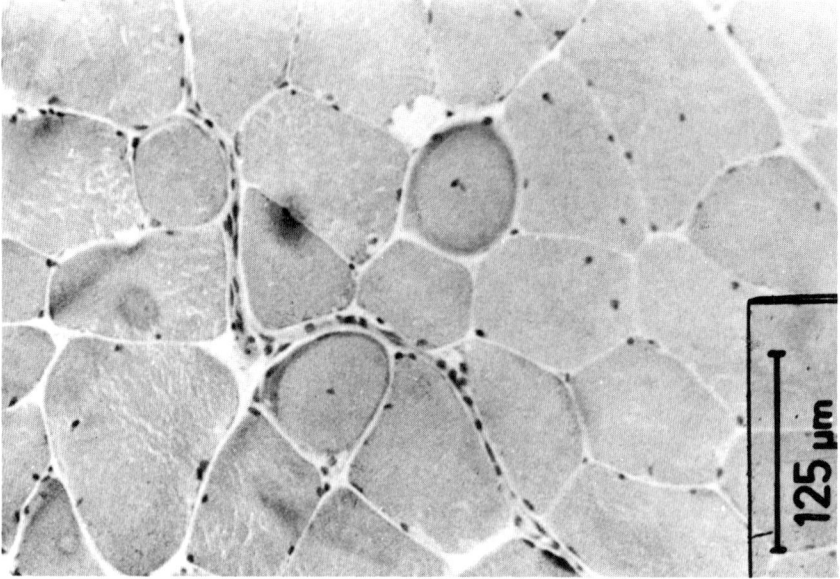

Fig. 28-5. Myotonic dystrophy. The pathologic features are ring fibers and internal nuclei (hematoxylin–eosin stain).

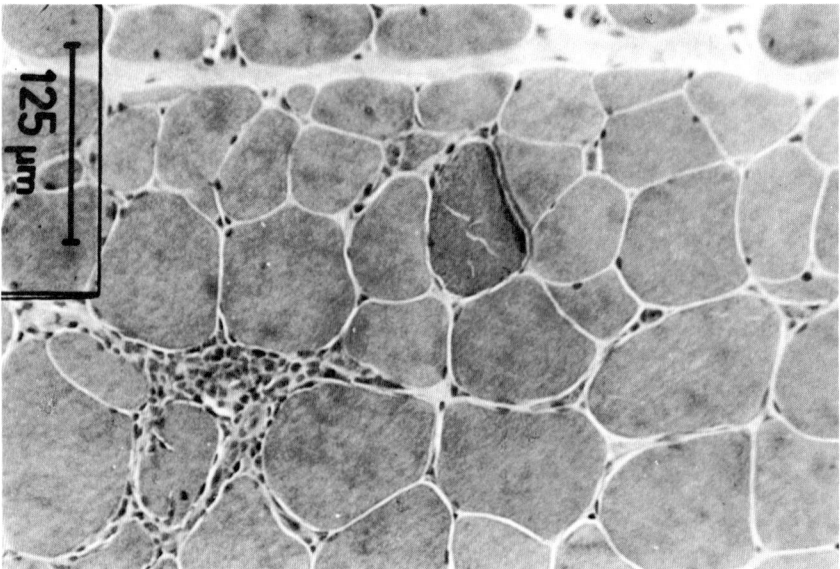

Fig. 28-6. Facioscapulohumoral dystrophy. The pathologic features are relatively minor. Note the small focal area of inflammation.

is a tendency toward diminished fertility with successive generations. There may be a number of minor endocrine disturbances, such as abnormal thyroid function, insulin activity, and menstruation.

The course is one of gradual deterioration over decades. Patients with an earlier onset have a worse prognosis. The diagnosis is made by EMG showing the characteristic high-frequency discharges (dive bomber). The CK may be mildly elevated and biopsy frequently shows type II fiber hypertrophy, ring fibers, and increased numbers of central nuclei (Fig. 28-5).

Facioscapulohumoral muscular dystrophy occurs with an incidence of approximately 5 in 100,000 and the onset is at any age, although it more frequently begins in late childhood or early adulthood. The early symptoms are secondary to facial weakness, with difficulty in blowing up balloons, sucking straws, and other such maneuvers. Marked shoulder weakness usually follows, with winging of the scapulae. Only later does the disease involve the lower extremities. There are no other distinctive clinical features. The laboratory diagnosis is not as specific as in other disorders. The CK may be mildly elevated and the EMG shows mild to moderate myopathic changes. The muscle biopsy is usually nonspecific but may show focal inflammation (Fig. 28-6). The dominant inheritance and the pattern of muscular involvement usually determine the diagnosis. diagnosis.

MYOTONIAS

Myotonia is continued active contraction of muscle fibers persisting after cessation of voluntary effort. It is a disorder of the muscle fiber and is not affected by neuromuscular blockade or peripheral nerve block. The present theory is that there is abnormal chloride conduction in the muscle membrane so that the membrane becomes unstable and tends to spontaneously depolarize.

Myotonic muscular dystrophy was described earlier. The primary clinical feature of the myotonias is painless stiffness of the muscles which is accentuated by rest, cold, or sudden movement. Often there is diffuse hypertrophy of muscles, particularly in myotonia congenita. In patients with paramyotonia, symptoms are most marked in cold weather and may worsen rather than improve with repeated muscle contraction. The Schwartz-Jampel syndrome is characterized by myotonia, skeletal deformities, and short stature, constituting somewhat of a specific syndrome diagnosis. Myotonia can be seen in some of the periodic paralysis.

METABOLIC MYOPATHIES

The periodic paralyses are summarized in Table 28-2. These are relatively rare disorders and are classified based upon the serum potassium level at the time of the attack. Characteristically there is episodic muscle weakness which may last from minutes to days. Although patients are normal between these attacks, there may be progressive weakness following repeated attacks.

The diagnosis can usually be made based upon the family history as well as the examination showing flaccid paralysis during a typical attack. Measurement of the electrolytes will also give a clue to the underlying etiology. Provocative tests should be performed with extreme caution. Challenging the patient with potassium, insulin, and glucose to simulate hyper- or hypokalemia should be performed in an intensive care setting by an experience examiner. The muscle biopsy may show the typical features of a vacuolar myopathy.

The treatment in the emergency situation is to correct the underlying electrolyte abnormalities. One must remember that other causes of hypokalemia may precipitate such attacks and in those cases the underlying disease should be treated. Periodic paralysis associated with hyperthyroidism is extremely rare in children but responds to treatment of the thyroid disease. The mainstay of treatment of familial periodic paralysis is acetazolamide. The dose is approximately 10 to 20 mg/kg/day and is highly effective in preventing attacks.

Glycogen Storage Disease

A number of inborn errors of carbohydrate metabolism have been described, with basically two presentations. The first is a progressive myopathy with storage of glycogen in muscle and occasionally in other tissues. Pompe's disease and debrancher deficiency are examples and are discussed in Chapter 20. The other presentation is one of symptoms with exercise, particularly cramps, weakness, or fatigue.

The other glycogen storage diseases present primarily with exercise induced symptoms and can best be categorized as disorders of energy production. Because of the defects in glycolysis, there is decreased energy production, especially with ischemic exercise. Symptoms are cramps on exercise, fatigue, and myoglobulinuria. If EMG is done during a cramp, it will be electrically silent. The cramp is not due to continued depolarization of the muscle but to the lack of adenosine triphosphate needed to relax the contraction of the actin and myosin. The diagnosis can be made during an ischemic exercise test by showing an inability to produce lactate because of the block in glycolysis. The muscle biopsy may show glycogen storage (Fig. 28-7). Histochemical stains are available for several of these enzymes and specific enzyme analysis can be done on muscle biopsy specimens. There is no specific treatment other than avoidance of strenuous activity and frequent feeding. Patients may experience the so-called second wind phenomenon, in which after fatty acid metabolism has been induced, alternative substrates for muscle fuel are available and the patient can proceed with activities without symptoms. After years of this disease a progressive myopathy may be superimposed on the exercise-related problems.

Disorders of Lipid Metabolism

Carnitine is necessary for the transport of fatty acid acylesters across the mitochondrial membranes. This is facilitated by specific transferases. Muscle carnitine deficiency presents with progressive weakness and cardiomyopathy.

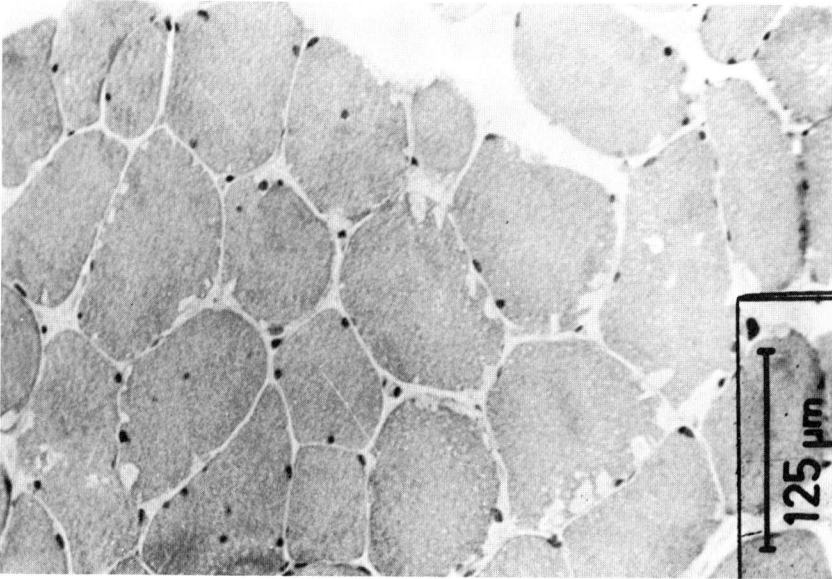

Fig. 28-7. McArdle's disease. Note the marked vacuolization of muscle fibers.

Systemic carnitine deficiency may present with repeated encephalopathies with hypoglycemia similar to Reye's syndrome. Muscle weakness is also present in the systemic type. Carnitine palmityltransferase deficiency has been described in a few patients with weakness and cramps on exercise. The symptoms are more likely to develop after prolonged strenuous exercise, fasting, or exposure to cold, when lipid metabolism is stimulated. The diagnoses of these disorders are made by measuring blood and tissue carnitine or tissue enzyme activities. Carnitine replacement has been helpful in some patients and avoidance of the situations mentioned above may be helpful in carnitine palmityltransferase deficiency.

Mitochondrial Myopathies

There are increasing numbers of infants reported with hypotonia, encephalopathy, and occasionally renal disease and lacticacidosis who are found to have abnormal mitochondria on electron microscopy of muscle. Rarely these patients with severe hypotonia improve with age. There is no known treatment.

Malignant hyperpyrexia can be a familial disease or complicate other myopathic diseases. It is a complication of general anesthesia, usually halothane and succinylcholine. It is characterized by high fever, rigidity, acidosis, and tachycardia. Muscle necrosis is the result and causes myoglobinuria. Intravenous dantrolene usually reverses the disorder. Other causes for myoglobinuria are listed in Table 28-3.

Table 28-3. Myoglobinuria in Childhood

Metabolic disorders
    Myophosphorylase deficiency (McArdle's disease)
    Phosphofructokinase deficiency and other defects of glycolysis
    Carnitine palmityltransferase deficiency
    Malignant hyperthermia
    Hypokalemic periodic paralysis
    Severe hypokalemia
    Diabetes acidosis
Toxins
    Alcohol
    Amphotericin B
    Gluphenazine
    Heroin
    Licorice
    Malayan sea snake venom
    Plasmocid
    Succinylcholine
    Toluene
Physical trauma or stress
    Crush injury
    Electric shock
    Intense muscle exertion
    Ischemia
    Heat stress
    Hypothermia
Inflammatory
    Acute idiopathic polymyositis
    viral myositis
Idiopathic or familial

INFLAMMATORY MYOPATHIES

Childhood dermatomyositis is a systemic disease of the endothelial cells of small arteries, capillaries, and veins. The major targets are skin and muscle and the pathogenesis is thought to be an immune-complex-mediated vasculopathy. It usually begins with generalized malaise, low-grade fever, weight loss, limb pain, and irritability. Contractures of the ankles may appear early and the rash may occur at any time. The rash is characterized by a maculopapular eruption primarily over the extensor surfaces of the limbs and in the malar area (Fig. 28-8). It can be subtle. There may be a violaceous discoloration around the eyes (heliotrope) and splinter hemorrhages under the nails. In some cases the rash will become eczematoid and generalized over the entire body. There is usually no significant muscle pain but children develop a severe weakness which is worse proximally while sparing the ocular and bulbar muscles. The symptoms progress over weeks to months. Untreated, the outcome is usually fatal. Complications include bowel infarctions, cardiac infarctions, and calcinosis universalis (Fig. 28-9). These complications can occur in treated patients.

The clinical diagnosis is made by the history, typical rash, and muscle weakness. The serum CK may or may not be elevated, but the EMG is almost always abnormal and may show both neuropathic and myopathic changes. The muscle biopsy is usually characteristic, showing fiber necrosis, inflammation, and per-

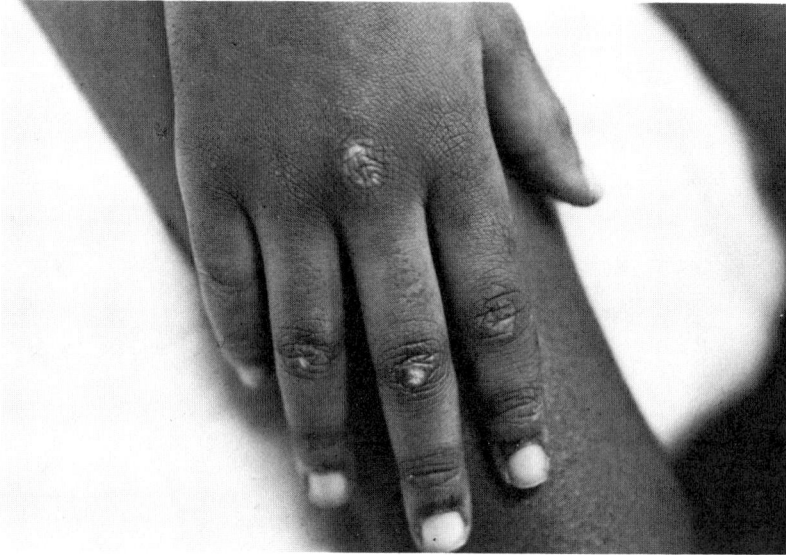

Fig. 28-8. Maculopapular rash over the knuckles in dermatomyositis.

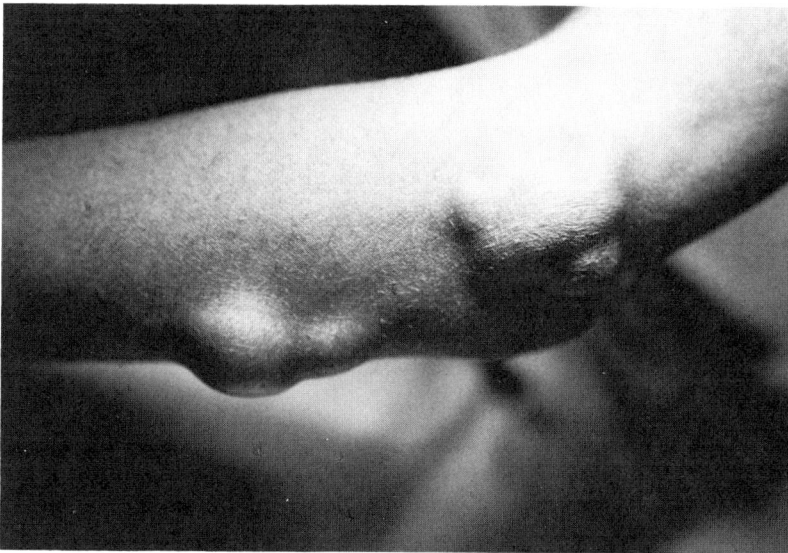

Fig. 28-9. Subcutaneous calcified nodules in a patient in remission with dermatomyositis.

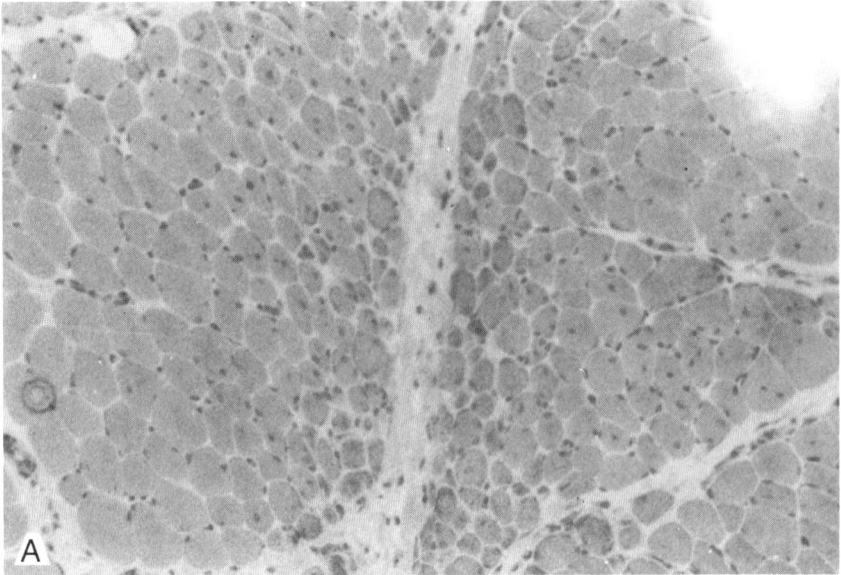

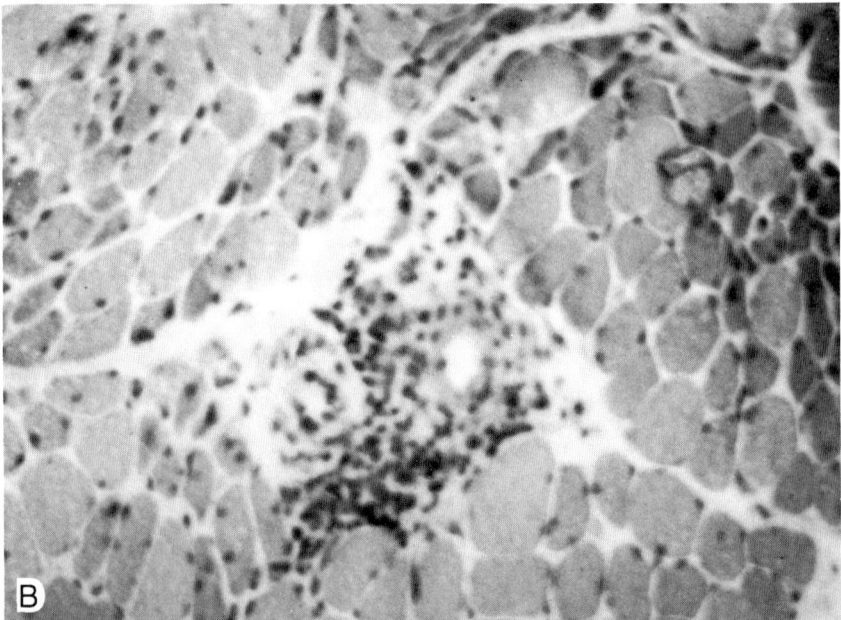

Fig. 28-10. (A) Dermatomyositis. Note the fiber atrophy at the edge of the muscle fasicle. (B) Dermatomyositis with perivascular inflammation.

ifascicular atrophy (Fig. 28-10). Electron microscopy demonstrates the endothelial vascular abnormalities.

The disease is treatable in many cases. Standard therapy is high doses of steroids (2 to 3 mg/kg/day prednisone) until the patient begins to improve or the CK lowers. Treatment can then be switched to alternate-day therapy and gradually tapered until the symptoms are suppressed. Thereapy frequently requires 2 to 3 years of low-dose prednisone (5 to 15 mg) every other day. Unresponsive patients may respond to immunosuppression with other chemotherapeutic drugs or plasmapheresis.

Polymyositis in children is extremely rare and presents with weakness without rash. It should be treated in the same manner. Muscle weakness can occur in association with other vascular diseases, such as lupus, but this is rarely an initial manifestation. Finally, dermatomyositis or polymositis associated with occult neoplasm rarely, if ever, occurs in children.

Other inflammatory myopathies include those due to infections or parasites. The most common infectious myositis is that associated with viral illnesses, particularly influenza. This is a monophasic illness usually following the onset of other symptoms of influenza and characterized by proximal weakness and elevation of CK. Toxoplasmosis and trichinosis can also cause inflammatory myopathies.

Continuous Muscle Contraction

Isaac's syndrome is a rare disorder of continuous fiber activity that causes the muscle to be constantly contracted and firm. Mobility is impaired. The "stiff man" syndrome is similar but more spasmodic and confined to adults. The "rigid spine" syndrome is actually a myopathic disorder but presents with stiffness of the spinal muscles. Dystonias and other extrapyramidal disorders enter into the differential diagnosis.

SELECTED READINGS

Carpenter S, Karpati G, Rothman S, Watters G: The childhood type of dermatomyositis. Neurology 26:952–962, 1976

Dickey RP, Ziter FA, Smith RA: Emery-Dreifuss muscular dystrophy. J Pediatr 104:555–557, 1984

DiMauro S, Bonilla E, Zeviani M: Mitochondrial myopathies. Ann Neurol 17:521–538, 1985

Dodge PR, Gamstorp I, Byers RK, et al: Myotonic dystrophy in infancy and childhood. Pediatrics 35:3–12, 1965

Dyken M, Zeman W, Rusche T: Hypokalemic periodic paralysis. Children with permanent myopathic weakness. Neurology 19:692–696, 1969

King JO, Demborough MA: Anesthetic induced malignant hyperpyrexia in children J Pediatr 83:37–43, 1973

Munsat TL, Pearson CM: The differential diagnosis of neuromuscular weakness in infancy and childhood. Part II. The dystrophic myopathies. Dev Med Child Neurol 9:319–323, 1967

Ringel SP, Carroll JE, Schold SC: The spectrum of mild X-linked recessive muscular dystrophy. Arch Neurol 34:408–412, 1977

Shaw RF, Dreifuss FE: Mild and Severe forms of X-linked muscular dystrophy. Arch Neurol 20:451–456, 1969

Slater GE, Swaiman KF: Muscular dystrophies of childhood. Pediatr Ann 7:170–193, 1977

Spencer CH, Hanson V, Singsen BH, et al: Course of treated juvenile dermatomyositis. J Pediatr 105:399–404, 1984

SECTION 7

Acquired Diseases of the Central Nervous System

There are two major signs of brain injury: focal loss of neurologic function and encephalopathy. Loss of function causes focal neurologic deficits such as hemiparesis. Encephalopathy is a general disturbance of the CNS causing altered consciousness, seizures, and/or behavioral disturbances. The etiologies of brain injury are diverse but the pathogenic mechanisms are relatively few: metabolic, toxic, or physical injury. Aside from seizures, which are discussed in Section 8, the diseases discussed in this section are the most common neurologic problems requiring acute management. More importantly, most of these disorders are treatable and an accurate diagnosis and therapy usually result in a favorable outcome.

29

DISORDERS OF CONSCIOUSNESS

Consciousness is a state of being awake, alert, and appropriately responsive to stimulation; coma is the opposite of consciousness. Between these two states is a continuum of altered states of consciousness (Table 29-1). A condition that causes altered consciousness is often called an "organic brain syndrome," but *encephalopathy* is a more appropriate term. Sleep is a special state of altered consciousness which is normal and most closely resembles stupor; however, the patient can be aroused to consciousness. Except for autonomic functions, consciousness is needed for all other normal activities of the brain, especially higher cortical functions. This chapter discusses the diagnosis and management of the unconscious child and the remainder of this section discusses specific etiologies in more detail.

PATHOPHYSIOLOGY

Altered consciousness results from either diffuse cortical dysfunction or interruption of the reticular activating system which modulates cortical activity. At the cellular level, consciousness is dependent upon the electrical activity of neurons. Interruption of this electrical activity or its transmission to other neurons is the final common pathway of altered consciousness. Neuronal metabolism enables this electrical activity to be processed and transmitted. As in other tissues, neuronal metabolism is involved in substrate utilization for energy production and the synthesis of proteins, lipids, and other complex molecules for cellular structure and metabolism. Neuronal metabolism differs from other cells because of the electrical properties of its cell membrane and the synthesis of neurotransmitters. Many encephalopathies are caused by cytotoxic injury that interferes with neuronal metabolism. Cytotoxic injury can result from direct poisoning of cellular metabolism or by substrate deprivation. Oxygen and glucose are the major substrates for energy production and are a function of cerebral blood flow. Lack of oxygen (anoxia), glucose, or blood flow (ischemia) disrupts energy production, which interferes with the neurons' ability to maintain membrane polarization, synthesize neurotransmitters, and other cellular functions. Cerebral ischemia accompanies many systemic diseases, such as cardiac arrest and shock, as well as CNS diseases, such as increased intracranial pressure and meningitis. Cerebral edema and increased intracranial pressure are common complications of cytotoxic injury.

Table 29-1. Alterations in Consciousness

Lethargy	Mild impairment of consciousness but with reactions and activity subdued
Obtundation	Impairment of consciousness that resembles drowsiness
Stupor	Unconsciousness with difficult arousal and purposeful reaction to stimulation
Coma	Unconsciousness with neither arousal nor purposeful reaction to stimulation
Delirium	Impaired orientation, perception, and reasoning with alertfulness

The other major mechanisms of encephalopathy are caused by alterations of the electrical properties of the cell membrane and interference with neurotransmission. Severe electrolyte disturbances especially interfere with membrane polarization. Toxins can depress or excite neuronal activity by altering the membrane polarization. Others block or enhance neurotransmission, which has the same effect.

Table 29-2 outlines the differential diagnosis of altered consciousness. Most cases of coma are caused by ingestions and acquired metabolic disturbances, as listed in Tables 29-3 and 29-4. One must never underestimate a child's ability to locate, open, and ingest medicines and other toxins located in the home.

DIAGNOSIS AND MANAGEMENT

In the child with altered consciousness, the physical and neurologic examinations are performed first for evidence of a rapidly reversible disorder. When time permits, a complete history is necessary. Historical evidence for injestion, toxic exposure, trauma, substance abuse, and infection are of particular importance. The history preceding the onset of altered consciousness may give

Table 29-2. Differential Diagnosis of
Altered Consciousness

Intoxications
    Accidental poisoning
    Substance abuse
Metabolic disorders
    Acquired
    Inborn errors of metabolism
Trauma
    Accidental
    Child abuse
Increased intracranial pressure
Infection
Postinfectious diseases
Vascular disorders
    Stroke
    Hypertensive encephalopathy
    Atypical migraine
Seizures
    Status epilepticus
    Nonconvulsive status
    Postictus
Hysteria

Table 29-3. Neurologic Signs and Symptoms of Toxic
Ingestions

Ataxia
  Alcohol
  Barbiturates
  Bromides
  Carbon monoxide
  Diphenylhydantoin
  Hallucinogens
  Heavy metals
  Organic solvents
  Tranquilizers
Convulsions and muscle twitching
  Alcohol
  Amphetamines
  Antihistamines
  Boric acid
  Camphor
  Chlorinated hydrocarbon insecticides (DDT)
  Cyanide
  Lead
  Organic phosphate insecticides
  Plants (lily-of-the-valley, azalea, iris, water hemlock)
  Salicylates
  Strychnine
  Withdrawal from barbiturates, benzodiazepines (Valium,
    librium), meprobamate
Coma and drowsiness
  Alcohol
  Antihistamines
  Barbiturates and other hypnotics
  Carbon monoxide
  Narcotic depressants (opiates)
  Salicylates
  Tranquilizers
Paralysis
  Botulism
  Heavy metals
  Plants (coniine in poison hemlock)
  Triorthocresylphosphate
Pupils
  Pinpoint
    Mushrooms (muscarine type)
    Narcotic depressants (opiates)
    Organophosphate insecticides
  Nystagmus on lateral gaze
    Barbiturates
    Minor tranquilizers (meprobamate, benzodiazepine)
  Dilated
    Amphetamines
    Antihistamines
    Atropine
    Barbiturates (coma)
    Cocaine
    Ephedrine
    LSD
    Methanol
    Withdrawal—narcotic depressants

(From Mofenson HC, Greensher J: The unknown poison. Pediatrics
54:336–341. Copyright American Acadmy of Pediatrics 1974.)

Table 29-4. Common Causes of
Metabolic
Encephalopathy

Fluid and electrolyte abnormalities
  Hypo-hypernatremia
  Hypo-hypercalcemia
  Hypo-hypermagnesemia
  Hyperosmolarity
  Water intoxication
Alterations of pH
  Acidosis (any cause)
  Alkalosis (any cause)
Intermediary metabolism
  Hypo-hyperglycemia
  Aminoacidurias
  Organic acidurias
  Lacticacidosis
Azotemia
Hepatic encephalopathy
Reye's syndrome
Endocrine disturbances
  Hypothyroidism
  Diabetic ketoacidosis
Hypothermia

clues to the etiology. Deterioration over days to weeks is often associated with increased intracranial pressure, infection, or chronic intoxication. Acute deterioration is more compatible with ingestions, cerebrovascular accidents, trauma, and metabolic disturbances. Symptoms of focal abnormalities prior to the onset of coma suggests an intracranial mass, cerebrovascular disease, or focal encephalitis. Metabolic and toxic encephalopathies cause diffuse neurologic dysfunction. The past medical history is explored for evidence of systemic disease, recurrent disorders, such as seizures and migraine, and metabolic diseases which can cause altered consciousness. A family history for migraine, epilepsy, or metabolic diseases is equally important.

The general physical examination is performed to determine signs of systemic disease, trauma, and infection. Breath odors, such as in ketosis and hydrocarbons, may lead to a specific diagnosis. Vital signs and measurements must be measured and recorded. The neurologic examination is amended for the degree of cooperation from the patient. The most important part is the documentation of the degree of consciousness. A written description is much more

Table 29-5. Glasgow Coma Scale

Best Motor Response		Verbal Response		Eye opening	
Obeys	6	Oriented	5	Spontaneous	4
Localizes	5	Confused conversation	4	To speech	3
Withdraws	4	Inappropriate words	3	To pain	2
Abnormal flexion/extensor response	3	Incomprehensible sounds	2	Nil	1
Nil	1	Nil	1		

(Modified from Jennett B, Teasdale G: Aspects of coma after severe head injury. Lancet 1:878–881, 1977.)

Table 29-6. Neurologic Signs of Herniation Syndrome

Herniation Syndrome	Pupils	Ocular Reflexes	Respiratory Pattern	Movement
Central herniation				
Forebrain	Small, reactive	Intact	Cheyne-Stokes	Appropriate or decorticate
Midbrain	Midposition, often irregular, nonreactive	Partially intact	Central neurogenic hyperventilation	Decerebrate posturing
Pons	Pinpoint, or midposition, reactive	Absent	Apneustic, cluster, ataxic	None or spinal reflexes
Medulla	Variable size, nonreactive	Absent	Gasping, absent	None
Transtentorial uncal herniation				
Early	Ipsilateral dilatation, reactive	Partially intact	Normal	Contralateral paresis
Late	Ipsilateral dilatation, nonreactive	Cranial nerve III paralysis	Cheyne-Stokes	Contralateral posturing

(Data from Plum F, Posner JB: The Diagnosis of Stupor and Coma. 3rd Ed. FA Davis, Philadelphia, 1982.)

valuable than words or phrases such as "semicomatose". The Glasgow Coma Scale (Table 29-5) is one method for objectively grading the degree of consciousness. One must modify the scoring for preverbal children. The neurologic examination also determines the presence and extent of cerebral swelling and brain herniation (Table 29-6). Asymmetry of neurologic signs usually indicates a structural or vascular lesion. Poisonings can be particularly difficult to diagnose from the examination. Table 29-3 summarizes the common toxic ingestions.

Table 29-7. Therapy-Directed Diagnosis in Nontraumatic Coma

Airway assessment and control
  If in coma: intubate and ventilate
  If seizure: intubate and ventilate (diazepam: 0.25–0.5 mg/kg iv)
Blood pressure and pulse assessment
  Intravenous lines
  If hypotensive: correct (prefer colloid over crystalloid)
More thorough physical and neurological exam
If etiology unclear or suspected abuse: immediate computed tomography
Simultaneous to placement of intravenous lines
  Blood samples: complete blood count, glucose, blood urea nitrogen, creatinine, electrolytes, calcium, magnesium, prothrombin time, serum glutamic-oxaloacetic transaminase, ammonia
  Immediately following administer G/W 50% (0.5–1.0 g/kg)
  Toxic screen or blood ethanol level as indicated
  Arterial blood gas sample
Indwelling bladder catheter
Arterial line placement
If infant with open fontanelle and not bulging: lumbar puncture. If closed skull or obvious intracranial pressure: computed tomography scan first

(From James HE: Coma in infants, children and adolescents. p. 45. In Nussbaum E (ed): Pediatric Intensive Care. Futura, New York, 1984.)

Table 29-8. Guidelines for the Determination of Brain Death

Cessation of brain function
  Absence of cerebral functions
    Coma
    Unresponsiveness (spinal reflexes may be present)
  Absence of brain stem functions
    Pupillary light reflex
    Corneal reflex
    Gag reflex
    Oculovestibular and oculocephalic reflexes
    Apnea: no spontaneous respirations with $PCO_2 > 60$ mmHg

Irreversibility
  Etiology known and sufficient to cause brain death
  No possible recovery
    Sedation, hypothermia, neuromuscular blockade, shock and other causes of reversible en-
      cephalopathy excluded
    Absence of cerebral blood flow if etiology is unknown
  Persistent signs of brain death for appropriate period of observation
    6 hours for known, irreversible etiology with objective laboratory studies: electrical silence
      on EEG or no cerebral blood flow by nucleotide scan or arteriography
    24 hours for known, irreversible etiology without objective laboratory studies
    24 hours for unknown etiology, reversible etiologies excluded, and confirmation by objective
      laboratory studies

(Data from President's Commission for the Study of Ethical Problems in Medicine and Biomedical and Behavioral Research: Guidelines for the determination of death: Report of the Medical Consultants on the President's Commission for the Study of Ethical Problems in Medicine and Biomedical and Behavioral Research. JAMA 246:2184–2186, 1981.)

Metabolic encephalopathies often have nonspecific signs such as seizures and coma. Their diagnosis is usually made by laboratory studies.

MANAGEMENT

If a specific etiology cannot be made by the initial assessment, then extensive laboratory testing is indicated (Table 29-7). In general, one should initiate these tests simultaneously rather than sequentially. If a probable cause is suspected, for example, meningitis, then a more streamlined approach can be taken. The unconscious child is a pediatric emergency. The principles of the initial management are the stabilization and support of the vital signs. Specific management of the various causes of altered consciousness are covered in subsequent chapters.

BRAIN DEATH

Legally, death is the irreversible cessation of all brain function. The guidelines for the determination of brain death apply primarily to adults. For want of alternative guidelines, however, the Presidential Commission guidelines are generally used to determine brain death in children as well (Table 29-8). It must be emphasized that all possible intoxications, metabolic abnormalities, and hypothermia must be corrected before such a diagnosis is made and the application of these guidelines to children less than 5 years of age has not been established.

IRREVERSIBLE COMA

Irreversible coma, or the persistent vegetative state, often follows acute coma. Spontaneous respirations, sleep–wake cycles, eye movement, and non-purposeful extremity movement return, but there is no conscious or purposeful activity. The prognosis for the persistent vegetative state is very poor if it lasts for longer than 1 month. The prognosis is better for patients whose etiology is secondary to metabolic disorders such as hepatic encephalopathy than those caused by trauma or other insults which structurally alter the brain.

LOCKED–IN SYNDROME

The locked-in syndrome is caused by brain stem death, usually from basilar artery infarction. The supratentorial portions of the brain are preserved, as well as the ability to open and close the eyes. To casual examination the patient appears to be comatose because of the absence of eye movement, breathing, and response to pain. Consciousness is preserved and the patient can learn to communicate with eye blinking.

SELECTED READINGS

James HE: Coma in infants, children and adolescents. p. 35. In Nussbaum E (ed): Pediatric Intensive Care. Futura, New York, 1984

James HE: Neurologic evaluation and support in the child with acute brain insult. Pediatr Ann 15:16–22, 1986

Jennett B, Teasdale G: Aspects of coma after severe head injury. Lancet 1:878–881, 1977

Lockman LA: Disorders of consciousness: the delirious states. p. 143. In Swaiman KF, Wright FS (eds): The Practice of Pediatric Neurology. CV Mosby, St. Louis, 1982

Lockman LA: Coma. p. 148. In Swaiman KF, Wright FS (eds): The Practice of Pediatric Neurology. CV Mosby, St. Louis, 1982

Margolis LH, Shaywitz BA: Outcome of prolonged coma in childhood. Pediatrics 65:477–483, 1980

Mofenson HC, Greensher J: The unknown poison. Pediatrics 54:336–341, 1974

Orlowski JP (ed): Pediatric intensive care. Pediatr Clin North Am 27:3, 1980

Plum F, Posner JB: The Diagnosis of Stupor and Coma. 3rd Ed. FA Davis, Philadelphia, 1982

President's Commission for the Study of Ethical Problems in Medicine and Biomedical and Behavioral Research. Guidelines for the determination of death. JAMA 246:2184–2186, 1981

Raichle ME: The pathophysiology of brain ischemia. Ann Neurol 13:2–10, 1983

30

INCREASED INTRACRANIAL PRESSURE

Increased intracranial pressure is a frequent complication of a variety of injuries and diseases of the brain and in many cases the intracranial pressure (ICP) itself is the major cause of morbidity and mortality. Early recognition and prompt medical intervention may ameliorate the effects of increased ICP on the brain.

PATHOPHYSIOLOGY

The calvaria is a rigid, spherical structure which contains three compartments: cerebrospinal fluid (CSF), blood, and cerebral tissue. Normally, these coexist in an equilibrium to maintain the ICP at approximately 18 mmHg or less. The relationship of the three spaces determines compliance: Expansion of one compartment has to be at the expense of another in order to maintain normal ICP. Increasing the volume of a space-occupying mass initially causes little change in the ICP because there is either an increase in CSF absorption and/or a decrease in blood volume. When the limits of these compensatory mechanisms are exceeded, then increasing ICP ensues (Fig. 30-1). If the ICP exceeds the venous pressure, then tamponade of the dural sinuses and veins occurs, causing venous obstruction and decreased perfusion. Ischemia causes cellular injury and swelling, which further increases the ICP. If the ICP exceeds the arterial pressure, then all cerebral blood flow ceases. A serious complication of increased ICP is displacement of the brain. Brain tissue cannot be compressed; so an expanding mass or edema will cause herniation of the brain across the tentorium, falx, or foramen magnum (see Table 29-6).

Increased ICP can be caused by a number of factors (Table 30-1). Any space-occupying mass such as a tumor or abscess can displace normal brain tissue and increase the tissue compartment. Alterations in the production or absorption of CSF can similarly increase the CSF compartment with resulting increased ICP. Excessive CSF is called hydrocephalus and has many causes (Table 30-2). Changes in the vascular space occur predominantly by intracranial hemorrhages, venous obstruction, or severe arterial hypertension. One of the most common causes of increased ICP is cerebral edema. There are three mechanisms of cerebral edema: Hydrostatic edema is caused by obstruction of venous drainage or an increase in arterial perfusion pressure; vasogenic edema results from a break-

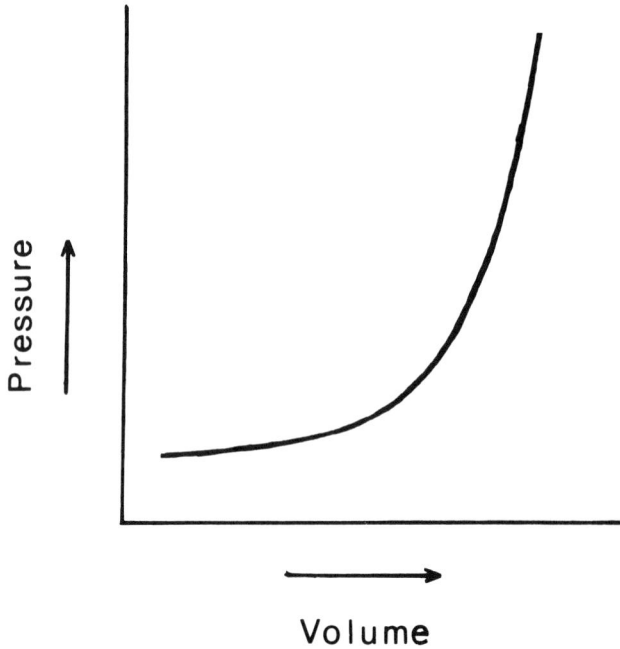

Fig. 30-1. Pressure–volume curve.

down of the blood–brain barrier, with leakage of fluid into the extracellular space; cytotoxic edema is caused by injury to cells with subsequent swelling. In most cases one or more factors contribute to cerebral edema and increased ICP.

CLINICAL MANIFESTATIONS

The clinical manifestations of increased ICP vary somewhat with age (Table 30-3). In the younger child prior to suture closure, increased ICP causes spreading of the sutures, bulging of the fontanelle, and an increasing head size. Early increased ICP in the infant causes irritability and vomiting and, with increasing pressure, lethargy and obtundation develop. If the ICP is extremely high, pulsation of the fontanelle is lost. The "cracked pot" sign (Macewen's) may be present upon percussion of the cranium but is not as useful as other signs. Papilledema is rare in the infant, probably because of the spreadability of the sutures. The "setting sun" sign (Fig. 30-2) caused by lid retraction can be seen in some children with increased ICP.

The preverbal toddler may show only vomiting, irritability, and changes of consciousness. Spreading of sutures is more difficult and papilledema is more apt to occur than in infants. Early papilledema takes approximately 24 to 48 hours to develop. Fully developed papilledema may take as long as a week (Fig. 30-3). Venous pulsations are a more sensitive funduscopic index of ICP pressure. Its presence indicates normal ICP. Absent venous pulsations can be found in

Table 30-1. Causes for Increased Intracranial
Pressure in Children

Cerebral edema
  Cytotoxic
  Vasogenic
  Hydrostatic
Intracranial mass
  Tumor
  Abscess
  Cyst
Intracranial hemorrhage
  Subarachnoid
  Subdural
  Intraventricular
  Epidural
  Intraparenchymal
Venous obstruction
  Dural sinus thrombosis
  Superior vena cava syndrome
  Polycythemia
Hydrocephalus (see Table 30-2)
Hepatic encephalopathy
  Reye's syndrome
Infection
  Meningitis
  Cerebritis
  Encephalitis
  Abscess
Trauma
  Contusion
  With Intracranial hemorrhage
  Childhood concussive syndrome
Generalized craniosynostosis
Hypertensive encephalopathy
Burn encepalopathy
Pseudotumor cerebri (see Table 30-5)
Chronic hypercapnia
Lead encephalopathy

Table 30-2. Classification of Hydrocephalus

A. Noncommunicating (intraventricular obstructive)
  1. Maldevelopments of the aqueduct [stenosis, forking ("atresia"), septum, gliosis]
  2. Obstruction due to mass lesions (neoplasm, cyst, hematoma, aneurysm of the vein of
     Galen)
  3. Obstruction secondary to exudate, hemorrhage, parasites, or acquired aqueductal septum
  4. Obstruction of the fourth ventricle outlet foramina (Dandy-Walker syndrome, arachnoiditis)
B. Communicating (extraventricular obstructive)
  1. Postinfectious, posthemorrhagic, or developmental adhesions of basilar cisterns or surface
     subarachnoid space
  2. Arachnoid villi obstruction by erythrocytes
  3. Communicating hydrocephalus with the Arnold-Chiari malformation
  4. Developmental failure of arachnoid villi
C. Communicating hydrocephalus due to excessive cerebrospinal fluid formation (choroid plexus
    papilloma)

(Reprinted with permission from Bell WE, McCormick WF: Increased Intracranial Pressure in Children. Diagnosis and Treatment. 2nd Ed. WB Saunders, Philadelphia, 1978.)

Table 30-3. Signs and Symptoms of Increased
Intracranial Pressure

Infants
  Full fontanelle
  Increasing head size
  Suture separation
Children
  Headache
  Papilledema
All ages
  Altered consciousness
  Nausea and vomiting
  False localizing neurologic signs

some normal children, but more often in those with pressures greater than approximately 18 mmHg.

In the verbal child, headache is the most common symptom. The headache is usually nonspecific but often worse in the morning and almost always associated with nausea or vomiting. Early morning headache and vomiting are the cardinal signs of increased ICP. Papilledema, false localizing signs, and alterations in consciousness are usually present, depending upon the rate of development and the severity of the increased ICP. Signs of herniation are a late manifestation. Altered respirations, bradycardia with hypertension (Cushing's reflex) may accompany central herniation, although the cardiovascular changes are not always classic in the child.

TREATMENT

The treatment of ICP depends upon the rate at which it develops: the more rapid the progression, the more aggressive the therapy. The general goals of therapy are to reduce ICP and preserve cerebral perfusion. If ICP can be main-

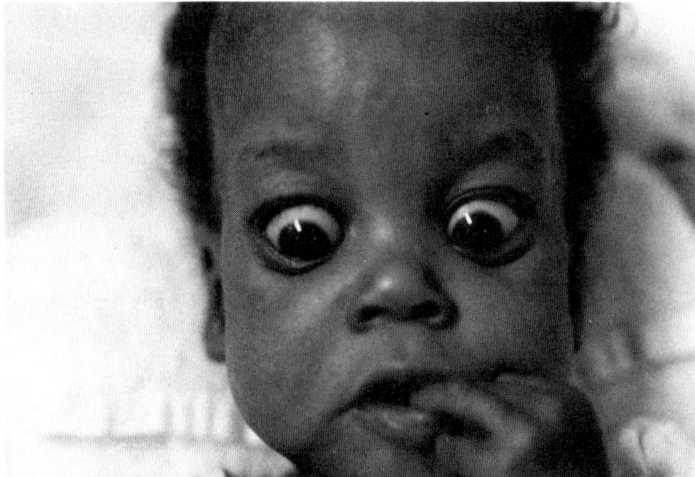

Fig. 30-2. "Sunset" sign in a child with hydrocephalus.

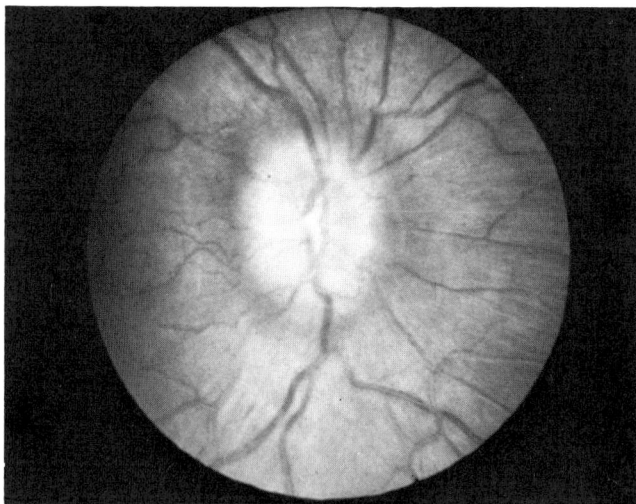

Fig. 30-3. Papilledema.

tained at 30 mmHg less than the mean perfusion pressure, the outcome is improved. Therapy for severe ICP can be hazardous and it is important that treatment be given only when appropriate. For this reason an ICP monitor can be useful. With a monitoring system one can determine the results of therapy and plan other strategies. Clinical signs of deterioration lag behind the increase in pressure so that early detection may prevent neurologic complications. Table 30-4 outlines the medical management of increased ICP.

The Glasgow Coma Scale has proved to be useful in judging the severity of intracranial hypertension (see Table 29-5). Patients who present with scores of 12 or greater have mild disease and can be treated with observation and fluid restriction. Patients with scores of 8 to 12 have significant but sublethal increased ICP and require aggressive therapy to prevent decompensation. Diuretics, fluid restriction, and steroids are begun, with careful observation for further deterioration. Patients with scores of 8 or less require vigorous therapy. These patients have obvious neurologic signs of ICP as well as altered consciousness. Controlled ventilation and intracranial monitoring are indicated and therapy is directed toward maintaining the ICP at less than 20 mmHg. Hyperventilation to maintain the PCO_2 at 23 to 25 mmHg is the most rapid method of lowering ICP. Osmotic diuretics, such as mannitol, may be needed if the ICP remains above 20 mmHg. This can be repeated every 4 to 6 hours as long as urine output is good and the serum osmolarity is less than 310. If the ICP does not respond to these measures, then hypothermia and/or barbiturate coma may be necessary.

Nursing care is equally important in the management of ICP. Patients are frequently in coma and may develop one or more organ system failures. All patients should have a urinary catheter to manage the large volumes of urine resulting from the use of osmotic agents. The patient should have the head of the bed elevated to 30° to reduce hydrostatic components of ICP. The use of

Table 30-4. Medical Management of Acute Intracranial Hypertension

Agent	Dose	Administration	Onset of Action	Peak Action	Advantages	Side Effects or Limitations
Passive hyperventilation	Reduce PCO_2 from 40 to 25 mmHg	Continuous	Minutes	2–30 minutes	Very prompt action; does not potentiate intracranial bleeding	Effect may not be sustained; cerebral ischemia
Mannitol	0.25–2.0 g/kg	Every 4–6 hours, iv	20–30 minutes	20–360 minutes	Prompt action	Rebound; dehydration; renal failure; intracranial bleeding
Glycerol	0.5–1.5 g/kg	Every 6 hours iv or orally	15–30 minutes	30 minutes (iv), 60–80 minutes (orally)	Prompt action by oral or iv route	Rebound may occur; dehydration; intracranial bleeding
Pentobarbital	3 mg/kg (loading dose: 5 mg/kg)	Every hour, iv	Minutes	Minutes	Prompt action; no rebound	Hypotension; renal failure; need for careful monitoring
Hypothermia	29–31°C	Continuous	Approx. 1 hour	2–3 hours	No rebound	Cardiac arrhythmias; need for careful monitoring
Dexamethasone	8 mg	Every 12 hours, iv	12–18 hours	12–24 hours	No rebound	Slow onset of action; uncertain efficacy in head injury; gastrointestinal hemorrhage

(Adapted from Rossman NP, Herskowitz J, Carter AP, O'Connor JF: Acute head trauma in infancy and children. Pediatr Clin North Am 26:707–736, 1979. Reprinted with permission from WB Saunders Co.)

Table 30-5. Clinical Disorders Associated with
Pseudotumor Cerebri

Idiopathic
Young, obese females
Menstrual dysfunction
Vitamin A deficiency
Delayed penicillin reaction
Addison's disease
Hypoparathyroidism
Iron deficiency anemia in adolescent girls
Galactosemia
Galactokinase deficiency
Congenital adrenal hyperplasia
Behçet's disease
Drugs
Tetracycline
Glucocorticoids
Vitamin A
Nalidixic acid

(Data from Bell WE, McCormick WF: Increased Intracranial Pressure in Children. 2nd Ed. WB Saunders, Philadelphia, 1978.)

controlled ventilation will necessitate endotrachial tube placement. Frequent suctioning can cause a marked Valsalva response which contributes to the ICP. For this reason most patients are paralyzed with pancuronium or a similar agent. In normal doses pancuronium does not interfere with pupillary reflexes but will abolish all other voluntary motor movements. Many clinical signs are therefore lost and one is dependent upon a monitoring system and the patient's vital signs.

A therapy of last resort is cranial decompression. Few centers use this procedure, but it may be indicated in some patients. It requires a relatively large craniotomy and a prolonged operative procedure.

PROGNOSIS

The prognosis for children with markedly increased ICP is relatively good if they survive the illness. Data from severe head trauma, Reye's syndrome, near-drowning, and meningitis suggests an overall mortality between 10 and 40 percent. Survivors of these illnesses do relatively well. Approximately 50 percent are normal, 30 percent have minor neurologic complications, and the remainder have significant neurologic complications. In some cases, the extent of injury is so great that even if the ICP is controlled, there is a bad outcome.

PSEUDOTUMOR CEREBRI

Pseudotumor cerebri, also called benign intracranial hypertension, has an unknown pathogenesis or definite etiology. It is associated with a number of clinical disorders and occurs more commonly in obese young females with menstrual dysfunction (Table 30-5). It can occur at any age and sex. The clinical features are headaches, vomiting, and papilledema. Visual disturbances include diploplia and visual obscurations consisting of temporary loss of vision. Prolonged increased ICP can cause optic atrophy and blindness. Aside from paresis of cranial nerve VI, focal signs are absent and the patients appear surprising well. There are no diagnostic tests except for an elevated CSF pressure on lumbar puncture. The computed tomographic scan is normal or may show small ventricles. Careful visual field mapping may show an enlarged blind spot. Skull radiographs may show spread sutures in the young child or an "empty sella."

The treatment is directed toward reducing the ICP. Acetazolamide at 10 to 20 mg/kg/day is started to reduce CSF production and daily lumbar punctures are performed to reduce the ICP to less than 18 mmHg until a remission is established. Some patients respond to steroids. If these measures are not effective, then a lumbar subarachnoid–peritoneal shunt is often effective.

OTITIC HYDROCEPHALUS

The association of otitis media or mastoiditis with raised ICP has been called otitic hydrocephalus. This is caused by lateral dural sinus thrombosis with venous obstruction.

SELECTED READINGS

Bell WE, McCormick WF: Increased Intracranial Pressure in Children. 2nd Ed. WB Saunders, Philadelphia, 1978

Blaauw G, Van Der Boss JL, Mus A: On pulsations of the fontanelle. Dev Med Child Neurol 16:23–26, 1974

Conn AW, Edmonds JF, Barker GA: Cerebral resuscitation in near drowning. Pediatr Clin North Am 26:691–701, 1979

Greer M: Benign intracranial hypertension (pseudotumor cerebri). Pediatr Clin North Am 14:819–839, 1967

Hahn JF: Cerebral edema and neurointensive care. Pediatr Clin North Am 27:587–591, 1980

31

HEAD TRAUMA

Trauma is one of the leading causes of death in children. Approximately 25 percent of trauma-related deaths are caused by head trauma. The risk of head trauma severe enough to cause loss of consciousness is about 1 in 10 throughout childhood. Head trauma is more often accidental but can be intentional, as in child abuse. It is more common in boys than in girls by a ratio of almost 2:1. Because of the high incidence and the need for early diagnosis and treatment of complications, head trauma is an important pediatric disease.

PATHOPHYSIOLOGY

Injury to the brain from trauma occurs via several mechanisms (Table 31-1). Significant head trauma usually causes concussion, which is loss of consciousness with amnesia. Retrograde amnesia is loss of memory of events prior to the injury, and antegrade amnesia is loss of memory following the injury. Loss of consciousness for less than 5 minutes is less likely to be associated with significant cerebral injury. The pediatric concussive syndrome is head trauma without loss of consciousness but with a variable period of being dazed or stunned followed by lethargy and nausea and/or vomiting. The mechanism of concussion is unknown but may be related to mechanical effects on the electrical properties of neurons or axonal injury. In the pediatric syndrome, hyperemia and vascular engorgement of the brain from disrupted vascular autoregulation have been implicated as a cause of cerebral edema and the signs of increased intracranial pressure. Concussion usually follows blunt injuries to the head.

Contusion, or bruising, of the brain may also follow blunt trauma. Coup injuries occur on the brain under the point of impact to the skull. Contracoup injuries are caused by the tips of the temporal, occipital, and frontal lobes being thrown against their bony encasement in the skull. These forces are usually angular. Contusions cause localized bruising, swelling, and neurologic deficits (Fig. 31-1).

Rapid acceleration/deceleration movements of the brain causes coup and contracoup contusions as the brain impacts on the bony confines of the skull. In addition to contusion, such movements produce shearing forces in the white matter, causing extensive axonal injury. This movement may also shear the delicate bridging vein and the surface of the brain, causing subdural hematoma (Fig. 31-2). The injury has been called the pediatric whiplash syndrome and occurs when the infant is vigorously shaken.

319

320 *Manual of Child Neurology*

Table 31-1. Pathogenesis of Cerebral Trauma

Primary cerebral injury
  Concussion
  Pediatric concussive syndrome
  Contusion
  Laceration
  Diffuse axonal injury
Secondary cerebral injury
  Cerebral edema
  Intracranial hemorrhage
  Intracranial infection

Lacerations are caused by penetrating wounds or depressed fragments of bone that physically disrupt the cerebral tissue and are usually associated with hemorrhage. The symptoms and signs are similar to those of contusion for the same reasons. The external signs of trauma are more obvious.

Secondary injuries to the brain are caused by complication of the trauma. Intracranial hemorrhage is the most common and most serious. Intraparenchymal, epidural, and subdural hemorrhages cause injury by compression of the brain, increased intracranial pressure (ICP), and vascular insufficiency. Intraparenchymal hemorrhages are caused by the rupture of blood vessels within the brain from contusion or laceration. Subdural hemorrhage is usually venous in origin from tearing of the bridging veins or dural sinuses and epidural hemorrhage from the meningeal arteries. Subarachnoid bleeding may occur in isolation or accompany other hemorrhages. If the hemorrhage is of arterial origin, the effects develop more rapidly than from venous sources. Infections can cause

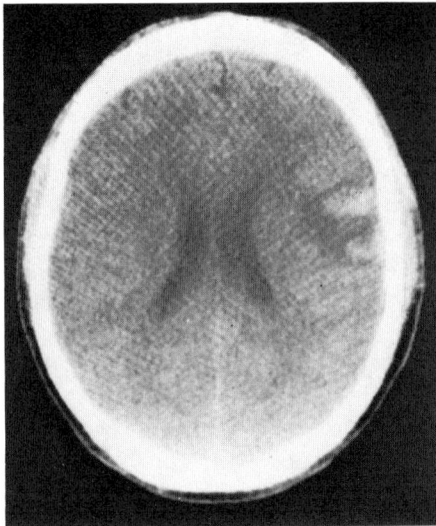

Fig. 31-1. Brain contusion.

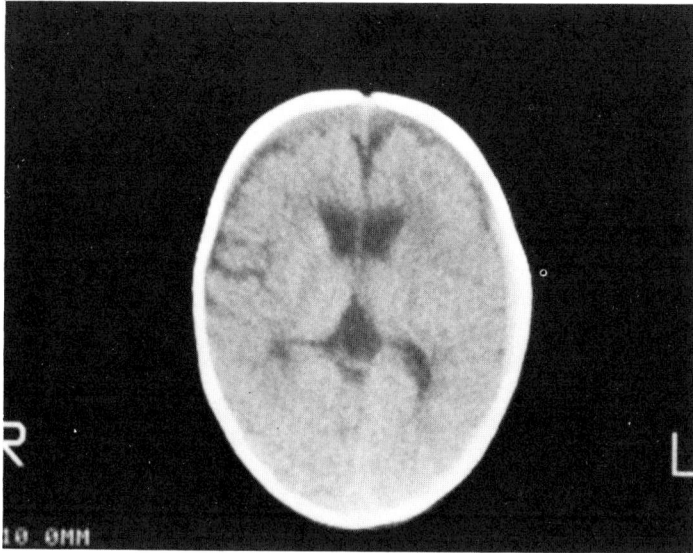

Fig. 31-2. Acute subdural hematoma from shake injury.

further injury by abscess formation and meningitis. Introduction of contaminated material from penetrating wounds and the creation of fistulas between the cerebrospinal fluid (CSF) space and contaminated air sinuses are the route of infection. Cerebral edema causes vascular ischemia and brain injury, as discussed in Chapter 30. Hyperemia, hemorrhage, and infection contribute to increased ICP.

Table 31-2. Initial Evaluation of Head Injuries

Physical examination
   Vital signs
   Airway and breathing
   Extracranial signs of trauma and bleeding
   Sinus and tympanic membrane bleeding or CSF drainage
   Signs of penetrating wounds in scalp, mouth, and ears
Neurologic examination
   Level of consciousness
   Funduscopic examination for hemorrhages
   Pupil size and reaction to light
   Symmetry of muscle movement and response to pain
   Symmetry of reflexes
History
   Type of injury
   Period of unconsciousness
   Postconcussive course
   Past history of neurologic or bleeding diseases
   Previous injuries or sibling injuries

Table 31-3. Clinical Features and Distinguishing Characteristics of Traumatic Intracranial Hemorrhages

	Acute Epidural Hematoma	Acute Subdural Hematoma
Supratentorial		
Frequency	Less	Greater
Skull fracture	75%	30%
Source of hemorrhage	Usually arterial	Venous
Age	Usually older than 2 years	Usually younger than 1 year
Laterality	Usually unilateral	Usually bilateral
Seizures	Less than 25%	75%
(Pre-)retinal hemorrhages	Less than 25%	75%
Incresed intracranial pressure	Present	Present
CT configuration	Usually lenticular	Usually crescentic
Mortality	25%	Less than 25%
Morbidity	Low	High
Infratentorial		
Frequency	Greater	Less than 25%
Skull fracture	Almost always	Usually
Source of hemorrhage	Venous	Venous

(From Rosman NP: Pediatric head trauma. Pediatr Ann 7:826–838, 1978.)

DIAGNOSIS AND EVALUATION

The diagnosis of head trauma is usually self-evident. Determining which children are at risk for serious complication is more difficult. All children with loss of consciousness for more than several minutes or stunned behavior lasting longer than 5 minutes should be evaluated by a physician. The initial evaluation

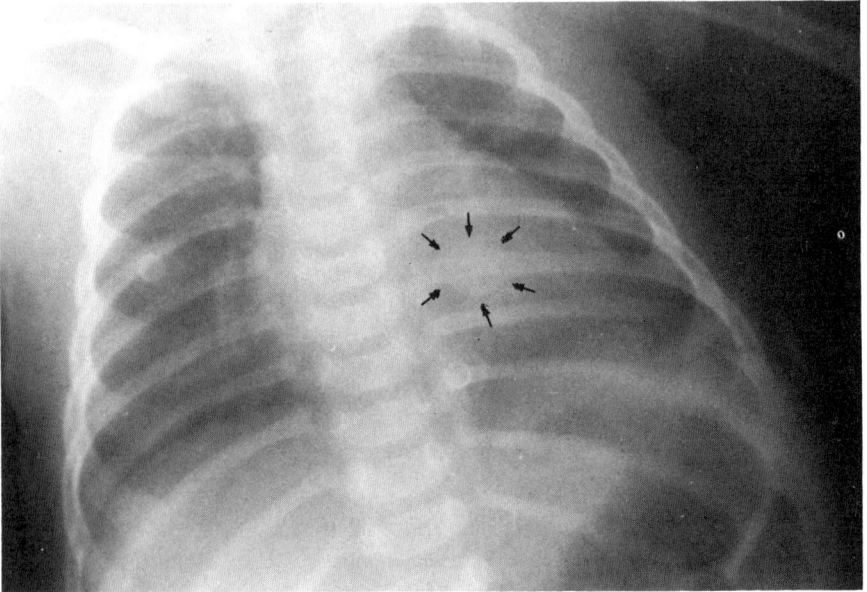

Fig. 31-3. Rib fracture from a shake injury.

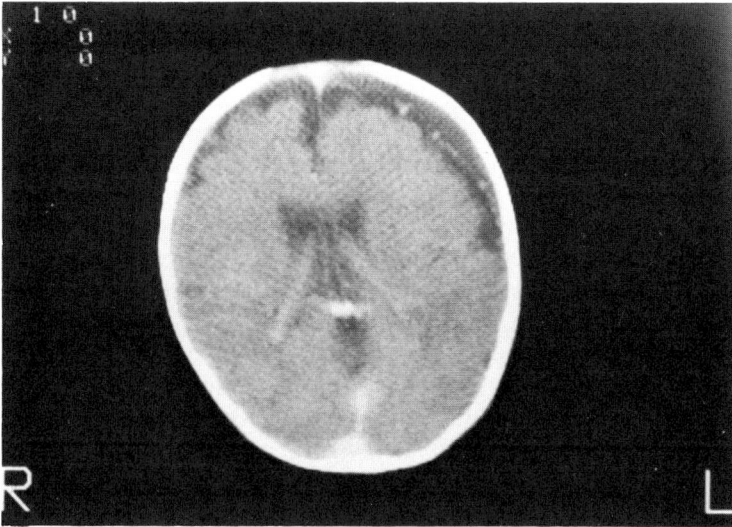

Fig. 31-4. Chronic subdural hematoma.

Table 31-4. Indications for Skull Radiographs Following Head Trauma

Historical
  Unconsciousness for more than 5 minutes
  Retrograde amnesia for more than 5 minutes
  Vomiting
  Gunshot or other penetrating wound
  Nonvisual focal symptoms
  Seizures
General physical examination
  Palpable bony malalignment
  Discharge from ear (CSF or blood)
  Discharge from nose (CSF)
  Eardrum discoloration or mastoid ecchymosis (Battle's sign)
  Bilateral black eyes (raccoon sign)
Neurologic examination
  Altered consciousness
  Apnea or abnormal breathing
  Asymmetric reflexes or Babinski sign
  Focal weakness or asymmetry in movement
  Sensory abnormality or asymmetry in response to pain
  Anisocoria as unreactive pupil
  Other cranial nerve abnormalities

(Data from Phillips LA: A study of the effect of high yield criteria for emergency room skull radiography. HEW Publication, FDA, 78-8089, 1978.)

is outlined in Table 31-2. Establishing an airway, treating shock, and other emergency procedures to maintain the vital signs are performed immediately. The neurologic exam must document the level of consciousness and the presence of focal or diffuse neurologic signs. The history is obtained after the examination to obtain the specifics of the injury and the relevant past history.

The initial assessment gives clues to the major head trauma syndromes. Brief loss or alterations of consciousness with prompt return to normal is a concussive syndrome with a low risk of complications, especially if there is no extracranial trauma. Contusions are more often associated with longer periods of unconsciousness and focal signs. Intracranial hemorrhage may show diffuse or focal signs and usually the neurologic status deteriorates with increasing ICP (Table 31-3). Evidence for complicated fractures and CSF leaks are usually obvious. Battle's sign (mastoid ecchymosis), racoon sign (periorbital ecchymosis), and blood behind the tympanic membrane suggest a basilar fracture. A special syndrome is encountered with child abuse. The "whiplash shake injury" should be suspected in any child with sudden onset of neurologic signs and retinal hemorrhages. The infants were shaken vigorously and excessively. Head instability causes acceleration/deceleration injury, with contusions, retinal hemorrhages, and subdural hematoma (Fig. 31-2). One can frequently find bruising on the chest and back or rib fractures or radiographs caused by vigorous squeezing of the infant (Fig. 31-3). The history usually does not explain the degree of injury. There is usually no evidence of trauma to the head and face. Some infants present months later with progressive head enlargement caused by chronic subdural hematomas (Fig. 31-4).

The skull radiograph may add to the diagnosis but is not necessarily indicated in every child with loss of consciousness. It is indicated if basilar, depressed, or compound fractures are suspected by the physician (Table 31-4). Documentation of a linear skull fracture adds little to the initial management except if the fracture is across the meningeal artery in older children. Perhaps more important is to ensure that there is no cervical spine injury. This can often be overlooked because of the cerebral injury. The computed tomography (CT) scan is the most important method of determining surgically correctable complications, especially intracranial hemorrhages. It is certainly indicated for persistent unconsciousness, focal signs, penetrating injuries, and late deterioration.

MANAGEMENT

The first management decision is to determine if the child has had significant head trauma to be at risk for developing complications (Table 31-5). These patients need hospitalization for immediate therapy, further tests, or observation. Patients with minor head trauma can be monitored at home if there is a responsible adult to observe the child, there are clear lines of communication to a physician familiar with the case, and the parents are given clear guidelines. The development of focal neurologic deficits, deterioration of consciousness, persistent vomiting, and the appearance of fever are indications to return for

Table 31-5. Indications for Hospitalization of Children with Head Trauma

Loss of consciousness for more than 5 minutes
Focal neurologic deficits
Compound, depressed, or basilar skull fractures and fractures
   across meningeal arteries
Bleeding or CSF drainage in sinuses or middle ear
Seizures
Deterioration of consciousness
Suspected child abuse
History of bleeding diathesis

Table 31-6. Neurosurgical Management of Head Trauma Complications

Depressed or compound skull fracture
   Surgical repair/debridement
   Tetanus prophylaxis
   Observation for other complication
Basilar skull fractures
   Antibiotics for fever
   Exploration and repair if CSF leaks for more than 2 weeks
   Observation for other complication
Intracranial hemorrhage with mass effect
   Surgical drainage
   Observation for other complications

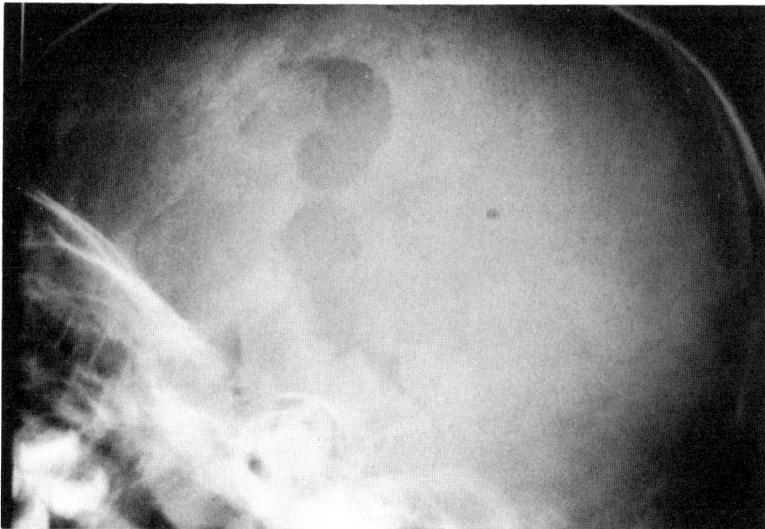

Fig. 31-5. Leptomeningeal cyst.

Table 31-7. Intensive Care Management of Head Trauma[a]

Coma score	Management
Greater than 8	Intensive care observation
	NPO
	Elevate head of bed to 10–15°
	Restrict fluids to 70% requirement iv
	Dexamethasone, 1 mg/kg
	Furosemide, 1 mg/kg
Less than 8	Intubation and controlled ventilation
	Nasogastric tube
	CT scan
	ICP monitor
	Foley catheter
	Central venous and aterial line
	Electrolytes, osmolarity, complete blood count twice daily
	For ICP >20
	Maintain PCO_2 at 23–25 mmHg
	Mannitol, 0.25–1.0 g/kg, every 4 hours, as necessary
	For refractory increased ICP
	Barbiturate coma
	Hypothermia

[a] Also see Chapter 30 for management of intracranial pressure.

further evaluation. Children sent home with known skull fractures should also return for repeat radiographs in 1 to 2 months to exclude a "growing fracture" from a leptomeningeal cyst (Fig. 31-5).

Hospital management is dependent upon the type and severity of the head injury. A baseline complete blood count, electrolytes, osmolarity, prothrombin time, partial thromboplastin time, urinalysis, liver enzymes, and chest radiograph should be obtained for every child admitted to the hospital. Complications that require neurosurgical intervention should be corrected when diagnosed (Table 31-6). Patients without neurosurgical complications need to be observed for development of those complications and cerebral edema. The Glasgow Coma Scale (see Table 29-5) can be useful in directing the management of head trauma (Table 31-7). In general, children with a score of 8 to 12 are observed, with fluid restriction and head elevation. If deterioration occurs or if the child is admitted with a score of less than 8, a CT scan should be obtained. The neurologic examination must be repeated every 4 to 6 hours or as necessary. Pupil reaction and consciousness can be documented with other vital signs. The medical management is similar to the plan discussed in Chapter 30 for increased ICP. If seizures develop, they should be managed with phenytoin, because it has fewer effects on consciousness than barbiturates.

PROGNOSIS

The prognosis for head trauma in children is generally good. Children with minor head trauma uniformly improved and return to normal activity. The most common long-term complication of mild to moderate head trauma is post-traumatic epilepsy. The incidence is about 2 percent for mild head trauma and 30 percent for brain laceration. The more severe the injury, the more likely the development of epilepsy. Seizures that occur within the first 48 hours are much less likely to cause epilepsy than those occurring after the first week. Prophylactic anticonvulsant therapy is indicated for this group. Children with severe head trauma (Glasgow score of less than 5) have a mortality of about 10 percent, 20 percent suffer from severe neurologic deficits, and the remainder have useful recovery.

Some patients develop a variety of symptoms following head trauma, such as anxiety, headaches, dizziness, poor attention, and personality changes. The estimated incidence is 30 percent, and the "postconcussive" syndrome may last for weeks to months. There is no specific therapy.

SPINAL CORD INJURIES

Injuries to the spinal cord present with diplegia and absent sensation distal to the injury. A hemicord lesion causes ipsilateral motor loss and contralateral loss of pain sensation (Brown-Séquard syndrome). Most cord injuries are associated with major trauma, although preexisting vertebral abnormalities, such as seen with Down's syndrome and others, may cause cord injury with less trauma. These patients must be stabilized and transported to a trauma facility as soon as possible.

SELECTED READINGS

Dershewitz RA, Kay BA, Swisher CN: Treatment of children with post traumatic transient loss of consciousness. Pediatrics 72:602–607, 1983

Jennett B: Trauma as a cause of epilepsy in childhood. Dev Med Child Neurol 15:52–62, 1973

Leonidas JC, Ting W, Binkiewicz A et al: Mild head trauma in children: when is a roentgenogram necessary? Pediatrics 69:139–143, 1982

Murten DF, Osborne DR: Craniocerebral trauma in the child abuse syndrome. Pediatr Ann 12:882–837, 1983

Rosman NP: Pediatric head injuries. Pediatr Ann 7:827–838, 1978

Rosman NP, Herskowitz J, Carter AP et al: Acute head trauma in infancy and childhood. Clinical and radiologic aspects. Pediatr Clin North Am 26:707–736, 1979

Shapiro K (ed): Pediatric Head Trauma. Futura, Mount Kisko, NY, 1983

Singer HS, Freeman JM: Head trauma for the pediatrician. Pediatrics 62:819–824, 1978

32

INFECTIONS OF THE NERVOUS SYSTEM

BACTERIAL MENINGITIS

If one considers its incidence, mortality, and morbidity, then bacterial meningitis is perhaps the most significant infectious disease in children. The risk of developing meningitis is approximately 1 in 1,000 during childhood and the mortality varies between 5 and 20 percent, depending upon age and the infecting organism. Morbidity is as high as 50 percent, with one-third showing significant neurologic sequelae. Early recognition, institution of appropriate antimicrobial therapy, and treatment of complications must be well studied by every physician who treats diseases of children.

Pathophysiology

Meningitis is an infection of subarachnoid space of the CNS. The portal of entry is by hematogenous spread in the vast majority of cases. Occasionally there is contiguous spread from other infected tissues or direct inoculation. One mechanism of neurologic injury is cerebral edema caused by toxic substances released from lysed bacteria and leukocytes, inappropriate antidiuretic hormone secretion, and vasculitis. Cerebral edema causes generalized neurologic dysfunction and can be so extensive as to cause herniation and death. Vascular injury is the second major mechanism for cerebral injury by thrombosis and ischemic infarction. Venous or arterial infarctions cause focal neurologic signs such as seizures, hemiparesis, and cranial nerve palsies. Greater than 95 percent of cases of meningitis in children are caused by a handful of organisms (Table 32-1). The incidence of the causative organism varies somewhat with age (Table 32-2). Host factors can also play a role in the type of infection encountered (Table 32-3).

Diagnosis

Common symptoms of meningitis are listed in Table 32-4. The clinical syndrome is relatively specific in showing a sick child with fever, vomiting, altered mental status, and nuchal rigidity. In the very young, those with septic shock, and those with advanced disease, signs such as meningism and irritability may

Table 32-1. Pathogens of Meningitis in Infants and Children

Cause	Incidence (%)
Hemophilus influenzae	57
Neisseria meningitidis	12
Streptococcus pneumoniae	8
Group B streptococci	7
Coliform bacilli	4.1
Listeria monocytogenes	0.8

(Modified from McCracken GH: New concepts in the management of infants and children with meningitis. Pediatr Infect Dis 1:S51–S55. © 1983 The Williams & Wilkins Co., Baltimore.)

be lost and replaced by coma. The definitive diagnostic test is examination of the cerebrospinal fluid (CSF) and every child with suspected meningitis should have lumbar puncture. Papilledema is sufficiently rare as a presenting sign of meningitis that its presence should make one suspect an alternative diagnosis, such as a brain abscess, venous sinus occlusion, or subdural/epidural empyema. In those who have papilledema, one should first obtain a computed tomographic (CT) scan. Occasionally the CSF results can be confusing. Partially treated meningitis attenuates but does not usually alter the basic characteristic of the CSF except to sterilize the cultures (Table 32-5). The major differential diagnoses are

Table 32-2. Causes of Bacterial Meningitis in Childhood[a]

Age Group	Hemophilus influenzae	Neisseria meningitidis	Streptococcus pneumoniae	Escherichia coli	Group B Streptococci	Other
<2 months	+	−	+	+ + +	+ + +	+ + +
2–12 months	+ + + +	+ +	+ +	−	−	+
1–4 years	+ + +	+ +	+ +	−	−	+
5–14 years	+ +	+ + +	+ +	−	−	+
15+ years	+	+ + +	+ + +	−	−	+
All ages	+ + +	+ +	+ +	+	+ +	+

[a] Symbols: − = less than 1 percent; + = less than 5 percent; + + = 5 to 25 percent; + + + = 25 to 50 percent; + + + + = more than 50 percent.

Table 32-3. Predisposing Disorders for Bacterial Meningitis

Severe burns
Immunodeficiency
Complement deficiency (meningococcus)
Diabetes
Renal insufficiency
Splenectomy, asplenia (pneumococcus)
Chemotherapy
Sickle cell disease (salmonella, pneumococcus)
Galactosemia (*Escherichia coli*)
Neurosurgical procedures
Head trauma (staphyloccus)
Congenital dermoid sinus or cribriform plate deformities
Subacute bacterial endocarditis

Table 32-4. Presenting Signs and Symptoms in Children with Bacterial Meningitis

Sign or Symptom	Incidence (%)
Fever	85
Vomiting	55
Meningism	50
Irritability	35
Obtundation	30
Convulsions	30
Anorexia	20
Headache	15

tuberculosis, fungal infections, and viral meningoencephalitis (Table 32-6). The routine CSF analyses are bacterial cultures, protein and glucose determinations, cell count and differential Gram stain, and, if available, detection of capsular antigens using counterimmune electrophoresis or other techniques. A reasonably accurate diagnosis can be made in 75 percent by Gram stain and antigen detection.

Treatment

Initial therapy for bacterial meningitis of unknown etiology is undergoing some changes with the introduction of the second- and third-generation cephalosporins. In the past, children older than 2 months received both ampicillin,

Table 32-5. CSF Characteristics in Initial and Final Lumbar Punctures in Children with Bacterial Meningitis

	Initial Lumbar Puncture		Final Lumbar Puncture
	Untreated	Pretreated	
Number of patients	50	38	88
CSF white blood cells ± SD	4,157 ± 4,747	4,552 ± 5,944	42 ± 10
Percentage of neutrophils ± SD	83.3 ± 26.5	79.5 ± 28.3	6 ± 13
Glucose (mg/dl) ± SD	33.7 ± 22.6	36.51 ± 26.8	47 ± 11
Protein (mg/dl) ± SD	279 ± 338	172 ± 271	53 ± 108
Culture positive (%)	92	68	0
Gram stain positive (%)	82	55	0

(Modified from Feigin RD, Dodge PR: Bacterial meningitis: newer concepts of pathophysiology and neurologic sequelae. Pediatr Clin North Am 23:541–556, 1976. Reprinted by permission from WB Saunders Co.)

Table 32-6. CSF Characteristics in Meningitis

	Bacterial	Tuberculous and Fungal	Viral
Cells	Usually >500	Usually <500	Usually <500
Cell type	Neutrophils	Mononuclear	Usually mononuclear (neutrophils early)
Lactate	Elevated	Elevated	Normal
Glucose	Low (<50% serum)	Low	Normal
Protein	Elevated	Elevated	Elevated
Gram stain, other stains, or antigen detection	Positive	Positive	Absent

Table 32-7. Initial Therapy for Bacterial Meningitis

Antibiotic	Dose (per kg/day)
Penicillin	250,000 U (q4h)[a]
Ampicillin and	400 mg (q4h)
chloramphenicol	100 mg (q6h)
Cefotaxime	150 mg (q4h)
Ceftriaxone	100 mg (q12h)
Cefoperazone	300 mg (q8h)
Moxalactam	150 mg (q4h)

[a] Dosage schedule

300 to 400 mg/kg/day, and chloramphenicol, 100 mg/kg/day, until culture sensitivities were obtained because of the 35 percent β-lactamase-positive *Hemophilus influenzae* isolates. Recently, however, cephalosporins have been advocated for single-drug therapy in the initial management (Table 32-7). Antibiotic therapy must be instituted as quickly as possible after the diagnosis is suspected.

The duration of therapy differs somewhat with the organism. In general, uncomplicated meningitis with gram-positive organisms or *H. influenzae* should be treated for approximately 10 days, and gram-negative organisms for approximately 21 days. If there is no clinical improvement in the first 48 to 72 hours, then lumbar puncture should be repeated. The cell count, glucose, and protein should be moving toward normal and the CSF should be sterile. The segmented neutrophils should be less than 50 percent if the therapy is effective. Children with *H. influenzae* or meningococcic meningitis need to be isolated for the first 24 hours. Household contacts require prophylaxis with rifampin, 10 mg/kg bid for 2 days for meningococcic disease and 20 mg/kg/day for 4 days for *H. influenzae,* for children younger than 4 years and their household contacts. The most recent advance in the therapy for bacterial meningitis is prevention. *Hemophilus* polysaccharide vaccine is available and recommended for all children 2 to 5 years of age. Children 18 to 24 months old in daycare facilities and children of any age with sickle cell disease, hemoglobin SC disease, or asplenia are at special risk and should be immunized.

Complications and Prognosis

Complications which frequently occur during the course of meningitis are listed in Table 32-8. Most will resolve without any specific therapy. The exception is hearing loss, where up to 10 percent of cases will develop permanent deficits. Other cranial nerve palsies almost routinely resolve with time. Cerebral edema is part of the syndrome and usually responds to simple fluid restriction. In fulminant meningitis, however, more specific measures, such as hyperventilation and mannitol, may be necessary. The syndrome of inappropriate antidiuretic hormone secretion occurs in about 30 percent of cases but is rarely persistent or clinically significant. Maintaining the child at 60 to 70 percent

Table 32-8. Acute Complications of Bacterial
Meningitis

Inappropriate secretion of antidiuretic hormone
Subdural effusions
Venous, arterial infarctions
Venous sinus thrombosis
Cranial nerve palsies
Seizures
Cerebral edema
Hydrocephalus

maintenance fluids for the first 48 to 72 hours or until the serum sodium returns to above 135 mEq/L is usually sufficient.

Subdural effusions occur frequently enough (approximately 40 percent of cases) that it should be considered as part of the syndrome complex (Fig. 32-1). This does not require therapy unless subdural empyema is suspected based upon recurrence of fever, bulging fontanelle, and progressive neurologic signs. Less than 1 percent of patients with effusions develop empyema. If it is diagnosed, repeated subdural taps are indicated until resolution. Cerebral infarctions, either venous or arterial, have no specific therapy. Seizures occur in 20 to 30 percent of children prior to diagnosis and in approximately an equal number after treatment has begun and should be treated with anticonvulsants. Unless the seizures persist beyond 72 hours, long-term therapy with anticonvulsants is not indicated. Thirty to forty percent of infants with meningitis will develop either a persistent fever which lasts beyond 10 days or a recurrent fever after

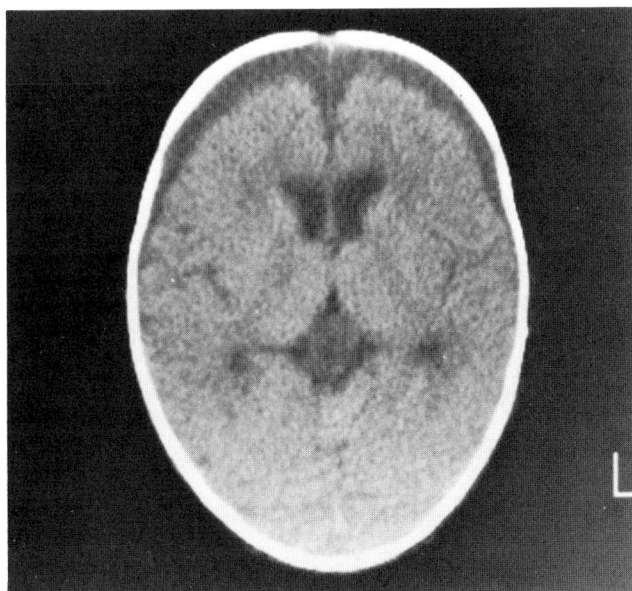

Fig. 32-1. A CT scan showing a subdural effusion in a child with bacterial meningtis.

Table 32-9. Cause for Recurrent or Persistent Fevers in Children with Bacterial Meningitis

Ineffective therapy
Phlebitis
Arthritis
Pericarditis
Mediastinitis
Subdural effusion/empyema
Osteomyelitis
Urethral catheter, tracheotomy tube, other foreign body
Tissue necrosis
Drug fever
Intercurrent illness
Unknown

the child has become afebrile on the second or third day (Table 32-9). Infants who have persistent fevers beyond 10 days are more likely to have an adverse outcome.

The prognosis varies somewhat with the organism. There is an overall mortality rate of approximately 5 to 20 percent (Table 32-10). The morbidity rate is relatively high. The most common neurologic sequelae are listed in Table 32-11. Of these, neurosensory hearing loss is the most common and distinctly more

Table 32-10. Mortality of Bacterial Meningitis in Children

Cause	Mortality (%)
Hemophilus influenzae	4.6
Neisseria meningitidis	6.5
Streptococcus pneumonia	9.2
Coliform bacilli	19.0
Group B streptococci	19.0

(Modified from McCracken GH: New concepts in the management of infants and children with meningitis. Pediatr Infect Dis 1:S51–S55. © 1983 The Williams & Wilkins Co., Baltimore.)

Table 32-11. Prognosis for Bacterial Meningitis

Sign or Symptom	Incidence (%)
Normal	60
Major handicaps	20
Deafness	
Mental retardation	
Motor deficits	
Ataxia	
Hydrocephalus	
Diabetes insipidus	
Cortical blindness	
Epilepsy	
Minor deficits	20
Learning disabilities	
Behavior disorders	

common following pneumococcal meningitis. Many of the complications of meningitis, such as behavioral disorders and learning disabilities, may not be apparent for years. Any child with recurrent meningitis should be examined carefully for immune deficiency, dermoid sinus, CSF leak, or other source of CSF contamination.

BRAIN ABSCESS

Brain abscesses result from hematogenous inoculation in patients with valvular or cyanotic congenital heart disease, contiguous spread from adjacent sinus and otitic infections, and rarely by direct inoculation from penetrating head injuries, compound skull fractures, or neurosurgical procedures. The association of brain abscess with cyanotic congenital heart disease is so frequent that such children who develop new neurologic signs or symptoms must be suspected of having a brain abscess until it is proven otherwise. The most common organisms are aerobic and anaerobic streptococci, although in large series many others have been isolated. Fungal abscesses are common as opportunistic infections. In the newborn period, gram-negative sepsis and meningitis can be complicated by abscess formation. About 30 percent of brain abscesses are located in the frontal lobes and the remainder are divided among the other major lobes of the brain and cerebellum; they are multiple in 15 percent.

The most common presenting signs and symptoms of brain abscess are signs of an intracranial mass, increased intracranial pressure, and fever. The mean duration of symptoms before diagnosis is 4 weeks, emphasizing the slow progression of this disease early in the course. Rapid decompensation can occur owing to growth of the mass and surrounding edema, and transtentorial and cerebellar herniation are the usual cause of death. The diagnosis is made by the clinical features and radiographic studies. A predisposing condition is usually evident and suggests the diagnosis. The chronicity of symptoms, focal signs, and papilledema are more compatible with an abscess than acute bacterial meningitis. The presence of fever and leukocytosis and the shorter duration of symptoms separate these children from those who have brain tumors (but not always).

The CT scan is the diagnostic study of choice. It should be performed both with and without contrast. The CT scan may be normal in a small abscess without much edema. In early abscess formation, there is a period of cerebritis in which there are no distinctive features on CT except for the presence of edema and mild contrast enhancement. After the abscess has becomes organized, the CT usually shows typical ring enhancement (Fig. 32-2). Tumors can also ring-enhance. The radionucleotide brain scan is also a good procedure for localizing a brain abscess. Lumbar puncture should not be performed if one suspects a brain abscess because of the risk of brain herniation.

Therapy includes supportive treatment of the vital signs and management of intracranial pressure. Antimicrobial therapy and neurosurgical intervention are definitive treatment. In the absence of bacterial identification, the initial choice of antibotics are penicillin G (250,000 U/kg/day in four divided doses)

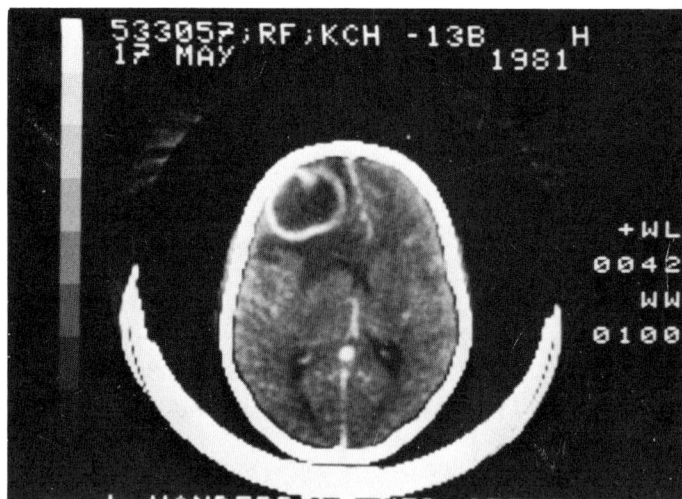

Fig. 32-2. A CT scan of a brain abscess.

and chloramphenicol (100 mg/kg/day iv in four divided doses). Patients can be managed medically if there is evidence of cerebritis only, without progressive mass effect, and the abscess shows definite reduction in size on serial CT scans. Most children will require surgery, not only because it is therapeutic but also to identify the organism and its antimicrobial sensitivities. Needle aspiration is recommended in children to lessen surgical trauma to the brain. The prognosis is a 10 percent mortality, 10 to 15 percent significant neurologic residual, and the remainder equally divided among normal and minor neurologic problems.

Epidural Cranial Abscess

Epidural abscesses are due to contiguous spread from an infected sinus or middle ear. The signs and symptoms are very similar to those of a brain abscess and frequently the two coexist. Additional features of an epidural abscess are the signs of the chronic sinus infection, such as swelling, redness, and tenderness to percussion of the infected sinus. Gradenigo's syndrome (apical petrositis, ipsilateral cranial nerve VI and cranial nerve V dysfunction) may complicate chronic middle ear disease. Otitic hydrocephalus is caused by lateral sinus thrombositis from similar infections. The diagnosis is usually apparent upon history and physical examination. The CT scan shows the subcranial location of an enhancing mass (Fig. 32-3). The treatment is similar to that for brain abscess but, in addition, the primary site of infection must be drained.

Epidural Spinal Abscess

Epidural spinal abscesses are rare in children under 10 years of age. The most common cause is due to hematogenous spread and less commonly contiguous infection from vertebral osteomyelitis. The location is usually thoracic

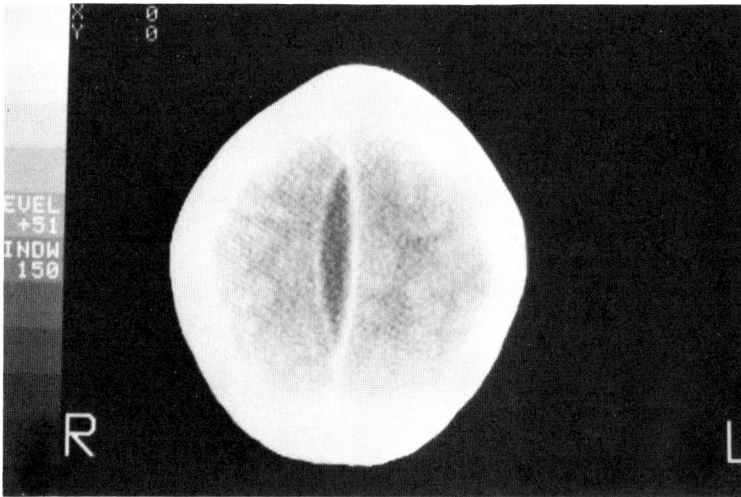

Fig. 32-3. A CT scan of an epidural abscess.

but can be in all regions. The causative organism is almost always *Staphylococcus aureus*. Rarely tuberculosis or fungal infections are encountered. The history may or may not indicate a prior injury or infection; often minor back trauma is reported. The most common symptom is severe back pain. Other signs and symptoms develop rapidly over several days (Table 32-12). The most significant sign is point tenderness over the site of the infection. Delay in diagnosis and treatment can result in permanent neurologic deficits such as paraplegia and loss of sphincter control.

The diagnosis is made by the history, physical examination, and selective laboratory tests. Most children appear ill with fever. Routine laboratory tests show a leukocytosis with a left shift and an elevated sedimentation rate. Ra-

Table 32-12. Progression of Symptoms and Signs of Epidural Spinal Abscess

Early
　Back pain
　Malaise
　Fever
　Irritability
Mid
　Severe back pain and tenderness
　Radicular pain
　Meningism
　Vomiting
Late
　Excruciating back pain or tenderness
　Paraparesis
　Bowel and bladder disturbances

Table 32-13. Differential Diagnosis and Clinical Features of Acute Paraparesis

Disease	Fever	Neutrophilic Leukocytosis	Elevated Erythrocyte Sedimentation Rate	Severe Pain	Bowel and Bladder Disturbance	Sensory Level
Epidural abscess	+	+	+	+	+	+
Transverse myelitis	−	−	−	−	+	+
Diskitis	+	−	+	+	−	−
Anterior spinal artery thrombosis	+	−	−	+/−	+/−	+
Epidural hematoma	−	−	−	+	+	+
Spinal cord tumor	−	−	−	+/−	+	+/−
Polio	+	−	−	−	−	−
Guillain-Barré syndrome	−	−	−	−	+/−	−
Hysteria	−	−	−	−	−	+/−

diographs of the spine are usually normal but may show vertebral osteomyelitis in a minority of patients. The differential diagnosis is listed in Table 32-13. The greatest confusion occurs in the diagnosis of acute transverse myelitis and diskitis. Myelography is the procedure of choice to diagnose an epidural spinal abscess and is normal in the other conditions. Transverse myelitis may not be resolved by clinical evaluation above without myelography. Diskitis causes intense back pain and refusal to walk but no neurologic deficits. Radiographs of the spine show a collapsed disk space and almost all children have an elevated sedimentation rate.

The treatment of spinal epidural abscess is a surgical emergency requiring decompression laminectomy and drainage. Antibiotics directed toward penicillin-resistant staphylococci should be instituted until cultures are available. A combination of choramphenical, 100 mg/kg/day, and methicillin, 200 mg/kg/day iv, or a similar antibiotic for 14 days is recommended. Longer therapy is indicated for coexistent osteomyelitits. The prognosis is excellent for full recovery if treatment is begun within 36 hours of the onset of weakness. Children with weakness for longer than 48 hours seldom recover without paraplegia.

Ventriculoperitoneal Shunt Infections

The incidence of shunt infections is 2 to 30 percent. The most common causes of shunt infections are *Staphylococcus epidermidis* (60 to 75 percent), *S. aureus* (20 to 30 percent), and grain-negative bacteria infrequently. The clinical signs are similar to those of increased ICP, with vomiting, lethargy, and irritability, but they can also be quite subtle. Fever is present in the majority of patients. Treatment requires intravenous antibiotics and removal of the shunt.

Table 32-14. Differential Diagnosis of Aseptic
Meningitis

Viral meningoencephalitis
Partially treated bacterial meningitis
Chronic granulomatous meningitis
Parameningeal bacterial infections
Brain abscess
Rocky Mountain spotted fever
Lyme disease
Sarcoidosis
Mucocutaneous lymph node syndrome
Acute disseminated leukoencephalitis
Amebic meningitis
Leukemic or carcinomatous meningitis
Systemic lupus erythematosis
Behçet's disease
Chemical meningitis
   Contrast myelography
   Rupture of dermoid cyst
Lead encephalopathy
Ventriculoperitoneal shunt infection
Mycoplasma
Neurosyphilis
Leptosporosis
Cat-scratch disease
Mollaret's disease

GRANULOMATOUS MENINGITIS

Chronic granulomatous infections should be considered if a child presents with meningitis or encephalitis with CSF pleocytosis, no growth on bacterial cultures, and failure to respond to antibiotic therapy and the CSF abnormalities and clinical signs persist. The differential diagnosis for chronic meningitis or persistent CSF pleocytosis is an important one (Table 32-14). Chronic infections are particularly common in the immunocompromised host. Specific antimicrobial therapy is available for most chronic granulomatous infections.

Tuberculous Meningitis

In children, tuberculous meningitis usually occurs with 3 to 6 months of primary pulmonary tuberculosis from hematogeneous spread during the miliary phase. The initial manifestations are very nonspecific, with fever, cough, malaise, and anorexia. Rarely there is direct inoculation from the middle ear or chronic mastoid infections. The neurologic manifestations of tuberculosis include meningitis, focal cerebral mass from tuberculomas or abscess, and osteomyelitis of the vertebra causing an epidural abscess and spinal cord compression (Pott's disease). Tuberculous meningitis can present fulminantly, similar to bacterial infections, or as a slowly progressive disease. If untreated, death will result within 3 to 5 weeks; it has a more rapid progression than other granulomatous infections. The clinical features are quite similar to those of acute bacterial meningitis

Table 32-15. Summary of Fungal Infections

Infection	Clinical Study	Primary Infection	Cerebral Infection	Treatment[a]
Actinomycosis	Opportunistic	Nasal sinuses	Abscess	P
Aspergillosis	Opportunistic	Pulmonary	Abscess	A, F
Blastomycosis	Sporadic	Pulmonary	Abscess	A
Candida	Opportunisitic	Indwelling catheters, skin mucosa	Chronic meningitis	A, F, M
Coccidioidomycosis	Sporadic	Pulmonary Disseminated	Chronic meningitis	A, M
Cryptococcal	50% opportunistic	Pulmonary	Chronic meningitis	A, F, M
Histoplasmosis	Sporadic	Pulmonary Disseminated	Chronic meningitis	A
Mucormycosis	Diabetes	Nasal sinuses	Abscess	A
Nocardia	50% opportunistic	Pulmonary	Abscess	S

[a] A = amphotericin B, F = 5-fluorocytosine, M = miconazole, S = sulfonamides, P = penicillin.

and fungal meningitis (Table 32-15). The granulomatous reaction is more intense in the basal subarachnoid space. Progressive strokes (Fig. 32-4), cranial nerve palsies, and extraventricular progressive hydrocephalus are the major pathogenic mechanisms of the neurologic disease.

The CSF is characteristically abnormal, with a pleocytosis of predominantly mononuclear cells which rarely exceed 500 cells/mm^3. The glucose is moderately depressed and the protein is elevated.

The diagnosis should be suspected in any child with progressive meningitis

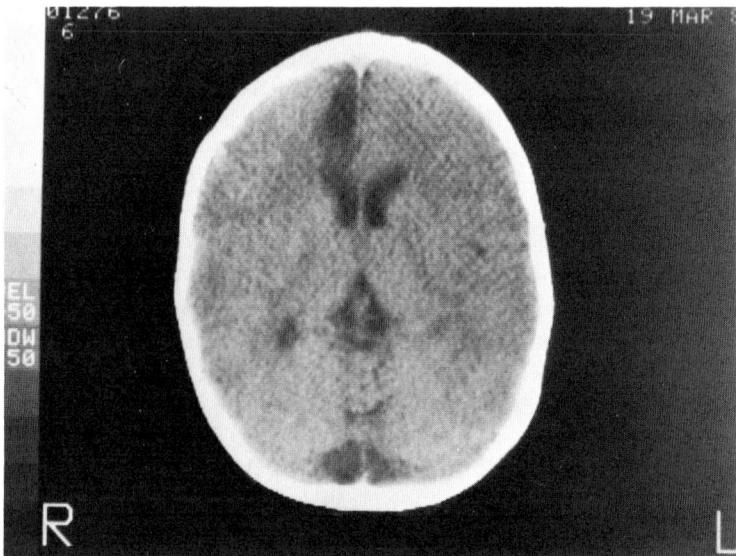

Fig. 32-4. A CT scan of multiple strokes in a child with tuberculous meningitis.

with negative bacterial cultures or CSF antigens. In almost every case an adult household contact will have active disease demonstrable on chest radiographs. The diagnosis is made by culturing organisms from the CSF. Because the time for the cultures to turn positive is relatively prolonged, initiation of therapy is indicated in suspected cases before culture-positive evidence is available. The skin test may or may not be positive. The differential diagnosis for chronic meningitis is listed in Table 32-14. Tuberculomas or tuberculous abscesses of the brain are extremely rare and present as a space-occupying mass lesions with focal signs and symptoms. An epidural spinal abscess with cord impingement is in the differential diagnosis of an acute compressive myelopathy.

The treatment consists of isoniazid (INH) at 20 mg/kg/day, up to a maximum of 300 mg, for 18 to 24 months. During the first 2 months of the illness streptomycin, 20 mg/kg/day, and rifampin, 15 mg/kg/day, are recommended. Mortality is 20 percent with therapy, and morbidity is approximately 20 to 30 percent.

FUNGAL INFECTIONS

A number of fungi are capable of producing neurologic disease (Table 32-15). Fungal infections present in two clinical situations. The first is during a primary pulmonary infection, with hematogenous spread to the CNS similar to tuberculosis. Often this is associated with disseminated disease of many organs. More common are fungal infections associated with the immunocompromised host in which an old infection is reactivated or an unusual organism causes opportunistic infection. Patients on glucocorticoid therapy or with cancer immunosuppression, diabetes, or other chronic diseases are more susceptible to fungal infections than healthy children. The clinical presentation of fungal infections consists of chronic meninigitis and focal infections of the brain. Rarely fulminant meningitis occurs, particularly in the immunosuppressed child.

The diagnosis of a CNS fungal infection is often difficult, particularly a primary infection not associated with immunosuppression. The major clinical features are listed in Table 32-16. The differential diagnosis of chronic meningitis is listed in Table 32-14. Except for cryptococcus, examination of CSF usually does not demonstrate the organism. The CSF India ink preparation can be diagnostic for cryptococcal meningitis. Several weeks are required for most fungi to be identified on appropriate culture media, except for *Candida,* which usually grows quite rapidly. Antigen detection and serologic studies are used for more rapid identification.

Amphotericin B is the major drug for the treatment of fungal infections (see Table 32-15). The dose is dependent upon the patient's tolerance of this nephrotoxic agent. It is initiated at approximately 0.1 mg/kg/day and increased, as tolerated, up to 1 mg/kg/day as an intravenous infusion over 4 to 6 hours. 5-Fluorocytosine, approximately 100 mg/kg/day orally every 6 hours, and miconazole, 30 mg/kg/day tid intravenously, are often used in conjunction with amphotericin B. The only exceptions are *Nocardia* infections, in which sulfonamides are the drug of choice, and actinomycosis, where penicillin is used.

Table 32-16. Clinical Features of
Granulomatous CNS
Infections in Children

Major clinical presentations
  Progressive meningitis
  Focal intracranial mass
  Epidural spinal mass
Clinical setting
  Glucocorticoid therapy
  Immunosuppresion
  Immunodeficiency
  Leukemia, lymphoma
  Indwelling catheters
  Uncontrolled diabetes
  Endemic exposure
  Chronic debilitating disease
Signs and symptoms
  Headache
  Meningism
  Vomiting
  Cranial nerve palsies
  Recurrent strokes
  Hydrocephalus
  Focal neurologic deficits
Laboratory abnormalities
  Persistent CSF pleocytosis
  Hypoglycorrhachia
  Elevated CSF protein

SPIROCHETAL INFECTIONS

The two major spirochetal infections are syphilis and leptospirosis. Syphilis is caused by *Treponema pallidum* and the infection is usually classified as primary, secondary, latent, or tertiary syphilis. A child can contract primary syphilis from sexual exposure, but more commonly syphilis in children is transmitted by trans-placental inoculation from the mother. If the mother has primary or secondary syphilis during pregnancy, stillbirth or fetal death usually results. With maternal latent or tertiary syphilis during pregnancy, however, the fetus may survive and have congenital syphilis. Children born with congenital syphilis may later de-velop the tertiary or neurovascular syphilis anywhere from 5 to 15 years after birth. The congenital manifestations are quite variable and presents from 2 to 8 weeks after birth. Signs at birth have a particularly poor prognosis. The major features include a rash, nasal discharge ("snuffles"), and other features to suggest a TORCH infection. The rash represents secondary syphilis and, unlike that in adults, is often bullous or vesicular. In addition, a papulosquamous reaction (condylomata), is often present in the genital region. Radiographs of the long bones may be particularly helpful in the diagnosis, in that the majority of patients shows metaphyseal osteochondropathy. Late manifestations of congenital syph-ilis include a number of dysmorphic features and signs such as Hutchinson's teeth.

Neurosyphilis is a late complication and follows a latent period of 4 years

Table 32-17. Laboratory Test for Syphilis

A. Nontreponemal antigen tests
    Flocculation (VDRL, Kahn, Kline)
    Complement fixation (Kolmer)
B. Treponemal antigen tests
    Complement fixation
      Reiter protein complement fixation
      Treponema pallidum complement fixation
    Agglutination
      Microhemagglutination (MHA-TP)
    Immobilization
      Treponema pallidum immobilization (TPI)
    Immunofluorescence
      Fluorescent treponemal antibody absorption (FTA-ABS)
      IgM-fluorescent treponemal antibody absorption (IgM-FTA-ABS)

(Reproduced with permission from Bell WE, McCormick WF: Neurologic Infection in Children. 2nd Ed. WB Saunders, Philadelphia, 1981.)

or more. Although rare in children, it should be considered in any child with a degenerative neurologic disease. There are four major presentations of neurosyphilis: meningiovascular syphilis, tabes dorsalis, general paresis, and focal neurologic symptoms secondary to gumma formation. Meningiovascular syphilis presents as a chronic meningitis without fever, recurrent cerebrovascular disease, and dementia. Tabes dorsalis is caused by vascular involvement of the dorsal root ganglia resulting in prominent posterior column signs with ataxia, a positive Romberg sign, and absent deep tendon reflexes. General paresis is a dementia associated with prominent psychiatric disturbances. Many of these patients often develop movement disorders as well. The Argyll Robertson pupil, a small irregular pupil with light–near reflex disassociation, may be present in any of these neurologic complications. Gumma formation is rare at any age but can present as a space-occupying mass.

The diagnosis of congenital syphilis is not difficult if the child has the typical clinical features of rash and snuffles. Long-bone x-rays and serologic testing will determine the diagnosis. Neurosyphilis may be difficult to diagnose but should be considered in the differential of the degenerative diseases in children. Features of congenital syphilis, abnormal CSF, and serologic testing of serum and CSF with the antigen-specific tests make the diagnosis (Table 32-17). Because the maternal IgG antibodies may confuse the diagnosis of congenital syphilis, a special IgM fluorescent treponemal antibody absorption test is available for the diagnosis in infants.

Treatment is with penicillin. If the mother is treated during the first trimester, it is unlikely the child will contract congenital syphilis. If the mother is treated later in the pregnancy, then the child is treated adequately as well. The child with congenital syphilis should be treated as if he had neurosyphilis. The dose of penicillin is 100,000 U/kg/day intravenously for 10 days. Often an exacerbation of the symptoms is noted (Herxheimer's reaction). Tertiary syphilis is treated with penicillin G at 600,000 U/day for 15 days. Repeated CSF examination is indicated to ensure eradication of the disease.

Leptospirosis

Leptospirosis is rare in young children and is primarily a disease of late adolescence and adulthood. The clinical features of leptospirosis are quite variable. The most severe infection is Weil's disease, which is characterized by fever, jaundice, azotemia, rash, headache, conjunctivitis, and abnormal liver function tests. Occasionally one sees a case of aseptic meningitis, with the typical features of headache, vomiting, meningism, and visual disturbances. There is usually a cellular pleocytosis of the CSF with mildly increased pressure and rarely a decrease in glucose. Some have considered this to be a postinfectious illness. The organismism can be cultured and diagnosed by serology. There are some questions as to whether penicillin alters the course of the disease. Lyme disease, another spirochetal infection, causes postinfectious complications (see Ch. 33).

RICKETTSIAL INFECTIONS

Of all the rickettsial infections, Rocky Mountain spotted fever is the most common cause of neurologic infections. This disease is geographically centered in the southern Atlantic and southern central United States. The organism infects the vascular epithelium. Seventy-five percent of affected children have a history of tick bite and the usual exposure time is May to September. The child may acquire the illness from a household pet or from direct invasion by walking in tick-infested woods. The clinical features are often nonspecific, with headache, malaise, anorexia, photophobia, and fever. After several days a rash which is more prominent on the extremities, including the hands and feet, and edema develop. Frequently the disease is confused with measles; purpura and a petechial rash at this stage may resemble meningococcemia.

Because there is a 15 to 40 percent mortality, an early diagnosis and prompt therapy are necessary. One should suspect the disease during the summer months of the year in a child with encephalitis associated with rash and a history of tick exposure. The diagnosis can be made by serology and the treatment is chloramphenicol, 100 mg/kg/day in divided doses for 10 to 14 days. Tetracycline at the same dose can be used in children following eruption of their permanent teeth.

Other rickettsial diseases are quite rare and their neurologic manifestations are milder. Most are associated with a rash.

MYCOPLASMAL INFECTIONS

The major pathogen of this group is *Mycoplasma pneumoniae,* which usually causes pulmonary infection or otitis media. The neurologic manifestations are primarily of two types. The first is an aseptic meningoencephalitis with a variable degree of severity. Although the disease might be quite severe, complete recovery is the rule. The second type of neurologic manifestation of myocoplasma consists of postinfectious complications. Mycoplasma has been implicated in transverse myelitis, acute cerebellar ataxia, Guillain-Barré syndrome, and leukoencephalitis. The diagnosis of mycoplasmal infections can be determined by serologic methods. Treatment, when indicated, is erythromycin.

PROTOZOAN INFECTIONS

The two major causes for neurologic protozoan infections are amebae and *Toxoplasma*. Amebae cause an amebic meningitis usually acquired from swimming in brackish water, stagnant lakes, and occasionally swimming pools. It can present as a chronic progressive meningoencephalitis or as an acute fulminating meningoencephalitis. It has features very similar to those of acute bacterial meningitis; however, the patient is unresponsive to antibiotics and the cultures are negative. Symptoms include headache, nausea and vomiting, fever, and meningism rapidly progressing to altered consciousness. Unless the disease is treated early in its course, it is usually fatal. It can be diagnosed by visualizing the organisms in the CSF.

The other major protozoan infection in children is acquired toxoplasmosis. This is usually a mild, asymptomatic illness with myalgia, rash, and symptoms similar to those of mononucleosis. Meningoencephalitis is a rare complication. In the immunocomprised host it can be a serious infection, with progressive deterioration resulting in coma and death. The CSF findings are usually mild and the protein modestly elevated.

PARASITIC INFECTIONS

Parasitic infections are quite rare in children. Perhaps the most significant parasitic infection of the nervous system in the United States is *Echinococcus* infection, which causes hydatid cysts in the CNS. In the southwestern states this is the most common cause of an intercranial mass in children. The presence of eosinophilia and focal neurologic signs suggest the diagnosis in the child from an endemic area. The CT scan will usually demonstrate the mass.

Many other parasitic diseases can cause neurologic infections. Eosinophilia and focal neurologic deficits are the most common signs.

VIRAL INFECTIONS

Viral infections of the nervous system cause three clinical syndromes: acute meningoencephalitis, "slow virus" infections, and postinfectious neurologic illnesses. The latter are covered in Chapter 32. The incidence of viral meningoencephalitis is greater than bacterial meningitis in children. Children are more likely to have neurologic complications of systemic viral infections rather than a primary infection of the CNS. The most common pathogens are the enteroviruses. They comprise greater than 90 percent of recorded viral infections of the nervous system.

Pathophysiology

The most common mode of CNS infection is hematogenous. Viral replication occurs at the primary infection site followed by a viremia. The virus enters the CNS through the choroid plexus and into the spinal fluid or by replication in the capillary endothelium of the brain. The other route of CNS inoculation is by contiguous spread through the peripheral nervous system into the CNS. The two common examples of this method are herpesvirus, along the trigeminal or olfactory nerves, and rabies, from peripheral nerves. Injury occurs by the process of viral replication and by vascular injury, which causes destruction of neurons and glial cells. The pathology of viral encephalitis demonstrates perivascular mononuclear cells (cuffing) and neuronal destruction. Intracellular and intranuclear inclusions are found, depending upon the specific infection.

Almost any virus can infect the CNS; however, some are more neurotrophic than others. In approximately 60 percent, a specific virus can be identified, by either culture or serology. Although there are some distinctive clinical features to suggest a specific infection, none are consistently present to distinguish one type of viral CNS infection from another. The geographic location, the age of the patient, the time of year, and community epidemiologic data are more likely to lead to a specific clinical diagnosis.

Clinical Presentation

The spectrum of viral neurologic diseases ranges from aseptic meningitis to encephalitis to chronic infection. Aseptic meningitis presents as a febrile illness with meningism; encephalitis is associated with altered consciousness, focal neurologic signs, and seizures. Many acute illnesses are characterized by meningoencephalitis with components of both meningitis and encephalopathy. The most common presenting symptoms are similar to those of bacterial meningitis. Myelitis causing flaccid paralysis is an occasional neurologic manifestation.

The clinical features of CNS infections of the major viral pathogens are listed in Table 32-18. Enteroviruses are the most frequent cause for aseptic meningitis and are often associated with rash and myalgia. Paralysis is characteristic of polio, although nonpolio enteroviruses can rarely cause paralysis. Poliomyositis is more likely to occur in the unimmunized during epidemics or in the immunocompromised child vaccinated with live attenuated poliovirus. Lymphocytic choriomeningitis is a typical aseptic meningitis except for the marked CSF lymphocytic pleocytosis.

Arbovirus infections are geographic and seasonal. Almost all occur in the summer and early fall months and are somewhat age related. California encephalitis and western equine encephalitis affect children and infants almost

Table 32-18. Viral Illnesses of Neurologic Importance

Virus	Syndrome[a]	Comment
DNA viruses		
Herpesviruses		
Herpesvirus hominis type I	EN	Common, sporadic
Herpesvirus hominis type II	AM	Genital herpes
Zoster varicellosus	EN, AM	Vesicular rash
Cytomegalovirus	EN	Congenital, immunosuppressed
Epstein-Barr	(EN, AM)	Mononucleosis
Adenoviruses	(EN)	Conjunctivitis, upper respiratory infection
RNA viruses		
Myxoviruses		
Rubeola	EN	Rash
Mumps	AM, EN (MY)	Parotitis
Togavirus		
Rubella	(EN)	Rash, congenital syndrome
Arboviruses		
California encephalitis	EN	Children, midwest
St. Louis encephalitis	EN	Adults
Eastern equine encephalitis	EN	Children, east and Gulf coast
Western equine encephalitis	EN	Children, west, midwest
Venezuelan encephalitis	(EN)	Rare
Colorado tick fever	(EN, AM)	Rare
Enteroviruses		
Poliovirus	AM, MY	Paralysis, immunosuppressed
Coxsackie	AM (EN, MY)	Rash, myalgia, viral syndrome
ECHO	AM (EN, MY)	Rash, viral syndrome
Arenavirus		
Lymphocytic choriomeningitis	AM	Marked lymphocytic pleocytosis
Rhabdovirus		
Rabies	EN	Animal exposure
? Mucocutaneous lymph node syndrome	AM	Adenopathy, stomatitis, rash

[a] EN = encephalitis, AM = aseptic meningitis, MY = myelitis. Parentheses indicate less common manifestations.

exclusively. On the other hand, St. Louis encephalitis is more likely to cause neurologic symptoms in adults than in children.

Herpes simplex encephalitis is the most common cause of nonepidemic encephalitis and occurs throughout the year. Herpesencephalitis has one of the worst prognoses for mortality and severe neurologic morbidity. Diagnosis should be suspected in any child with acute encephalitis, focal seizures or neurologic signs, and nonpurulent CSF. The spinal fluid may be normal, however. Periodic lateralizing epileptiform discharges on the EEG and temporal lesions on the CT or radionucleotide scan support the diagnosis.

Mumps encephalitis is a frequent complication of parotitis. As many as 50 percent of children with mumps demonstrate a CSF pleocytosis, but far fewer show frank encephalitic symptoms, which are usually mild. Occasionally encephalitis may be the only manifestation of the mumps infection. The incidence of this disorder is decreasing owing to immunizations.

Rabies is an almost universally fatal disease with a very long incubation period of 1 to 2 months. It is contracted from a bite or skin abrasion from an infected animal. Carriers include the bat, skunk, cat, fox, and raccoon and the infected domestic dog. Initial symptoms are usually abnormal sensation at the area of the scratch or bite followed by generalized malaise. This progresses over days with persistent fever, hypersensitivity to noises and light, hyperexcitability, autonomic dysfunction with increased lacrimation, perspiration, and salivation, followed by hydrophobia. Death occurs 3 to 8 days after the onset of the encephalitic signs. Because of the long incubation period, the encephalitis can be prevented if treatment is begun early. Human diploid rabies vaccine in conjunction with hyperimmune serum is the accepted method of postexposure treatment.

Diagnosis

An acute febrile illness, encephalopathy and/or meningsm, and a compatible CSF suggest the diagnosis of viral meningoencephalitis. Table 32-6 lists the CSF characteristics of viral and bacterial infections. In most viral infections, neutrophils predominate the CSF cells in the first 36 hours. In almost all instances, however, this reverts to a lymphocytic pleocytosis over the next 36 hours. It is rare for bacterial meningitis, even treated, to revert to a lymphocytic meningitis within the first 72 hours. The CSF protein tends to be much higher in bacterial disease, and hypoglycorrhachia is almost a constant feature. Distinguishing between early bacterial meningitis and viral meningoencephalitis can be difficult. Repeating the lumbar puncture after 12 hours in doubtful cases will usually clarify the issue. Serum antibody titers can be obtained for many of the neurotrophic viruses, although they are seldom available during the acute illness.

Treatment

Acyclovir (10 mg/kg every 8 hours) has been shown to reduce the mortality and serious morbidity of herpesencephalitis if instituted early in the course of the disease. There is no convincing evidence that its use will favorably affect the course of other viral infections of the brain. The treatment of rabies was discussed above.

SLOW VIRUS INFECTIONS

Table 32-19 lists the causes for slow virus infections in humans. Only a few are of clinical significance in children. Subacute sclerosing panencephalitis (Dawson's disease) and rubella panencephalitis are similar disorders. With the advent of immunization both are becoming less common. Subacute sclerosing panencephalitis is more likely to occur in children who had measles early in childhood than in those who had it at a later age. It is characterized by a relatively long latency period of 5 to 10 years. Initial symptoms are often a change in

Table 32-19. Chronic Viral Infections in Humans

Kuru	Tremulousness, ataxia; transmitted by cannabilism
Jakob-Creutzfeldt disease	Dementia, ataxia, extrapyramidal signs, myoclonus, spasticity
Progressive multifocal leukoencephalitis	Multifocal, asymmetric deficits, dementia; caused by papovavirus in the immunocompromised host
Subacute sclerosing panencephalitis	Dementia, myoclonic seizures, spasticity; caused by rubeola
Progressive rubella panencephalitis	Dementia, ataxia, seizures, spasticity; caused by rubella
Chronic enterovirus encephalitis	Dementia, seizures; associated with IgG deficiency
Chronic poliomyelitis	Late reactivation of poliomyelitis

personality or deterioration in school performance followed by the onset of myoclonic seizures, dementia, and ataxia. The disease is universally fatal but may follow a rapid, slowly progressive, or saltatory course. The diagnosis can be made by demonstrating increased specific anti-measles antibodies in the CSF. The EEG shows a characteristic burst supression pattern early in the course of the disease. There is no effective therapy. Rubella panencephalitis has been described in children with congenital rubella. It has an earlier onset than subacute sclerosing panencephalitis but similar clinical features.

Children with agammaglobinemia cannot eradicate enteroviral infections of the CNS, which results in a persistent infection with progressive neurologic decline. Progressive multifocal leukoencephalitis also occurs in the immunosupressed, with symptoms of progressive focal neurologic deficits and a CT scan revealing multiple hypodense regions in the cerebral white matter. This disease has only rarely been described in children. Mollaret's disease is recurrent meningoencephalitis of unknown etiology but has the clinical and CSF characteristics of a viral infection.

SELECTED READINGS

Balagtas RC, Levin, S, Nelson KE et al: Secondary and prolonged fevers in bacterial meningitis. J Pediatr 77:957–964, 1970

Bell WE: Current therapy of acute bacterial meningitis in children. Part I. Pediatr Neurol 1:5–14, 1985

Bell WE, McCormick WF: Neurologic Infections in Children. 2nd Ed. WB Saunders, Philadelphia, 1981

Dodge PR, David H, Feigin RD et al: Prospective evaluation of hearing impairment as a sequela of acute bacterial meningitis. N Engl J Med 311:869, 1984

Fenichel GM: Neurological complications of immunizations. Ann Neurol 12:119–128, 1982

Grose C, Henle W, Henle G et al: Primary Epstein-Barr infections in acute neurologic diseases. N Engl J Med 292:392–396, 1975

Haynes RE, Sanders DY, Cramblett HG: Rocky Mountain spotted fever in children. J Pediatr 76:685–691, 1970

Jadavji T, Humphreys RP, Prober CG: Brain abscess in infants and children. Pediatr Infect Dis 4:394–398, 1984

Lerer RJ, Kalavsky SM: Central nervous system disease associated with *Mycoplasma pneumoniae.* Pediatrics 52:658–668, 1973

Lewis EB: Partially treated meningitis. Am J Dis Child 12:145–150, 1973

Kaplan SL: Current management of common bacterial meningitides. Pediatr Rev 7:77–87, 1985

McCracken GH: New concepts in the management of infants and children with meningitis. Pediatr Infect Dis 1:S51–S55, 1983

Menkes JH: Viral neurologic infections in children. Hosp Pract 13:101–109, 1977

Schaad UB, Nelson JD, McCracken GH, Jr.: Recrudescence and relapse in bacterial meningitis of childhood. Pediatrics 67:188, 1981

Sell SH: Long term sequelae of bacterial meningitis in children. Pediatr Infect Dis 2:90–93, 1983

Sumaya CV, Simek M, Smith MHD et al: Tuberculous meningitis in children during the isoniazid era. J Pediatr 87:43–49, 1975

Taylor HG, Michaels RH, Mazur PM et al: Intellectual, neuropsychological, and achievement outcomes in children six to eight years after recovery from *Haemophilus influenzae* meningitis. Pediatrics 74:198, 1984

Townsend JJ, Barringer JR, Wolinsky JS et al: Progressive rubella panencephalitis: late onset after congenital rubella. N Engl J Med 292:990–993, 1975

Whitley RJ, Alford CA, Hirsch MS et al: Vidarabine versus acyclovir therapy in herpes simplex encephalitis. N Engl J Med 314:144–149, 1986

Wilfert CM, Buckley RH, Mohanakumar T et al: Persistent and fatal central nervous system ECHO virus infections in patients with agammaglobulinemia. N Engl J Med 296:1485–1489, 1977

Yoger R: Cerebrospinal fluid shunt infections: a personal view. Pediatr Infest Dis 4:113–118, 1985

33

PARAINFECTIOUS NEUROLOGIC DISEASE

Parainfectious neurologic diseases are complications of the immune response to the infectious agent or other indirect pathogenic mechanisms rather than by direct injury by the infection itself. Different organisms can be associated with strikingly similar parainfectious syndromes and often the syndromes are not associated with any known previous infectious diseases. This chapter discusses monophasic parainfectious diseases of the CNS and specific infectious diseases with characteristic parainfectious neurologic complications.

POSTINFECTIOUS ENCEPHALOMYELOPATHIES

Postinfectious encephalomyelopathies (vasculomyelinopathies) are diseases which affect primarily the CNS, focally or diffusely, follow an infectious illness or immunization, and are associated with vascular injury, perivascular inflammation, demyelinization and occasionally hemorrhage. A number of terms have been used to describe these disorders (Table 33-1). The severity of the preceding infectious illness is not correlated with the severity of the neurologic syndrome. Because the pathologic picture is similar to that of experimental allergic encephalomyelitis, cell-mediated immunity against myelin basic protein appears to be the pathogenic mechanism. The typical pathologic lesion consists of small areas of perivascular inflammation, demyelinization, and edema. The lesions range from small and discrete to large confluent areas of necrotic injury with hemorrhage and liquefaction. White matter is involved to a greater extent than gray matter. Several clinical syndromes are recognized, although there may be considerable clinical overlap.

Disseminated Encephalomyelitis

Disseminated encephalomyelitis has been associated with the common viral exanthems, other viral infections, mycoplasma, bacterial infections, serum sickness, leptospirosis, drugs, vaccinations, and immunizations. It was particularly common when measles epidemics were widespread, with an incidence of about 1 in 1,000 cases. The illness occurs from several days to weeks following contact with the infectious disease or immunization. Progression may be acute or subacute over days to weeks. The syndrome consists of fever, seizures, meningism,

351

Table 33-1. Descriptive Terms for the
Vasculomyelinopathies

Acute disseminated encephalomyelitis
Acute disseminated vasculomyelinopathy
Acute hemorrhagic leukoencephalitis
Acute hemorrhagic leukoencephalopathy
Allergic encephalomyelitis
Demyelinating encephalopathies
Disseminated vasculomyelinopathy
Infectious encephalomyelitis
Parainfectious encephalomyelitis
Perivenous encephalitis
Postinfectious encephalitis
Postinfectious encephalomyelitis
Postinfectious leukoencephalitis
Postvaccinial encephalitis
Postvaccinial meningoencephalitis

(From Evans OB: Parainfectious neurologic diseases. Semin
Neurol 5:288–297, 1985.)

and altered mental status. Focal neurologic signs are common, particularly
ataxia. The cerebrospinal fluid (CSF) usually shows a mononuclear pleocytosis
and an elevated protein concentration. The computed tomographic (CT) scan
may show focal cortical enhancement and low-density white matter lesions.
Death occurs in 10 to 20 percent of patients, and an equal number remain
neurologically impaired. Many cases are mild and present as an aseptic
meningitis.

Acute Hemorrhagic Leukoencephalitis

Acute hemorrhagic leukoencephalitis (AHL) or Hurst syndrome, can occur
at any age but is more common in adults. Often there is no preceding illness.
The clinical features are similar to those of disseminated encephalomyelitis but
more severe and often associated with focal neurologic signs. In many cases an
expanding hemispheric mass is suspected and brain abscess or herpesencephalitis
is mistakenly diagnosed. Acute hemorrhagic leukoencephalitis is probably one
of the causes of the acute hemiplegia syndrome of childhood. Myelitis may also
be a prominent feature. Laboratory studies in AHL show a neutrophilic leukocytosis as high as 30,000/mm³; proteinuria is also common. There is a CSF
neutrophilic pleocytosis, xanthochromia, and elevated protein concentrations.
The CSF is normal in 10 to 20 percent of cases. The CT in AHL often shows
large, hypodense areas in the subcortical white matter with mass effect which
resolve if the patient survives. The majority of the patients die within several
days. There is no convincing evidence that corticosteriods are effective, although
some advocate their use.

TRANSVERSE MYELITIS

Transverse meylitis is probably an immune-mediated disease within the
spectrum of the vasculomyelinopathies, although the majority of cases have no
preceding infection. The clinical features are remarkably constant. Numbness

Table 33-2. Infections Associated with
Acute Cerebellar Ataxia

Coxsackievirus
ECHO-virus
Epstein-Barr virus
Influenza
Mumps
Pertussis
Poliovirus
Rubella
Rubeola
Scarlet fever
Typhoid fever
Vaccinations
  Smallpox
  Measles
Varicella

(From Feldman W, Larke RPB: Acute cerebellar ataxia associated with isolation of coxsackie virus type A9. Can Med Assoc J 106:1104–1107, 1972.)

and tingling in the feet often coincide with the onset of fever. Progressive loss of function in the lower extremities and difficulty in voiding follow. Back pain is a frequent complaint and some patients have meningism. Paraparesis and a sensory level are found on examination, with the sensory level usually at the midthoracic area. Often there is a band of hyperesthesia at the level of involvement. Pain and temperature loss are greater than position and vibratory sensory loss. Hyperreflexia and Babinski signs appear later. Rarely the cervical cord is involved, causing quadriplegia and respiratory compromise. The CSF may show a mononuclear pleocytosis of less than 100 cells and an elevated protein with normal glucose concentrations.

Cord compression by an epidural abscess and other causes of acute paraparesis should be considered in every patient (see Table 32-13). The illness progresses over several days in the majority of cases and then stabilizes. Improvement begins at 2 to 12 weeks, especially in children. If there is no improvement by 3 months, then the prognosis is poor; about one-third will have permanent deficits. About 3 to 6 percent of patients with transverse myelitis will ultimately be diagnosed as having multiple sclerosis because of recurrent demyelinating events.

ACUTE CEREBELLAR ATAXIA

Acute cerebellar ataxia (ACA) is a childhood disease with onset between 1 and 10 years, but the majority of patients are less than 3 years of age. Acute cerebellar ataxia can follow a number of viral infections, especially varicella (Table 33-2); in 50 percent there is no prodromal illness. The child is often recovering from the previous illness and then rapidly develops severe truncal and limb ataxia, titubation, nystagmus, occasionally lethargy, and rarely vom-

Table 33-3. Differential Diagnosis of Acute Cerebellar Ataxia

Postinfectious disorders
  Acute cerebellar ataxia
  Fisher syndrome
  Guillain-Barré syndrome
  Acute sensory neuropathy
  Myoclonic encephalopathy
Intoxications and ingestions
  Anticonvulsants
  Piperazine
  Cytosine arabinoside
  Other drugs
  Heavy metals
  Tick paralysis
Trauma
  Cerebellar contusion
  Posterior fossa subdural hematoma
  Postconcussive syndrome
Tumor
  Cerebellar astrocytoma, medulloblastoma
  Pontine glioma
  Ependymoma
  Remote effect of neuroblastoma
Meningitis
Acute hydrocephalus
Vascular
  Brain stem or cerebral stroke
  Cerebellar hemorrhage
  Basilar migraine
  Benign paroxysmal vertigo of childhood
Familial recurrent ataxia
Multiple sclerosis
Ataxia associated with episodic metabolic diseases

iting. The signs progress over several days until the disease reaches a maximum deficit and then plateaus for days to weeks. Recovery over weeks to months can be anticipated, although some children will have permanent mild ataxia. In general, the more severe the cerebellar signs, the longer the recovery and the more likely there will be persistent deficits. There are no specific diagnostic tests. The CT scan is normal but should be obtained in most cases to exclude tumor, unless the syndrome follows a typical varicella infection. Ingestions should always be considered in the differential diagnosis of acute cerebellar ataxia (Table 33-3). The CSF shows a mononuclear pleocytosis of 15 to 100 cells, but following varicella infection the predominant cell type may be the neutrophil. The CSF protein and glucose concentrations are usually normal.

The Fisher syndrome consists of ophthalmoplegia, ataxia, and polyneuropathy. It combines several features of both ACA and Guillain-Barré syndrome. The CSF shows albuminocytologic dissociation.

The ataxia/opsoclonus syndrome (myoclonic encephalopathy) is similar to ACA. Patients with this syndrome have polymyoclonus in addition to the violent eye movements. Many of these patients have an occult neuroblastoma, although most will not. In all such cases, however, a thorough search for tumor should be pursued with a chest and abdominal CT scan and measurement of urine catecholamines.

SYDENHAM'S CHOREA

Sydenham's chorea occurs between 7 and 30 days following group A streptococcal infection and can have a rather abrupt onset, although it is usually more insidious. The pathogenesis is unknown. Generalized chorea, emotional lability, and hypotonia are the major clinical features. Hemichorea occurs in 18 percent of cases. The chorea and hypotonia may be severe, but the emotional lability may be the most handicapping component. The syndrome persists for several weeks followed by improvement over several months. Most children will recover within 6 months, although some may have persistent signs, and relapses can occur, especially during pregnancy. Sydenham's chorea is found in one-third of patients with rheumatic fever, and in 10 percent it is the only manifestation. One-third of patients with isolated Sydenham's chorea ultimately develop other features of rheumatic fever. The anti-streptolysin O titer is normal in one-third of patients without other signs of rheumatic fever. The anti-DNAase B and anti-NADase titers may be helpful if the anti-streptolysin O titer is not distinctly elevated. Chorea may respond to haloperidol and, because of the high association with carditis, patients with Sydenham's chorea must have pencillin prophylaxis.

CAT-SCRATCH DISEASE

Cat-scratch disease is a relatively common disorder and is typically a mild illness with malaise, low-grade fever, anorexia, headaches, and regionally lymphadenitis 3 to 30 days following a cat scratch or bite. Ten percent of cases have neurologic complications after several weeks when the adenopathy begins to resolve. The neurologic manifestations range from aseptic meningitis to acute confusion, stupor, and convulsions. The neurologic signs are hypo- or hyperreflexia, extensor plantar responses, weakness, altered mental status, decerebrate posturing, nuchal rigidity, and occasionally optic neuritis. Complete recovery can be anticipated in almost all patients. An immune-mediated pathogenesis is suspected, although unproven, and the etiology of cat-scratch disease is unknown. The disease can be diagnosed by application of cat-scratch antigen prepared from lymph nodes of affected individuals. There is no therapy.

PERTUSSIS

Pertussis infections (whooping cough) is one of the most contagious of the infectious diseases and has a 3 percent mortality. It is particularly severe in infants and the unimmunized. Pertussis encephalopathy occurs during the paroxysmal stage, with acute onset of convulsions, stupor, and hemiplegia or quadriplega

Table 33-4. Guidelines Deferring Pertussis Immunization

Considerations to defer pertussis immunization
  Children with a personal history of convulsions
  Children with neurologic conditions that might predispose to seizures
Contraindications for pertussis immunization
  History of previous severe neurologic reaction following a previous pertussis immunization
  Persistent inconsolable screaming for 3 hours or more following a previous pertussis
    immunization
  Hyporesponsive shocklike state following a previous pertussis immunization
  Fever of 105° or more within 24 hours following a pertussis immunization not explained by
    other causes
  Convulsion within 48 hours following a previous pertussis immunization
  Allergic reaction to the vaccine

(Data from Committee on Infectious Diseases: Pertussis vaccine. Pediatrics 74:303–305, 1984.)

and is caused by hypoxemia associated with the paroxysmal coughing and airway obstruction. There is controversy concerning pertussis immunization and the selection of patients for pertussis immunization. The risk for severe neurologic complications with pertussis immunization is about 1 in 310,000 and consists of fever, encephalopathy, and seizures. The natural disease is associated with a much higher risk of neurologic injury and death than the risk involved with immunization. Guidelines published by The American Academy of Pediatrics recommend deferring pertussis immunization for certain patients (Table 33-4).

REYE'S SYNDROME

Reye's syndrome is characterized by encephalopathy and fatty infiltration of the liver. Reye's syndrome is not thought to be immune mediated. It follows many viral illnesses, most frequently influenza B and varicell (Table 33-5). The disease begins with persistent vomiting and lethargy several days after the viral illness. Somnolence and occasionally combativeness follow and may progress to stupor and coma. At this stage decorticate or decerebrate posturing appear with other signs of increased intracranial pressure. Liver dysfunction is apparent by elevations in serum enzymes (serum glutamic-oxaloacetic transaminase, serum glutamic-pyruvic transaminase) and a prolongation of the prothrombin time. Other metabolic abnormalities include hypoglycemia, hyperammonia, lacticacidosis, and hyperlipidemic. Hyperbilirubinemia does not occur and, if present, one should consider other causes for hepatic encephalopathy. The CSF is normal except for elevated pressure. The characteristic pathologic finding in Reye's syndrome is a generalized mitochondropathy. Fatty accumulation in the liver and cerebral edema are characteristic. The mitochondrial injury causes the metabolic abnormalities and probably the neurologic injury.

There is no specific therapy, and treatment consists of general support and reduction of the increased intracranial pressure. Staging of the disease is helpful in directing therapy (Table 33-6). The liver injury is usually nonfatal and im-

Table 33-5. Viral Infections Associated with Reye's Syndrome

Adenovirus
Coxsackie A and B
Epstein-Barr
ECHO
Herpes simplex
Herpes zoster
Influenza A and B
Parainfluenza
Polio
Reovirus
Rubella
Rubeola
Vaccinia
Varicella

(From DeVivo DC, Keating JP, Haymond MW: Acute encephalopathy with fatty infiltration of the viscera. Pediatr Clin North Am 23:527–540, 1976.) Reprinted with permission from WB Saunders Co.)

proves prior to resolution of the encephalopathy. Mortality is about 30 percent; however, the majority of survivors are neurologically intact.

Epidemiologic data from several studies have suggested an association of Reye's syndrome with prior salicylate use in varicella or influenza infections. The American Academy of Pediatrics has recommended that children with these infections not be given salicylates.

ACQUIRED IMMUNE DEFICIENCY SYNDROME

Approximatly 30 percent of adults with acquired immune deficiency syndrome (AIDS) have neurologic signs. Reports of children with AIDS also indicate a high incidence of neurologic involvement. The neurologic signs usually follow

Table 33-6. Staging of Reye's Syndrome

	Stage I	Stage II	Stage III	Stage IV	Stage V
Level of consciousness	Lethargy, follows verbal commands	Combative stupor, verbalizes inappropriately	Coma	Coma	Coma
Posture	Normal	Normal	Decorticate	Decerebrate	Flaccid
Response to pain	Purposeful	Purposeful or nonpurposeful	Decorticate	Decerebrate	None
Pupillary reaction	Brisk	Sluggish	Sluggish	Sluggish	None
Oculocephalic reflex (doll's eyes)	Normal	Conjugate deviation	Conjugate deviation	Inconsistent or absent	None

(From National Institutes of Health Consensus Development Summary: The Diagnosis and Treatment of Reye's Syndrome. Vol. 4, No. 1. National Institutes of Health, Bethesda, MD, 1983.)

the systemic manifestations of failure to thrive, lymphadenopathy, hepatosplenomegaly, parotitis, and recurrent infections. Developmental delay is the initial neurologic sign. Encephalopathy is the most common complication and can mimic a progressive degenerative disease or an acute illness. Microcephaly, pyramidal tract signs, dementia, and seizures are common features. Some children appear not to have progression. A CT scan shows cortical atrophy, calcifications, and ventricular dilatation. Postmortem studies have shown cytomegalovirus infections in some children, but no etiology in others, despite evidence of vasculopathy and white matter injury.

Most children with AIDS are born to mothers who have AIDS or pre-AIDS. The etiology of the maternal disease consists of intravenous drug abuse, sexual exposure to high-risk groups, or Haitian hereditary extraction. A small percentage of children have contracted AIDS from contaminated blood products. The disease is caused by a retrovirus, human T-cell lymphotrophic virus type III (HTLV-III). Serologic assays have been developed that detect antibodies to HTLV-III.

SELECTED READINGS

Belman AL, Ultman MH, Horoupian D et al: Neurological complications in infants and children with acquired immune deficiency syndrome. Ann Neurol 18:560–566, 1985

Berman M, Feldman S, Alter M et al: Acute transverse myelitis: incidence and etiologic considerations. Neurology 31:966–971, 1981

Bird, MT, Polks H, Prensky AC: A follow-up study of Sydenham's chorea. Neurology 26:601–606, 1976

Byers RK: Acute hemorrhagic leukoencephalitis: reports of three cases and review of the literature. Pediatrics 56:727–735, 1975

Committee on Infectious Diseases. Aspirin and Reye syndrome. Pediatrics 69:810–812, 1984

Committee on Infectious Diseases. Pertussis vaccine. Pediatrics 74:303–305, 1984

Cotton DG: Acute cerebellar ataxia. Arch Dis Child 32:163–188, 1957

DeVivo DC, Keating JP, Haymond MW: Acute encephalopathy with fatty infiltration of the viscera. Pediatr Clin North Am 23:527–540, 1976

Doughtry RA: Lyme disease. Pediatr Rev 6:20–25, 1984

Evans OB: Parainfectious neurologic diseases. Semin Neurol 5:288–297, 1985

Grose C, Henle D, Henle G et al: Primary Epstein-Barr virus infections in acute neurologic diseases. N Engl J Med 292:392–395, 1975

Lerer RJ, Kalavsley SM: Central nervous system disease associated with *Mycoplasma pneumoniae* infection. Report of 5 cases and review of literature. Pediatrics 52:658–668, 1973

Poser CM: Disseminated vasculomyelinopathy. Ann Neurol 8:550, 1980

Weiss S, Carter S: Course and prognosis of acute cerebellar ataxia in children. Neurology 9:711–721, 1959

34

CEREBROVASCULAR DISEASE

Stroke is a relatively rare disorder in children, especially when it occurs as an isolated event. It is more frequently seen as a complication of other diseases such as cyanotic congenital heart disease and hemoglobinopathies. Atherosclerotic disease is the most common cause of stroke in adults but is extremely rare in children. One can divide strokes into those which are caused by thrombosis of cerebral arteries or veins, by intracranial hemorrhage, and by embolic disease.

PATHOPHYSIOLOGY

The neurologic manifestations of cerebrovascular disease are the result of brain infarction and focal edema or mass effect from hemorrhage. Thrombotic infarction is usually associated with diseases of the vessel walls which cause narrowing and sludging of blood flow. The factors that affect the viscosity of blood and its flow also contribute to the pathogenesis of thrombotic stroke, such as is found in sickle cell disease and polycythemia. Hemorrhage is usually caused by congenital structural defects of cerebral vessels. Embolic strokes are almost always of cardiac origin due to valvular heart disease or paradoxical embolus in cyanotic congenital heart disease.

The clinical progression of the stroke reflects the pathophysiology. Thrombotic infarction frequently progresses in a crescendo manner. There is a sudden onset of a mild deficit which progresses to a maximum deficit over hours as the thrombus propagates, thereby increasing the affected vascular territory. There is usually no headache or seizure. An embolus causes a sudden deficit with maximal loss of function at the onset. The embolus frequently will fragment and dislodge with clinical improvement. Hemorrhage is almost always associated with a severe headache at the onset because of the sudden increase in intracranial pressure. The neurologic deficits tend to be quite variable with hemorrhage and not as anatomically localizing as with the other causes of stroke.

Regardless of the cause, the pattern of neurologic deficits can lead to neuroanatomic localization. The distribution of the middle cerebral artery is the most common distribution of infarction, although others can occur. Table 34-1 outlines the major stroke syndromes. When small vessels are involved, partial expression of the stroke syndrome can occur. Strokes in children have an overall favorable prognosis. The majority of cases will improve if not completely resolve their deficits, depending upon the extent of the lesion and any underlying diseases. Repeated strokes, however, are additive. Young children have a better

Table 34-1. Stroke Syndromes

Anterior cerebral artery	Contralateral hemiparesis with legs > arms > face
Left middle cerebral artery	Contralateral hemiparesis with arm = face > leg, contralateral homonymous hemianopsia contralateral cortical sensory deficits, asphasia
Right middle cerebral artery	Contralateral hemiparesis with arm = face > leg, contralateral homonymous hemianopsia, contralateral cortical sensory deficits, constructional apraias
Posterior cerebral artery	Contralateral homonymous hemianopsia
Carotid artery	Combined features of individual branches
Vertebral-basilar	"Crossed" signs: ipsilateral cranial nerve and cerebral deficits, contralateral long tract signs "Locked in" syndrome: preserved consciousness and eye blink but no other voluntary movement

prognosis than other children or adults, probably because of the plasticity of the developing brain.

THROMBOTIC INFARCTION

Table 34-2 lists the causes of thrombotic stroke in childhood, most of which are quite rare. Traumatic causes are associated with three major syndromes. The first occurs in the young child who falls with an object in his mouth which penetrates his posterior pharynx and injures the carotid artery. Symptoms may not develop for up to 24 hours. The second syndrome is one of trauma to the neck which injures either the internal carotid artery or more commonly the vertebral arteries. Anomalies of the cervical spine may predispose one to such an injury. The infarction is caused by kinking or compression of the vessel associated with cervical fractures, hyperextension rotation injuries, and chiropractic manipulation of the neck. Head trauma is also a cause for thrombotic stroke, although more commonly hemorrhage is encountered.

Sickle cell disease is the most common cause of stroke in centers which have a large population of patients with this disorder. Approximately 25 percent of patients with sickle cell disease with develope neurologic symptoms, and of these 15 to 20 percent will be cerebrovascular accidents. The etiology is related both to intimal hyperplasia and to sluding of blood during a sickle cell crisis. Some children have repeated strokes, whereas many children never have any. Strokes do not occur with sickle cell disease at an incidence higher than that in the normal black population. Hematologic disorders that cause hypervicosity and stroke include polycythemia, thrombocytosis, and leukemic blastic crisis. Stroke can also be a complication of disseminated intervascular coagulopathy.

Thrombotic strokes can occur with cyanotic congenital heart disease, although embolic disease is more common. Polycythemia is a contributory factor. Vascular headaches appear to be more common in children with congenital heart disease, which also may be additive. The rare extracranial vascular diseases

Table 34-2. Thrombotic Cerebrovascular Disease in Children

Arterial thrombosis
   Traumatic
      Penetrating injury of the oropharynx or neck
      Cervical fracture
      Hyperextension–rotation of the neck
      Head trauma
   Hematologic
      Sickle cell disease
      Leukemic blastic crisis
      Polycythemia
      Disseminated intravascular coagulopathy
      Thrombocytosis
   Cardiovascular
      Cyanotic congenital heart disease
      Fibromuscular dysplasia
      Dissecting aneurysm
      Moyamoya
      Atherosclerosis
   Neurocutaneous syndrome
      Neurofibromatosis
      Sturge-Weber
      Tuberous sclerosis
   Infections
      Retropharyngeal abscess
      Acute bacterial meningitis
      Chronic meningitis (tuberculous, fungal)
      Herpes simplex ophthalmicus
      Meningovascular syphilis
   Arteritis
      Systemic lupus erythematosis
      Periarteritis nodosa
      Schönlein-Henoch purpura
      Cat-scratch encephalitis
      Isolated cerebral arteritis
   Drug-induced
      Oral contraceptives
      Ergotism
      L-asparinginase
      Intravenous amphetamine
      α-aminocaproic acid
      Phenylpropanolamine
      Ephedrine
   Metabolic
      Homocystinuria
      Fabry's disease (trihexosidase deficiency)
   Other
      Acute infantile hemiplegia
      Radiation induced vasculopathy
      Migraine
      Associated with neoplasms
      Hyperosmotic coma

Venous thrombosis
   Infections
      Bacterial meningitis
      Parameningeal infections
      Infections of ears, nose, face
   Hematologic
      Leukemia
      Polycythemia
   Other
      Cyanotic congenital heart disease
      Severe dehydration
      Nephrotic syndrome
      Lead encephalopathy

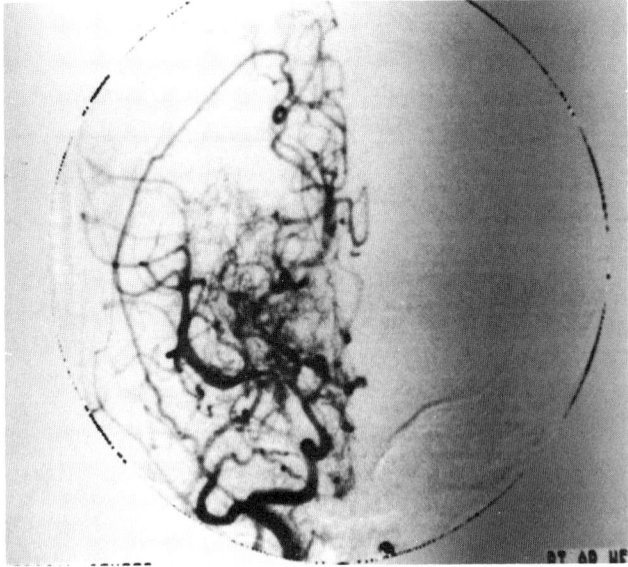

Fig. 34-1. Digital subtraction angiography in a child with moyamoya. Note the intense proliferation of collateral vessels arising from the proximal middle cerebral artery.

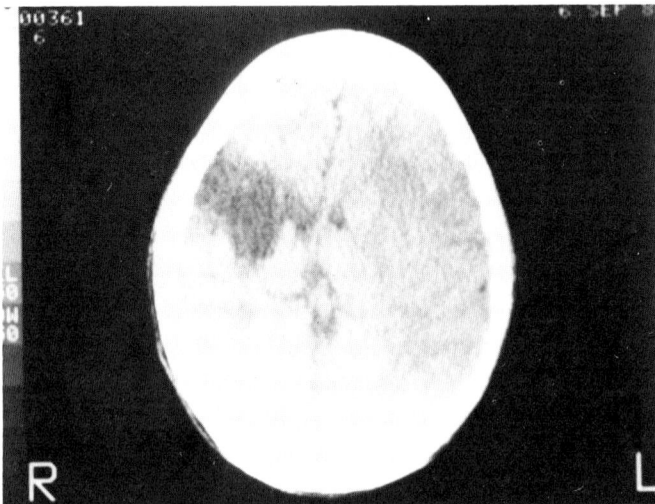

Fig. 34-2. A CT scan of an acute thrombotic stroke of the right middle cerebral artery.

Table 34-3. Hemorrhagic Cerebrovascular Disease in Children

Vascular malformation
  Aneurysm
    Congenital
      Idiopathic
      Associated with coarctation
      Associated with polycystic kidney disease
    Mycotic
    Myxomatous
    Traumatic
  Arteriovenous malformations
    Congenital
      Cerebral
      Vein or Galen malformation
      Spinal
      von Hippel-Lindau
    Traumatic

Other
  Hemorrhagic infarction
  Tumor hemorrhage
  Thrombocytopenia
  Anticoagulation therapy
  Perinatal intraventricular hemorrhage
  Traumatic
  Hemophilia
  Schönlein-Henoch purpura
  Leukemia
  Hereditary hemorrhagic telangiectasia
  None

include fibromuscular dysplasia of the carotid arteries, dissecting aneurysms, and extremely rarely atherosclerosis in such diseases as progeria and familial hypercholesterolemia. Moyamoya is becoming increasing recognized as a common cause of stroke of young children. It is also called progressive alternating hemiplegia and begins with either transient neurologic deficits or a strokelike episode without full recovery. Repeated strokes lead to multiple neurologic handicaps, retardation, and seizures. The disease affects the large arteries at the base of the brain. Compensatory collaterals are luxuriant and appear to dense on arteriograms as to give the impression of smoke (moyamoya; Fig. 34-1). Thrombotic stroke is rarely associated with neurofibromatosis and other phakomatoses.

Thrombotic stroke is frequently a complication of infections, particularly bacterial and tuberculous meningitides. Both veins and arteries are located in the subarachnoid space and traverse within the purulent material. The resultant vasculitis and thrombosis account for most of the focal neurologic deficits encountered in bacterial meningitis. Other infectious causes are quite rare and include retropharyngeal abscess with compression of the carotid artery, vasculitis associated with herpes simplex, and meningovascular syphilis.

Systemic arteritis, such as periarteritis, causes a vascular disease in many organs in which the brain is just one target. Isolated cerebral arteritis is the exception and can be very difficult to diagnose without biopsy. Of the remaining

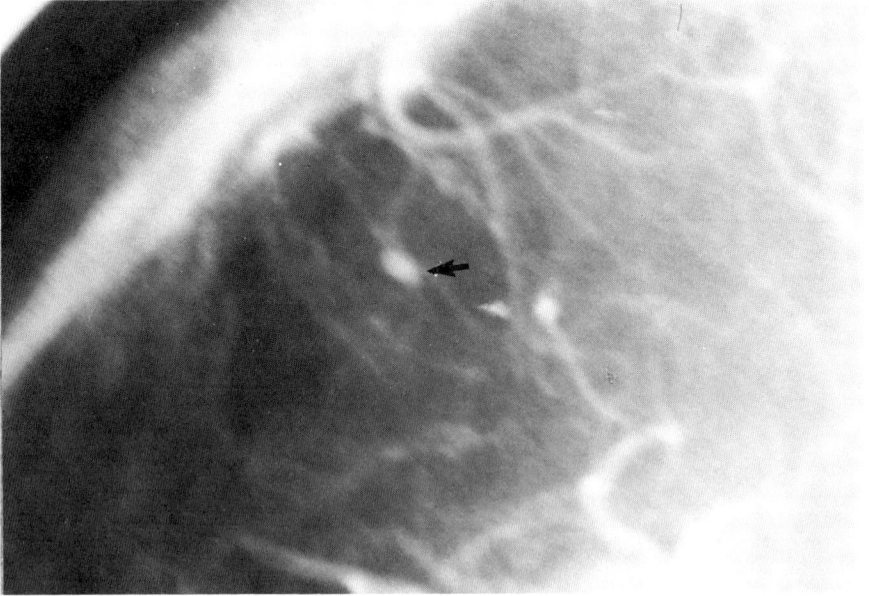

Fig. 34-3. Arteriogram showing a mycotic aneurysm.

causes of thrombotic stroke, none are common, particularly the drug-induced and metabolic causes. Radiation-induced vasculopathy occurs months to years after the exposure and causes an intimal hyperplasia. Neoplasms can cause compression of vessels in the neck or the brain and thrombotic stroke can occur with hyperosmotic coma. This often occurs in the setting of diabetic ketoacidosis or a hyperosmotic coma. Stroke as a complication of migraine is extremely rare and is more likely to occur in females who are on birth control pills.

Acute hemiplegia of childhood is a syndrome occurring in children less than 10 years old and characterized by an onset of hemiconvulsions, hemiplegia, and coma. The illness can be associated with a variety of disorders, as described above, but often the etiology cannot be determined. The neurologic deficits tend to be severe and persistent.

Venous infarctions occur almost exclusively with severe systemic diseases such as sepsis, meningitis, or severe dehydration. Dural sinus thrombosis is usually associated with meningitis, parameningeal infections, and ear, nose, and throat infections. Venous and dural sinus thrombosis causes both hydrocephalus and infarction. The clinical syndrome is one of dense deficits, seizures, and altered consciousness. The prognosis is uniformly poor. Increased intracranial pressure associated with lateral sinus thrombosis has been called otitic hydrocephalus.

The sudden onset of neurologic signs and the clinical setting usually suggest the diagnosis of thrombotic stroke. The computed tomographic (CT) scan can be particularly useful in confirming the diagnosis (Fig. 34-2). The therapies for

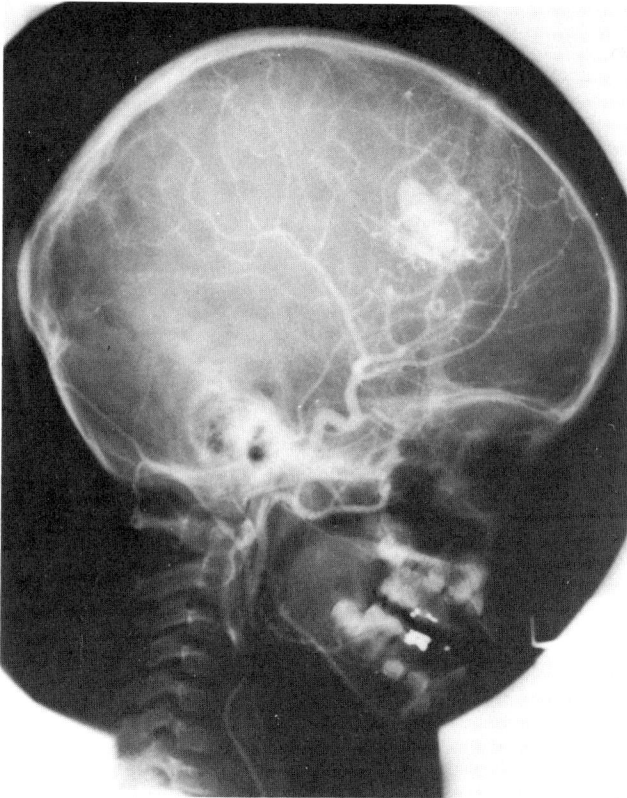

Fig. 34-4. Arteriogram of an arteriovenous malformation.

thrombotic stroke are aimed at correcting the underlying illness. There is no evidence that anticoagulation modifies the natural course of thrombotic stroke in childhood. Anticoagulation is contraindicated in venous infarctions because of hemorrhagic complications. Therapy for sickle cell disease has been shown to lessen the incidence of stroke. Hypertransfusion to maintain sickle cell hemoglobin at less than 30 percent has been shown to reduce the recurrence rate of stroke. The duration for such therapy has not been established, but 2 to 3 years is the normal period. The treatment of moyamoya is evolving with the sophistication in microsurgical techniques. Temporal artery bypass may improve blood flow to ischemic portions of the brain.

INTRACRANIAL HEMORRHAGE

Table 34-3 outlines the major causes of intracranial hemorrhage. The most common are those associated with prematurity, which are discussed in Chapter 9. In the older child, most hemorrhages occur as a result of either trauma or rupture of vascular malformation. One-third of children with a brain hemor-

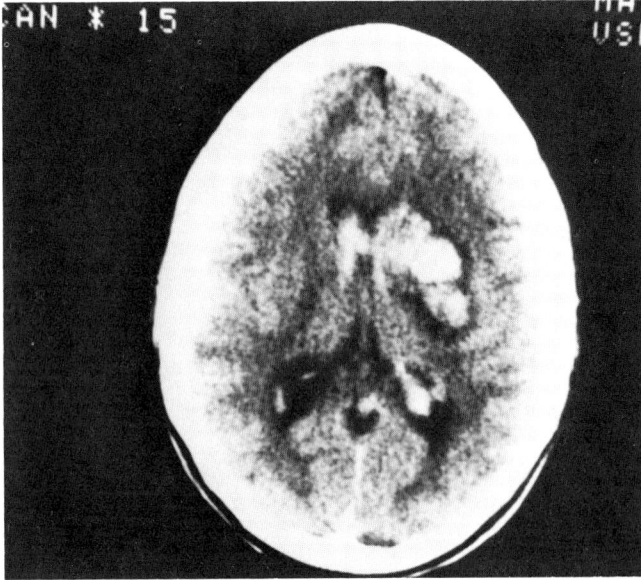

Fig. 34-5. A CT scan of an intraparenchymal and intraventricular hemorrhage from a ruptured AVM.

rhage have a ruptured aneurysm, one-third have a ruptured arteriovenous mal-formation (AVM), and one-third of cases have no discernible cause. Aneurysms are rare in young children. It has been reported in infants as young as 4 months but in the majority of cases occurs in the 10- to 20-year age group. Aneurysms can occur as an isolated disorder or can be associated with coarctation of the aorta or polycystic kidney disease. Berry aneurysms in children differ from those in adults in that they tend to be more distally located and are less likely to be

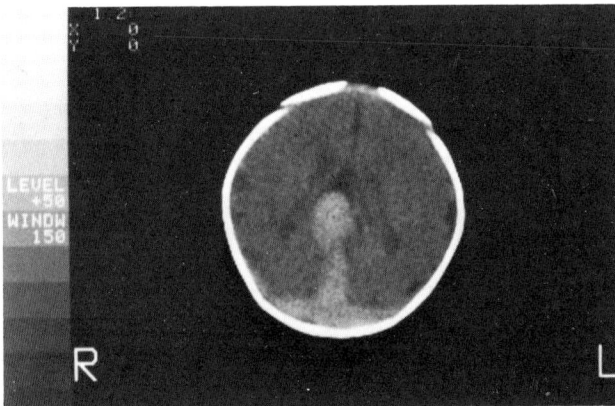

Fig. 34-6. Aneurysm of the vein of Galen.

Table 34-4. Embolic Cerebrovascular Disease in Children

Rheumatic heart disease
Subacute bacterial endocarditis
Atrial fibrillation
Myocardial infarction
Congenital heart disease with paradoxical embolus
Carotid atherosclerosis
Complications of cardiac bypass
Air or platelet embolism from surgery or catheterization
Fat embolism from fracture
Tumor embolism from atrial myxoma

multiple. Mycotic aneurysms as a cause of hemorrhage are extremely rare (Fig. 34-3).

Arteriovenous malformations (Fig. 34-4) present more frequently in the pediatric age group than in any other age. The most common presentation is a hemorrhage; less common are seizures and headaches. The headaches may be similar to migraine headaches. The AVMs are more likely to be in the parenchyma of the brain, as opposed to the leptomeninges, and usually cause intraparenchymal hemorrhages (Fig. 34-5). Rarely they can hemorrhage into the subarrachnoid space with little, if any, focal neurologic deficits. Intraparenchymal hemorrhage causes both focal neurologic deficits and increased intracranial pressure and frequently a fatal outcome. Malformations of the great vein of Galen usually present in the newborn with prominent scalp veins, signs of a mass lesion, heart failure, and hydrocephalus (Fig. 34-6).

Hemorrhage into a tumor presents as an acute deterioration of preexisting neurologic signs, although tumors can be clinically silent until hemorrhage occurs. Hemorrhage is often associated with head trauma, particularly with underlying conditions such as thrombocytopenia, anticoagulant therapy, and hemophilia.

EMBOLIC INFARCTIONS

Embolism to the brain almost always occurs as a complication of heart disease (Table 34-4). The most common causes are paradoxical emboli from cyanotic congenital heart disease with right–left shunting and emboli associated with valvular heart disease. Embolic stroke can be a complication of cardiac surgery and arterial catherization. Either thrombus formation at the site of invasion or an accidental introduction of air causes the embolic stroke. Fat embolism from long-bone fractures and tumor embolism from atrial myxomas are rare causes of embolic stroke.

DIAGNOSIS AND EVALUATION

The diagnosis of a cerebrovascular accident is usually obvious from the history and neurologic examination. The differential diagnoses are Todd's paralysis, complicated migraine, intracranial mass, and hysteria. The evaluation is

```
History          ─────────▶ Obvious etiology: infection, dehydration,      ─────▶ Diagnosis
Examination                                   trauma, leukemia, etc.
Routine laboratory       │
                         │
                  No etiology ─────▶ CT scan: tumor, abcess,                ─────▶ Diagnosis
                                              trauma, etc.
                                  │
                                  ▼
                         CT scan: infarction
                                  ↓
                                  EKG, Echo
                                  ESR, ANA, Anti-DNA
                                  hemoglobin
                                    electrophorsis
                                  urine nitroprusside
                                  VDRL
                                  LP                                         ─────▶ Diagnosis
                                  │
                                  │
                                  arteriography                             ─────▶ Diagnosis


                         CT scan: hemorrhage
                                  ↓
                                  PT, PTT, platelets                        ─────▶ Diagnosis
                                  │
                                  arteriography                             ─────▶ Diagnosis


                         CT scan: normal
                                  ↓
                                  LP                                        ─────▶ ?Diagnosis
                                  observe
                                  reevaluate
```

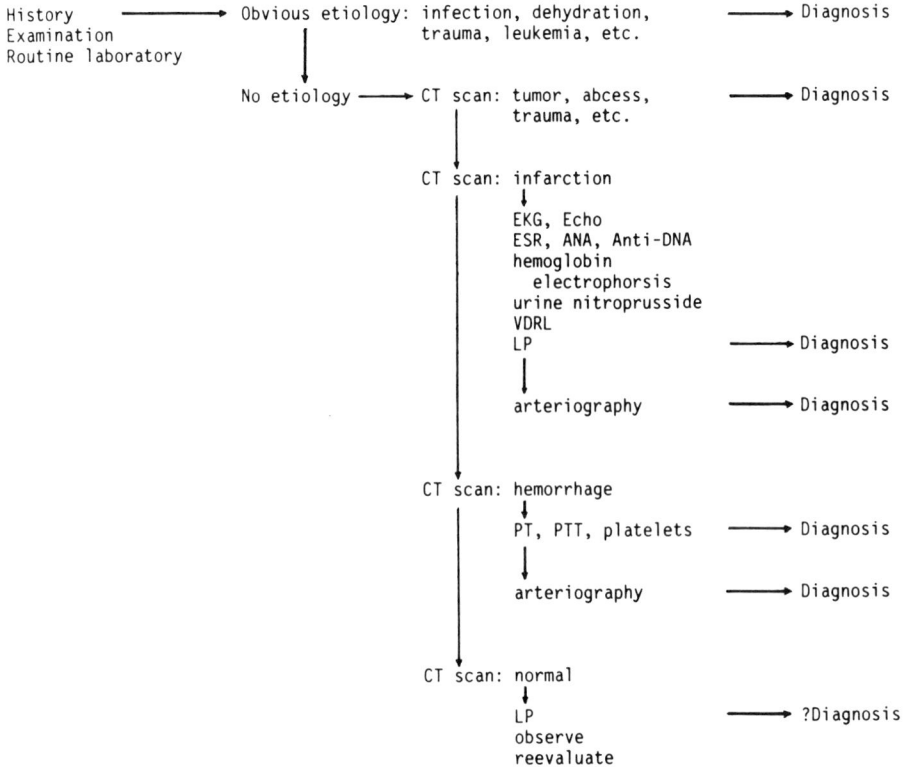

Fig. 34-7. Evaluation outline for cerebrovascular disease in children.

outlined in Fig. 34-7. The CT scan is the most important test, although a child with thrombotic or embolic stroke may not show any abnormalities on the CT scan in the early phases. Later hypodense areas appear which often contrast-enhance because of luxuriant perfusion. After resolution of the stroke, the hypodense lesion persists. The CT scan can easily determine the presence and location of intraparenchymal hemorrhages. Subarachnoid hemorrhages are less easily identified, particularly if they are small. In such cases the lumbar puncture may be more diagnostic.

Cerebral arteriography is indicated for all patients with brain hemorrhage and for thrombotic infarction if the etiology cannot be determined. The risk of arteriography is relatively small in skilled hands. If large-vessel disease is suspected or if the child is an infant, then digital subtraction angiography can be utilized with less risk. If the etiology is completely unknown, then four-vessel arteriography is often required (see Ch. 6).

The treatment of cerebrovascular disease is directed to the underlying disease, if known. Physical therapy is necessary to prevent contractures and to improve muscle strength. Rehabilitation should start as soon as the patient is stable. The goals of rehabilitation are to restore ambulation, teach self-help skills (e.g., eating, toileting, dressing), and speech therapy if necessary.

SELECTED READINGS

Aicardi J, Amsilli J, Chevvie JJ: Acute hemiplegia in infancy and childhood. Dev Med Child Neurol 11:162–174, 1969

Carlson CB, Harvey FH, Looper J: Progressive alternating hemiplegia in early childhood with basal arterial stenosis and telangiectasia (moya moya syndrome). Neurology 23:734–739, 1973

Cottrill CM, Kaplan S: Cerebral vascular accident in cyanotic congenital heart disease. Am J Dis Child 125:484–487, 1973

Harwood-Nash DC, McDonald P, Argent W: Cerebral arterial disease in children. Am J Roentgenol 3:672–686, 1971

Kelly JJ, Jr., Mellinger JF, Sundt TM, Jr.: Intracranial arteriovenous malformations in childhood. Ann Neurol 3:338–343, 1978

Lagos JC, Riley HD, Jr.: Congenital intracranial vascular malformations in children. Arch Dis Child 46:285–290, 1971

Long DM, Seljeskog EL, Chou SN, French LA: Giant arteriovenous malformations of infancy and childhood. J Neurosurg 40:304–312, 1974

Gold AP, Carter S: Acute hemiplegia of infancy and childhood. Pediatr Clin North Am 23:415–433, 1976

Grindal AB, Cohen RJ, Saul RF et al: Cerebral infarction in young adults. Stroke 9:39–42, 1978

Portnoy BA, Herion JC: Neurological manifestations in sickle-cell disease. Ann Intern Med 76:643–652, 1972

Roach ES, Garcia JC, McLean WT: Cerebrovascular disease in children. Am Fam Physician 30:215–227, 1984

Rodin AE, Chabali R, Minella PA et al: Cerebral berry aneurysm in a child. J Pediatr 100:156–159, 1982

Russel MD, Goldberg HI, Reis L et al: Transfusion therapy for cerebrovascular disease. J Pediatr 88:382–387, 1976

Seeler RA, Royal JE, Powre L et al: Moya moya in children with sickle cell anemia and cerebrovascular occulsion. J Pediatr 93:808–810, 1978

Wright TL, Bresnan MJ: Radiation induced cerebrovascular disease in children. Neurology 26:540–543, 1976

35

TUMORS OF THE NERVOUS SYSTEM

BRAIN TUMORS

Brain tumors are the most common solid tumors in children and constitute 20 percent of all neoplasms. The incidence of brain tumors pales in comparison with that of more common neurologic problems such as migraine, epilepsy, and developmental disorders, yet the brain tumor is still the most feared diagnosis by parents, even though the chance for cure is much better than for most neuromuscular or degenerative diseases. With modern neuroimaging techniques, the exclusion of a diagnosis of brain tumor can often bring immediate relief to concerned parents and children. This chapter discusses the clinical presentation of neoplasms of the CNS and the diagnosis and treatment.

Epidemiology

The incidence of primary brain tumors is 2 to 3 per 100,000 in children. The incidence remains relatively constant throughout childhood and has a male predominance. There is a much higher incidence of certain types of brain tumors in children than in adults (Table 35-1). Meningiomas and other nonglial tumors are very rare in children, whereas gliomas of the cerebellum, pons, optic nerves, and diencephalon are more common in children than in adults. The majority of tumors in children are located in the posterior fossa. In the adult population most tumors are supratentorial. About 50 percent of all brain tumors in adults are metastatic, whereas metastatic tumors in children are quite rare. Solid tumors that do metastasize in children are neuroblastoma, rhabdomyosarcoma, and Wilms' tumors. Leukemias can metastasize to the CNS and cause leukemic meningitis or multifocal leukemic nodules.

Clinical Presentation

The clinical presentation of a brain tumor depends entirely upon its location and, to a lesser extent, the tumor type. Table 35-2 lists the most common symptoms and signs of tumors in childhood. Clinically one can divide brain tumors into three groups: posterior fossa tumors, diencephalic tumors, and tumors of the cerebral hemispheres (Table 35-3).

Table 35-1. Approximate Distribution of Brain Tumors in Children and Adults

Tumor Type	Younger than 15 years (%)	Older than 15 years (%)
Cerebellar astrocytoma (spongioblastoma)	25	3
Ependymoma	15	4
Meduloblastoma	15	2
Other gliomas	13	12
Pontine	9	
Optic	4	
Craniopharyngioma	9	3
Oligondendroglioma	4	9
Pituitary adenoma	2	8
Meningioma	2	22
Ganglioma	2	<1
Pineal tumors	2	<1
Teratoma	1	<1
Angioblastoma	<1	3
Neurinoma	<1	10
Glioblastoma	<1	18
Choroid plexus papilloma	<1	<1
Other	<10	4

Posterior fossa tumors are those which are located in the posterior fossa itself or along the aqueduct. They have two major features: obstruction of the ventricular system by occlusion of the aqueduct or the fourth ventricle and compression of brain stem structures. The features of ventricular obstruction include headache, vomiting, personality changes, and changes in sleep habits. Findings may be seen with either small or large tumors, because either can completely obstruct the cerebrospinal fluid (CSF) drainage system. Interference with structures in the brain stem depend upon the tumor type. Brain stem gliomas, for example, usually involve cranial nerves quite early, whereas tumors located in the cerebellum present more often with long-tract signs and ataxia. The constellation of progressive cranial nerve palsies, long-tract signs, ataxia, and signs of increased intercranial pressure in a child is considered a posterior fossa tumor until proven otherwise.

Tumors of the hypothalamic region often present with endocrinologic disturbances. Although pituitary tumors are relatively rare in children, hypothalamic gliomas, craniopharyngiomas, and other rare tumor types frequently interfere with normal neurohumoral control of the endocrine system. Diabetes insipidus, accelerated or delayed sexual development, hypothyroidism, and growth disturbances are early features. Because of the tumor's location, there may be disturbances in the visual fields, particularly with craniopharyngiomas and optic gliomas. The major neurologic complication of histiocytosis is diabetes insipidus from parasellar bony involvement.

Cerebral hemisphere tumors are often difficult to diagnose. Depending upon the degree of malignancy, the tumor may be slow growing over many years and only be associated with seizures or headaches. The diagnosis is often made when the tumor grows to such a size as to cause increased intracranial pressure or

Table 35-2. Presenting Symptoms amd Signs of Brain Tumor

Symptoms
  Headache
  Nausea or vomiting
  Gait disturbance
  Visual disturbance
  Personality changes
  Developmental regression or declining school performance
  Speech disturbance
  Lethargy or drowsiness
  Enlarging head size
  Seizures
Signs
  Head
    Macrocephaly
    Bulging fontanelle (infant)
    Split sutures
  Eyes
    Papilledema
    Ptosis
    Asymmetric pupils
    Paralytic squint
    Visual loss
  Coordination
    Ataxia, dysmetria
  Reflexes
    Hyperreflexia, Babinski signs
  Motor
    Facial asymmetry
    Hemiparesis
    Diplegia
  Mental status
    Confusion
    Lethargy
    Somnolence
    Stupor or coma
  General exam
    Growth disturbance
    Precocious or delayed sexual development
  Other
    Head tilt
    Meningism

uncontrollable seizures. Other tumors, because of their location, manifest themselves relatively early with focal neurologic deficits. Seizures are a frequent sign of cerebral hemisphere tumors, although tumors are extremely rare in patients who have seizures. The presence of seizures and an acquired focal neurologic deficit suggest the diagnosis of a cerebral hemisphere tumor.

Regardless of location, tumors present differently, depending on their rate of growth. Rapidly enlarging tumors or tumors located in strategic locations where a small amount of growth may cause a significant amount of CSF obstruction may present over a few weeks or even a few days. Hemorrhage into a tumor can precipitate an acute presentation. Rarely, the tumor may be located so that it causes intermittent symptoms, such as an intraventricular tumor which intermittently obstructs the ventricular system. Most tumors are subacute in their

Table 35-3. Tumor Syndromes in Children

Location and Tumor Type	Predominant Clinical Features
Posterior fossa and pineal tumors	Signs of obstructive hydrocephalus and
Cerebellar astrocytoma	increased intracranial pressure (headache,
Ependymoma of the fourth ventricle	vomiting, etc.)
Medulloblastoma	Ataxia
Pontine glioma	Cranial nerve palsies Spasticity
Pinealomas and teratoma	Gaze paralysis
Diencephalon	Short stature
Hypothalamic glioma	Failure to thrive (diencephalic syndrome)
Optic gliomas	Visual field deficits
Craniopharyngioma	Visual disturbances
Pituitary adenomas	Visual loss
Colloid cysts	Optic atrophy
Cerebral hemisphere	Endrocrinologic disturbances
Astrocytomas	Parahypopituitarism
Glioblastomas	Diabetes insipidus
Oligodendrogliomas	Cushing's disease
Ependymomas	Acromegaly
	Abnormal sexual development
	Seizures
	Hemiparesis
	Language disturbances
	Headache
	None

progression, with signs and symptoms existing for months before a diagnosis is made. This is true especially in infants, because spreading sutures can more easily accommodate an expanding tumor. Occasionally there are chronic tumors which are present for years before becoming clinically apparent. These tumors are often located in the deep frontal structures and are of such low malignancy and slow growth that they do not cause any serious disturbance of underlying cerebral function.

The malignancy of a tumor depends upon its histology, location, and response to therapy. All of these characteristics must be considered when making

Table 35-4. Tumors Associated with Degenerative and Systemic Diseases

Disease	Tumors
Neurofibromatosis	Gliomas
	Meningiomas
	Neurilemomas
Tuberous sclerosis	Giant cell astrocytomas
Wiskott-Aldrich syndrome	Gliomas
	Lymphoreticular tumors
Basal cell nevus syndrome	Medulloblastomas
Ataxia-telangiectasia	Medulloblastomas
	Lymphoreticular tumors
Von Hipple-Lindau syndrome	Hemangioblastomas
Renal transplantation	Reticulum cell sarcomas

a prognosis. Certain tumors, such as medulloblastomas and ependymomas, can metastasize to the CSF space, causing spread to the spinal cord. Extra-CNS metastasis is rare and occurs most frequently with medulloblastomas. Some tumors are associated with certain degenerative and systemic diseases, especially the neurocutaneous syndromes (Table 35-4).

Diagnosis

If a brain tumor is suspected because of the history or examination, appropriate studies should be performed as soon as possible. Skull radiographs may show separation of sutures and other signs of increased intercranial pres-

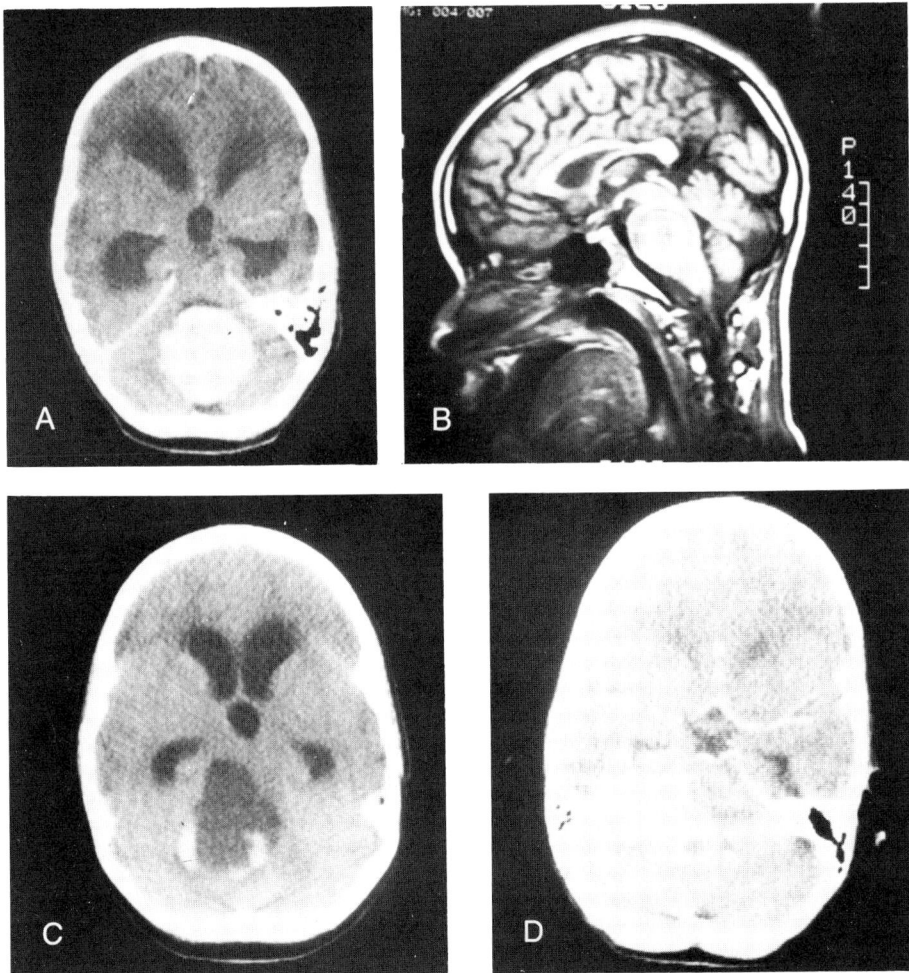

Fig. 35-1. Common pediatric brain tumors. (A) Medulloblastoma (CT). (B) Pontine glioma (MRI). (C) Cystic astrocytoma (CT). (D) Ependymoma (CT).

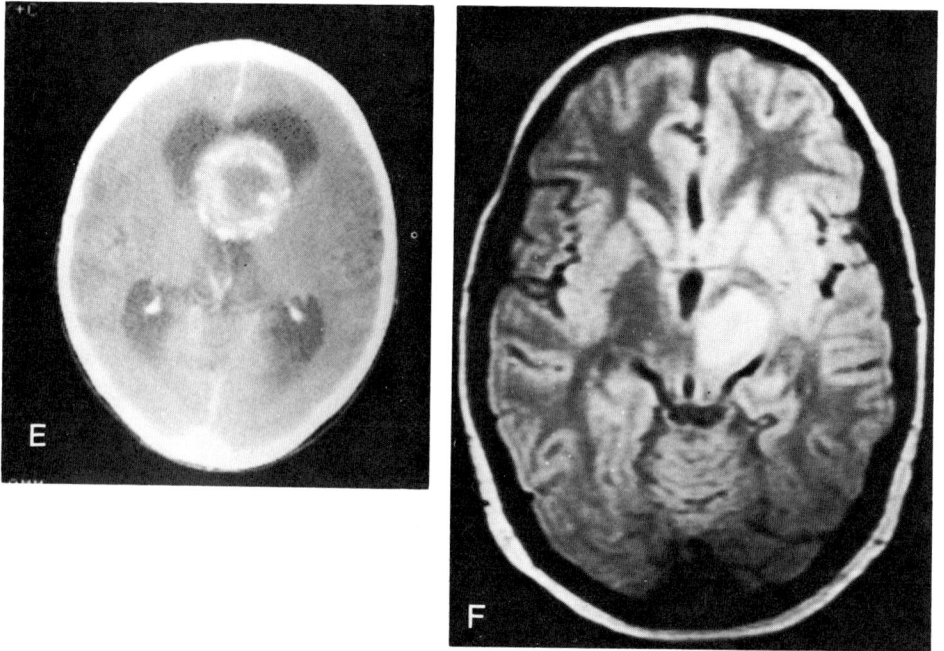

Fig. 35-1(Continued).   (E) Craniopharyngioma (CT). (F) Brain stem glioma (MRI).

sures, calcifications, or erosion of the sella and other signs of bony erosion. The pineal gland does not calcify until after 16 years of age in most children and its visualization before this age suggests a tumor. The computed tomographic (CT) scan with contrast enhancement will identify most tumors, but in some instances magnetic resonance imaging (MRI) or a technetium brain scan may be indicated if the CT scan fails to show an abnormality (Fig. 35-1). Electroencephalography, lumbar puncture, and evoked responses should not be used to make a primary

Table 35-5. Differential Diagnosis of Brain Tumors in Children

Infections
  Brain abscess
  Chronic meningitis
  Hydatid cyst
  Arachnoid cyst
Vascular malformations
  Arteriovenous malformations
  Aneurysms
Hydrocephalus
Chronic subdural hematoma
Pseudotumor cerebri
Degeneerative and metabolic diseases
Leukemia with CNS involvement
Lead encephalopathy

Table 35-6. Treatment and Prognosis of Common Childhood Brain Tumors

Tumor	Treatment	Five-year survival (%)
Medulloblastoma	Resection, focal and cranial irradiation, ? chemotherapy	40–50
Cystic astrocytoma	Resection, focal irradiation	75
Ependymoma	Resection, focal and craniospinal irradiation	50
Brain stem gliomas	Focal irradiation, ? chemotherapy	
High grade		0
Low grade		30
Pineal tumors	Focal and craniospinal irradiation, ? surgery, ? chemotherapy	50[a]
Astrocytomas (high grade)	Surgical resection, focal irradiation, ? chemotherapy	<20
Oligodendrogliomas	Surgical resection	>75
Optic gliomas	None[b]	>75
Craniopharyngiomas	Surgical resection	>75

[a] Depending on the tumor type. Germinomas are extremely radiosenstive.
[b] Resection indicated for patients with proptosis.

diagnosis but may be needed in the further evaluation to determine the extent of the tumor and clarify its location. Polyamines are elevated in the CSF of children with medulloblastomas and α-fetoprotein and chorionic gonadotrophins are elevated in teratomas and other germ-cell tumors. Arteriography is often performed to determine the vascular supply.

The differential diagnosis of brain tumor is presented in Table 35-5. The major considerations are other space-occupying masses and hydrocephalus. Whenever possible, a histologic diagnois should be obtained in any intracranial mass.

Treatment and Prognosis

The treatment of brain tumors should be performed by an experienced team specialized in neurosurgery, onocology, and radiation therapy. In general, surgical resection should be attempted unless the tumor is inoperable because of its location. The more tumor that can be resected, the better the prognosis. Stabilizing the patient medically and reducing edema are attempted before surgery. Frequently one must shunt obstructed ventricles prior to excision of the tumor, although there is a small risk of upward herniation with posterior fossa tumors.

Radiation is the mainstay of medical therapy, with 4500 to 6500 rads to the craniospinal axis for medulloblastoma, pineal tumors, and ependymoma. Radiation may retard the growth of other tumors. Chemotherapy is still experimental. A number of agents have been tested that show promise when used in conjunction with surgical excision and irradiation. Medulloblastoma has been the most extensively studied tumor and is perhaps the most chemosensitive.

The overall survival rate for brain tumor patients is about 50 percent, but the prognosis depends upon several factors. Females and older children have a better prognosis, as do supratentorial tumors and tumors with low-grade malignancy. Table 35-6 summarizes the treatment and prognosis.

SPINAL CORD TUMORS

Spinal cord tumors occur at approximately one-fifth the incidence of brain tumors, or approximately 0.4 per 100,000 per year. Spinal cord tumors can be generally divided into extradural and intradural tumors. Intradural tumors are either extramedullary or intramedullary in location in reference to the spinal cord or in the subarachnoid space (Table 35-7). Spinal cord tumors in children differ from those in adults in that there is a higher percentage of gliomas and congenital tumors. These latter tend to congregate in the upper cervical and lower lumbar regions near the embryonic neuropores.

Clinical Presentation

The most common symptom is back pain and the most common sign is a gait disturbance. In infants and small children, the inability to communicate symptoms and their immature motor abilities obscure the diagnosis. Irritability and inactivity may be the major complaints. One should consider a spinal cord tumor in any child with regression of development, particularly loss of bowel

Table 35-7. Tumors of the Spinal Cord	
Intramedullary	35%
Astrocytoma	
Ependymoma	
Hemangioblastoma	
Intradural-tetramedullary	30%
Congenital tumors	
Dermoid	
Epidermoid	
Lipoma	
Neuroenteric cyst	
Meningocele	
Neurinoma	
Extradural	30%
Neuroblastoma	
Lymphoma	
Sarcoma	
Congenital tumors	
Subarachnoid	5%
Medulloblastoma	
Ependymoma	
Pinealoma	
Papilloma	
Primitive neuroectodermal tumors	

(From Millorat TH: Pediatric Neurosurgery. FA Davis, Philadelphia, 1978)

or bladder control and/or an increasing gait disturbance. Back pain is a sufficiently infrequent complaint in children that it should be taken seriously and may lead to an early diagnosis of a spinal cord tumor.

It is difficult to determine clinically whether the tumor location is intramedullary or extramedullary. Extramedullary tumors are more likely to cause back pain and unilateral segmental deficits. Intramedullary tumors frequently cause early bilateral sensory and motor loss in a segmental distribution and disrupt the myelinated tracts, causing diplegia, sensory loss, hyperreflexia, and loss of bowel and bladder control. Of more importance is the rapidity of the tumor growth. Rarely a spinal cord tumor presents acutely, similar to an epidural abscess (see Ch. 32). Chronic tumors, such as those of congenital origin, interfere with growth of the back and extremities and result in asymmetric growth of the extremities, torticollis, and scoliosis, depending upon the location.

Congenital tumors may cause a tethered cord syndrome and often have skin abnormalities on the back and occult spina bifida (see Ch. 12). The cauda equina syndrome is caused by a mass in the spinal roots distal to the cord. Drop metastases from cerebral tumors (e.g., medulloblastoma, ependymoma) frequently present this way. The roots extent beyond the conus at L1 to their respective vertebral foramina. A tumor arising from a spinal root or encroaching from the dura distal to L1 can compress some roots and spare others, resulting in patchy neurologic signs in the lower extremities rather than the symmetric diplegia commonly found in cord tumors.

Diagnosis

A suspected diagnosis is made based on the physical findings and history. The differential diagnosis is relatively broad. In the acute spinal syndrome, the major differential considerations are transverse myelitis, ischemic cord injury from ateriovenous malformation or thrombosis of the anterior spinal artery, and epidural abscess (see Table 32-13). Extremely rarely a central herniated disk will produce similar symptoms. Other causes for the symptoms and signs seen in the chronic cord syndromes include brain tumors and hydrocephalus, congenital diseases such as a spinal cerebellar ataxia, and syringomyelia. A syrinx is a cavitary lesion in the spinal cord that presents with segmental sensory loss, scoliosis, and long-tract signs. It is frequently associated with a tumor or Arnold-Chiari malformation.

The key to diagnosis is radiography. Plain radiographs of the spine are positive in approximately 40 to 50 percent of children who have cord tumors, showing a widened canal or bony erosion. Myelography is the diagnostic method of choice (Fig. 35-2). Metrizamide is the contrast used most frequently in children, not only because it is soluble but also because it can be used in conjunction with CT scans to obtain better resolution. Anterior, lateral, and oblique views are necessary for a complete study. If no obvious tumor is present, the level of the conus should be determined to exclude the diagnosis of tethered cord. Delayed CT is indicated if one is considering a syrinx, although an MRI scan is more sensitive for this than CT (Fig. 35-3).

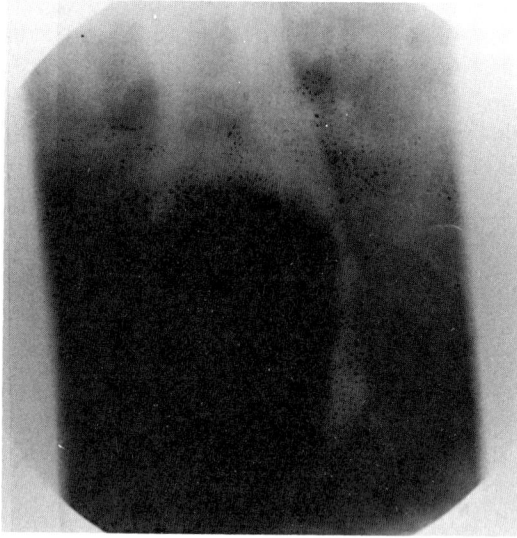

Fig. 35-2. Myelography of a congenital spinal tumor.

Treatment and Prognosis

The acute cord syndrome is a neurologic emergency and decompression laminectomy following myelography should be performed as soon as possible to avoid permanent neurologic deficits. In a chronic cord syndrome, one should

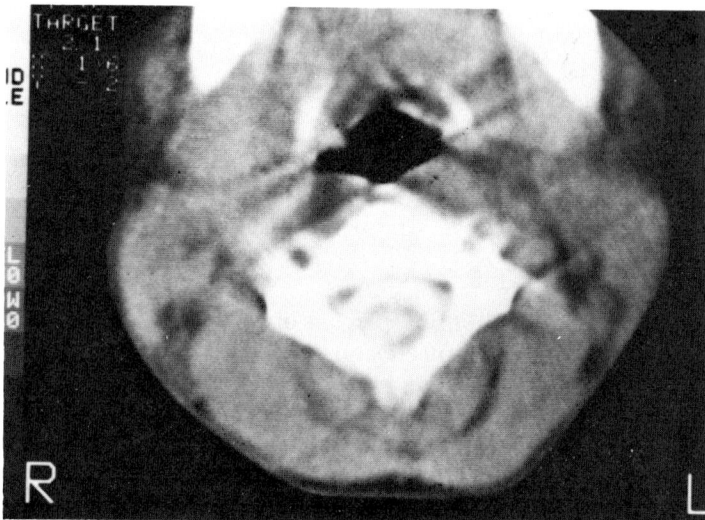

Fig. 35-3. Delayed CT scan of the spine following metrizamide myelography showing central cord enhancement of a syrinx.

first exclude the possibility of metastatic diseases or spread from contiguous structures, which might respond better to treatment directed toward the primary cause. With intrinsic cord disease, however, operative resection or decompression is the treatment of choice. Few spinal tumors respond to radiation. The prognosis for spinal cord tumors is relatively good; 50 percent have long-term survival. Even if the tumor cannot be completely resected, many additional years of ambulation and continence can be gained by early therapy.

TUMORS OF THE PERIPHERAL NERVOUS SYSTEM

Peripheral nervous system tumors arise from primitive neuroectoderm and neural crest cells. Tumors of segmental and peripheral nerves arise almost entirely from Schwann cells and are of two types: the schwannoma, or neurilemoma, and the neurofibroma. The schwannoma is an encapsulated spherical tumor composed of Schwann cells and collagen. Axons do not run through the tumor but are displaced to one side. The schwannoma may be an isolated tumor or it may be found in patients with neurofibromatosis and multiple tumors. Rarely does it degenerate into a fibrosarcoma.

Neurofibromas are unencapsulated fusiform swellings of nerves and have nerve axons embedded within them. The isolated neurofibroma is a slow-growing tumor and rarely undergoes malignant degeneration. It is commonly found in patients with neurofibromatosis.

There are a number of neurocutaneous syndromes in which neurofibromas and less frequently schwannomas occur at multiple sights. The best example is neurofibromatosis or von Recklinghausen's disease. Some families are more prone to get tumors of the cranial nerves, such as acoustic neuromas, whereas other families are more prone to get peripheral nerve tumors. The tumors may be small and subcutaneous or gigantic. Other variations of the tumors in neurofibromatosis include the plexiform neurilemomas and elephantiasis neuromatosa, which cause giant soft tissue tumors and the bony overgrowth seen in some patients with this disease.

Isolated peripheral nerve tumors may arise from any segmental peripheral or cranial nerve. They cause symptoms by compression of the nerve and usually present as a painless swelling but later develop into a painful, tender mass and may cause loss of function due to compression.

The treatment is excision for cosmetic reasons or if compression is compromising adjacent structures. If a peripheral nerve tumor undergoes rapid enlargment suggesting malignant degeneration, then radical excision is indicated. Malignant neurilemomas arising from these tumors can metastasize widely.

NEUROLOGIC COMPLICATION OF NEOPLASTIC DISEASE

Although neoplasms do metastasize to the CNS in children, other neurologic complications also occur. Some of the manifestations are listed in Table 35-8.

Table 35-8. Neurologic Complications of Cancer and
Cancer Chemotherapy

Metastatic effects
  Neoplastic meningitis
  Metastatic tumors
  Leukemic nodules
  Cranial nerve palsies
Remote effect of neoplasms
  Cerebellar atrophy
  Peripheral neuropathy
  Ataxia–opsoclonus–myoclonus syndrome
  Central pontine myelinosis
Secondary effects of therapy
  Radiation
    Decreased academic performance
    Acute edema amd encephalopathy
    Growth retardation
    Arteritis
  Immune suppression
    Opportunistic infections
    Progressive multifocal leukoencephalitis
    Chronic enteroviral infections
  Cytotoxic medications
    Vincristine: polyneuropathy
    Intrathecal methotrexate: arachnoiditis, myelitis (with
      irradication), subacute leukoencephalopathy
    L-Asparinginase: stroke

SELECTED READINGS

Allen JC, Epstein F: Medulloblastoma and other primary malignant neuroectodermal tumors of the CNS. J Neurosurg 57:446–451, 1982

Allen JC, Nisselbaum J, Epstein F, Rosen G et al: Alphafetoprotein and human gonadotropin determination in cerebrospinal fluid. J Neurosurg 51:368–374, 1979

Blume WT, Girvin JP, Kaufmann JCE: Childhood brain tumors presenting as chronic uncontrolled focal seizure disorders. Ann Neurol 12:538–541, 1982

Broadbent VA, Barnes ND, Wheeler TP: Medulloblastoma in childhood. Cancer 48:26–30, 1981

Dohrmann GJ, Farwell JR, Flannery JT: Glioblastoma multiforme in children. J Neurosurg 44:442–448, 1976

Dohrmann GJ, Farwell JR, Flannery JT: Ependymomas and ependymoblastomas in children. J Neurosurg 45:273–283, 1976

Goldberg TD, Bloomer WD, Dawson DM: Nervous system toxic effects of cancer therapy. JAMA 247:1437–1441, 1982

Haft H, Ransohoff J, Carter S: Spinal cord tumors in children. Pediatrics 23:1152, 1959

Jooma R, Kendall BE: Diagnosis and management of pineal tumors. J Neurosurg 58:654–665, 1983

Lyen KR, Grant DB: Endocrine function, morbidity and mortality after surgery for craniopharyngioma. Arch Dis Child 57:837–841, 1982

Marton LJ, Edwards MS, Levin VA et al: Predictive value of cerebrospinal fluid polyamines in medulloblastoma. Cancer Res 39:993–997, 1979

Merten DF, Goodnig CA, Newton TH et al: Meningiomas of childhood and adolescence. J Pediatr 84:696–700, 1974

Panitch HS, Berg BO: Brain stem tumors of childhood and adolescence. Am J Dis Child 119:465, 1970

Richardson FL: A report of 16 tumors of the spinal cord; the importance of spinal rigidity as an early sign of disease. J Pediatr 57:42, 1960

Wilson CB: Diagnosis and treatment of childhood brain tumors. Cancer 35:950, 1975

SECTION 8

Paroxysmal Disorders

The most common neurologic problems in children are the paroxysmal disorders. In most instances, the child is normal betweeen episodes. Seizures are by far the most common cause for neurologic consultation, but other paroxysmal disorders cause equal concern for children and their parents. At least 10 percent of all children will experience a seizure, severe headache, or other paroxysmal event. Fortunately, most of these disorders have a benign outcome and can be successfully managed if properly diagnosed and treated.

36

SEIZURES AND EPILEPSY

A seizure is an abrupt change in neurologic behavior and may be as dramatic as a generalized motor convulsion or as subtle as momentary inattentiveness. Seizures are the result of paroxysmal electrical discharges from the brain that supersede normal behavior. Seizures can complicate an acute encephalopathy or can be recurrent, in which event the case is called a seizure disorder or epilepsy. Approximately 3 to 5 percent of children will experience a seizure during childhood. Except for status epilepticus or seizures associated with acute encephalopathy, the physician will rarely observe an actual seizure. One must rely solely upon the history in order to make the diagnosis.

CLASSIFICATION

One must be familiar with the clinical characteristics of the various seizure types in order to recognize a seizure by another's description. A seizure episode is divided into three phases. The seizure itself is the ictus and can be convulsive, with motor activity, or nonconvulsive, with an interuption of activity, inattentiveness, or unresponsiveness (absence). The ictus occurs during the epileptic discharge of the brain. Symptoms just prior to the seizure form the aura, which is actually the first manifestation of the ictus. The symptoms reflect the functions of the brain involved with the seizure. They may be complex, with visceral or psychic experiences, or may consist of simple sensory sensations. The post-ictus follows the seizure and is a period of normalization of the electrical activity. The postictal features vary with the type of seizure and are characterized by inactivity. Generalized seizure activity is followed by generalized inactivity with altered consciousness similar to stupor. Partial seizures are followed by partial inactivity, such as a paralysis of an extremity following a focal motor seizure (Todd's paralysis) or confusion following a partial complex (psychomotor) seizure.

A classification of the seizure types is outlined in Table 36-1. Generalized seizures are those which eminate from deeper structures of the brain and involve the cerebral cortex more or less simultaneously. The generalized motor seizure may begin with a vague abdominal discomfort or dizziness. The ictus consists of generalized motor activity. This may involve generalized tonic contractions of the muscles, clonic rhythmic contractions, or a combination of both (grand mal). There is an autonomic component consisting of excessive salivation, tachycardia, sweating, and frequently urinary or bowel incontinence. The seizure may last for seconds but is usually longer and may interfere with normal respiration

387

Table 36-1. Classification of Epileptic Seizures

Generalized	
Tonic	Generalized muscle contraction
Clonic	Semirhythmic generalized muscle contractions
Tonic–clonic (grand mal)	Generalized muscle contraction followed by rhythmic contractions
Atonic	Brief loss of muscle tone
Myoclonic	Brief muscle jerks, generalized or focal
Absence (petit mal)	Loss of responsiveness and awareness, may have automatisms and changes in muscle tone
Partial	
Simple	Focal motor, sensory, or psychic symptoms and signs without impairment of consciousness
Complex (psychomotor)	Complex motor, sensory and psychic symptoms and signs with impairment of consciousness
Secondarily generalized (Jacksonian)	Partial seizures progressing to a generalized seizure
Unclassifiable	

(Adapted from Dreifuss FE: Proposal for revised clinical and electroencephalographic classification of epileptic seizures, Epilepsia 22:489, 1981.)

such that the patient becomes cyanotic. Following the seizure, there is postictal phase which is one of stupor with gradual recovery taking minutes to hours. During the postictal period there may be some neurologic signs, such as the extensor plantar response or posturing when stimulated. As the patient recovers he may become combative or seem confused. When awakened, the patient is amnesic for the event. The EEG during the generalized motor seizure shows generalized discharges involving both cerebral hemispheres simultaneously (Fig. 36-1). The interictal EEG can show paroxysmal spikes or spike wave discharges or can be normal.

The minor motor seizures are generalized seizures that are characterized by momentary changes in postural tone. One of the more common types in childhood is the infantile spasm (salaam, jackknife, giant myoclonic seizure). This occurs in children 3 to 18 months of age and is characterized by sudden flexion of the trunk and limbs. Extension occurs in a minority of patients. The seizures tend to be repetitive over several minutes. The most frequent time of occurrence is upon arising from sleep. Frequently parents mistake this for colic or other abdominal disorders. Many children with infantile spasms will have a characteristic EEG of generalized disorganization and high-amplitude multispiked wave discharges, called hypsarrhytmia (Fig. 36-2).

Atonic seizures are characterized by brief loss of muscle tone. This may vary from eye blinking to head nodding to completely falling. The EEG may show rhythmic spiked wave discharges (atypical petit mal). Myoclonic seizures are brief contractions of muscles or groups of muscles and may precede generalized motor seizures. The EEG in patients with minor seizures can show generalized disorganization, multifocal cortical discharges, or secondary generalization of a focal discharge.

Absence seizures, or petit mal, are characterized by brief staring episodes. Petit mal seizures usually last about 5 to 10 seconds, during which time the patient becomes inattentive but appears awake. There is rarely a change in pos-

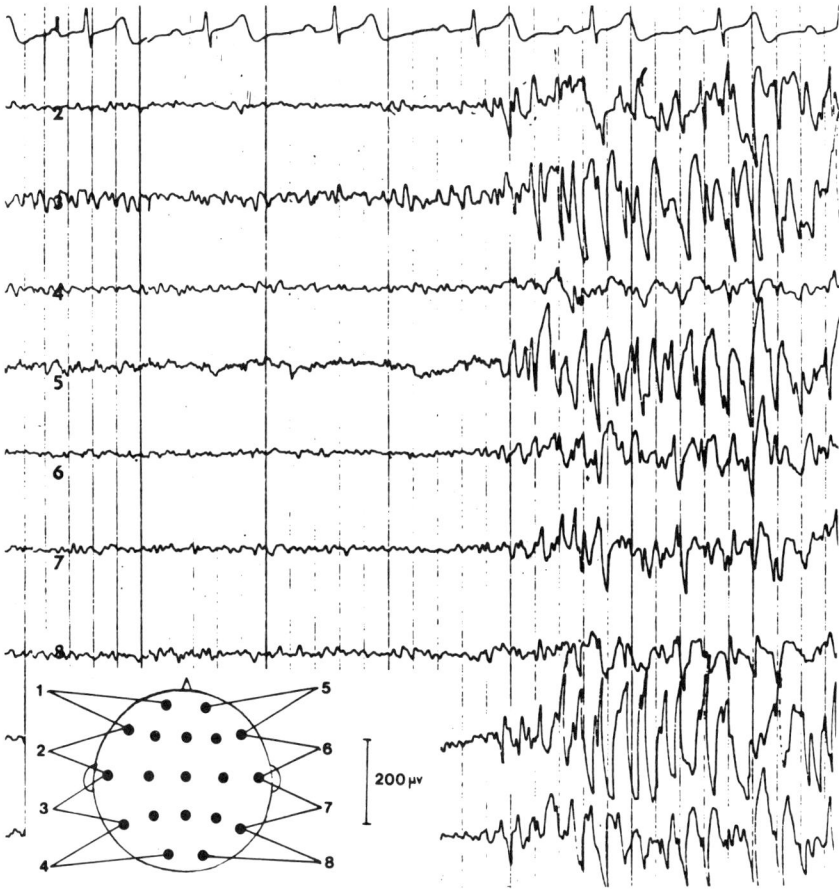

Fig. 36-1. Ictal EEG of a generalized motor seizure.

tural tone but occasionally the patient will make eye-blinking or mouthing movements. Other automatisms have been described. Frequently the child interrupts speech or other activities and then resumes the activities following the seizure. There is no significant aura or post-ictus. Children with petit mal epilepsy can have a few or a hundred such episodes a day, to the extent that it interferes with school performance. Absence seizures characteristically show three spike and wave discharges per second (Fig. 36-3). The latter can often be precipitated by having the child hyperventilate for 3 minutes.

The other major category of seizures are partial seizures. Unlike generalized seizures, partial seizures arise from a focal area of the cerebral cortex (Fig. 36-4). The ictus often begins with an aura that reflects that part of the brain which initiates the convulsion. Sensory and psychic experiences are common. If the discharge spreads, surrounding structures of the brain become involved in the seizure. The most classic example is that of the Jacksonian seizure, in which a

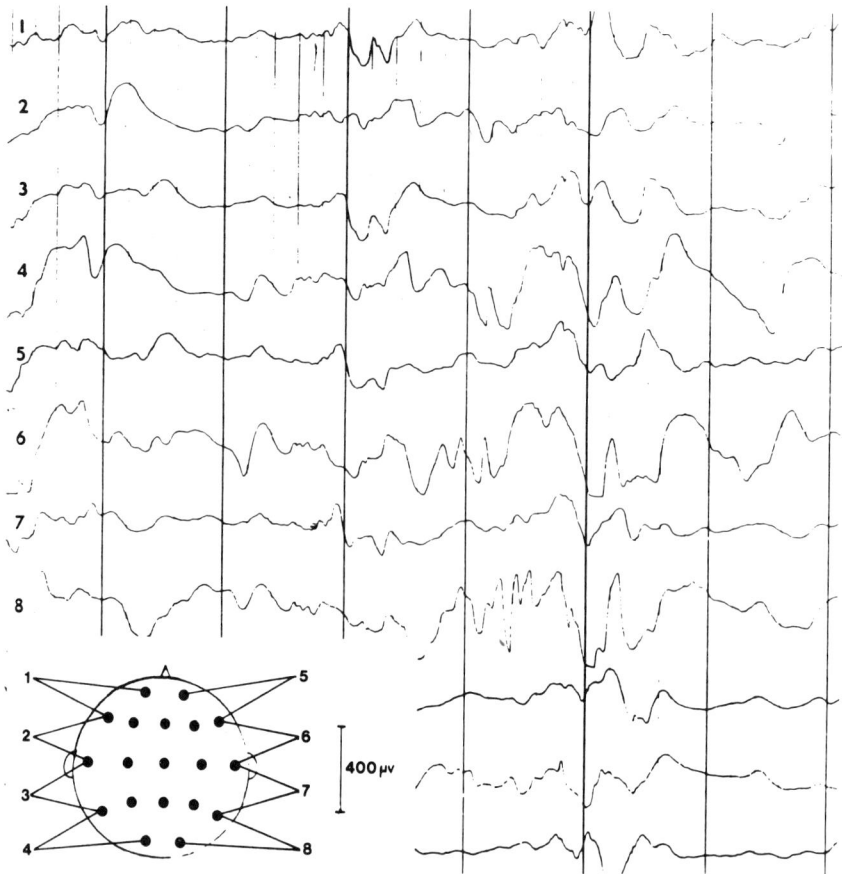

Fig. 36-2. Hypsarrhythmia.

focal motor seizure spreads in a marching fashion from one part of the body t ᴐ adjacent parts. A partial seizure may become generalized if it crosses the inteɪ - hemispheric connections and involves the opposite side of the brain. Descriptioɪ of the early part of the seizure, such as eye deviations or motor activity of one limb, may disclose its focal origin. Focal sensory or focal motor seizures are called partial simple seizures because the patient remains conscious. Rolandic epilepsy is a benign disorder in children arising from the motor cortex and frequently occurs during sleep (Fig. 36-5).

A partial complex seizure implies an alteration in consciousness. This is a focal seizure which involves those parts of the brain having to do with behavior and orientation and is also called a psychomotor seizure. These seizures frequently originate from a temporal lobe but may originate from other parts of the brain. During such spells there is abnormal behaviorism that is inappropriate to the child's situation. Symptoms range from staring to complex automatic movements such as chewing, vocalizing, or ambulating. The patient is amnesic for the seizure but may remember the aura.

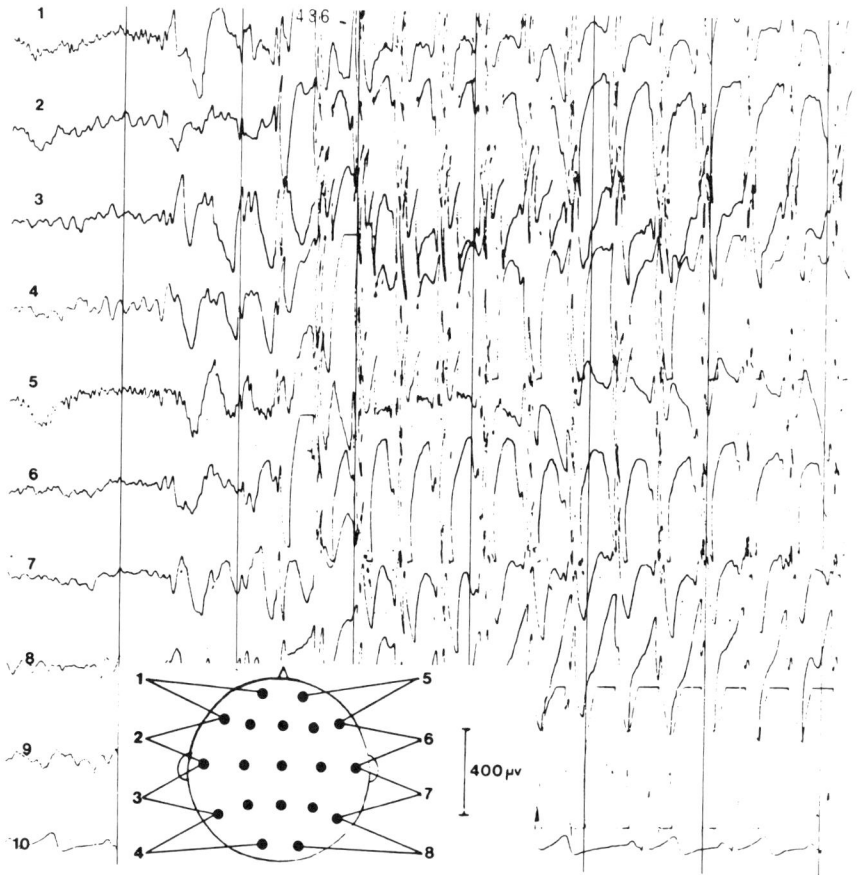

Fig. 36-3. Ictal EEG of absence (petit mal) seizure.

The post-ictus following a partial simple seizure with focal motor convulsion may consist of Todd's paralysis which normally resolves within a few minutes to hours but occasionally lasts as long as 24 hours. The EEG in partial seizures frequently demonstrates a focal cortical discharge from the appropriate part of the brain of the seizure origin.

THE EPILEPSIES

The epilepsies are based upon the seizure type and clinical features, such as age of onset, etiology, and pathology, that form specific epileptic syndromes and the basis of classification (Table 36-2). Some epileptic syndromes include more than one seizure type. The two major categories of the epilepsies reflect the classification of seizures: generalized and partial. The frequencies of the epilepsies in childhood are listed in Table 36-3.

Generalized epilepsies are either primary (idiopathic) or secondary (symp-

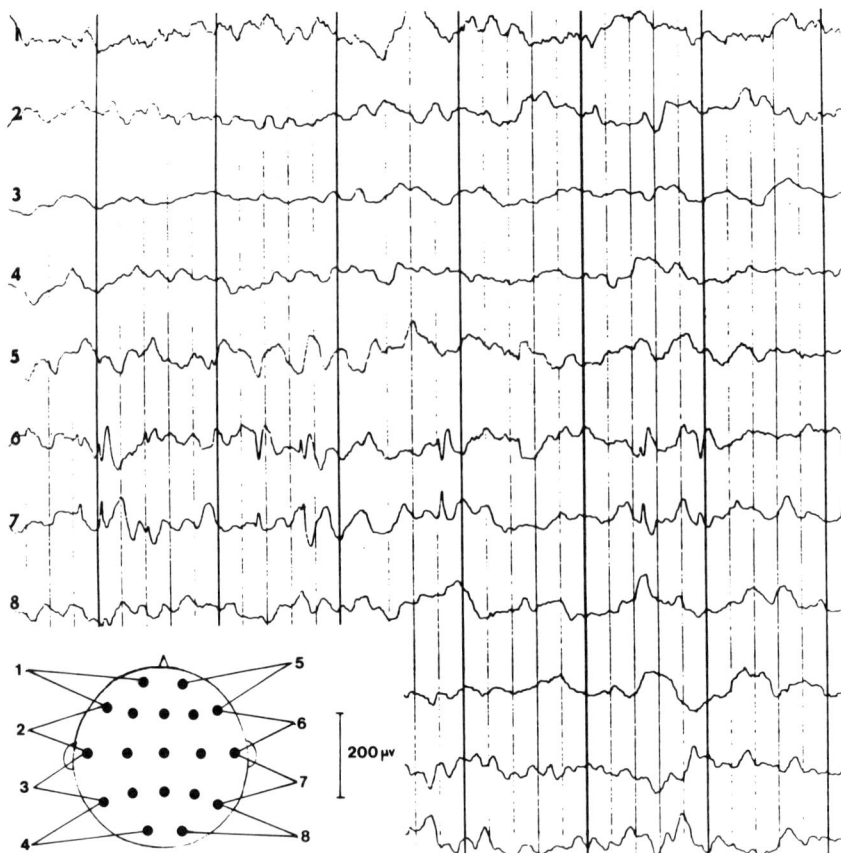

Fig. 36-4. Interictal EEG showing a right mid-temporal discharge in a patient with partial complex seizures.

tomatic). The primary epilepsies have a strong genetic tendency and are less common than other types. Idiopathic tonic–clonic epilepsy rarely begins before 6 months of age and is not usually associated with other neurologic dysfunction. Absence epilepsy is rare before 2 years of age and is also not associated with other neurologic diseases. Some children with absence epilepsy will also have generalized motor seizures. Generalized motor seizures must be differentiated from secondarily generalized partial seizures, and absence seizures from partial complex seizures. The other primary generalized epilepsies are rare and the major features are described in Table 36-2.

Many of the generalized epilepsies can occur as either a primary or secondary disorder. Such primary epilepsies are often called cryptogenic, and infantile spasms are a typical example. Whether cryptogenic or symptomatic, children with infantile spasms have a worse prognosis than those with other epilepsies. Half of the patients with cryptogenic infantile spasms wil be retarded and most will continue to have seizures. Infantile spasms secondary to other

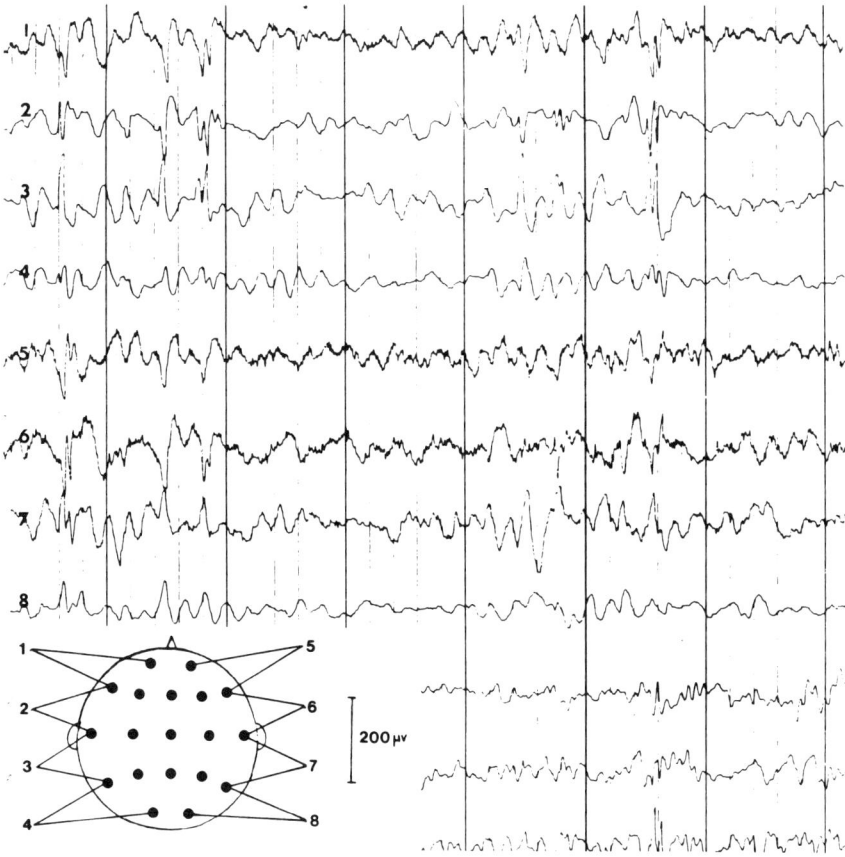

Fig. 36-5. Interictal EEG in a patient with rolandic epilepsy.

diseases have a worse prognosis. The West syndrome consists of infantile spasms, developmental regression, and hypsarrhythmia and has many etiologies (Table 36-4). Astatic-myoclonic seizures have a similar prognosis. Most, but not all, have a diagnosable etiology. The association of a mixed seizure disorder, including astatic–myoclonic, absence, and other seizures, with mental retardation and slow spiked wave discharges on EEG is called the Lennox-Gastaut syndrome or atypical absence (Fig. 36-6). Symptomatic generalized seizures are found in a variety of chronic encephalopathies, both static and progressive. Except for typical absence, all generalized seizures may be a sign of underlying brain disease.

The partial epilepsies are secondary or symptomatic of focal or multifocal brain disease. The exception is rolandic epilepsy, which is a benign disease with focal motor partial seizures and focal discharges on EEG from the frontolparietal area of the brain and is often nocturnal.

There are some epilepsies that are difficult to classify. Some children only have seizures with high fevers (febrile convulsions) and others only following

Table 36-2. Clinical Features and Classification of the Epilepsies

Classification	Age of Onset	Seizure Type	Etiology	Prognosis (Percent Remission)
Generalized epilepsies				
Primary				
Familial neonatal	Birth	Clonic	Familial	90
Infantile spasms	0–18 months	Infantile spasms, others	Idiopathic, secondary	<50
Myoclonic–atonic	1–5 years	Petit mal, tonic–clonic, myoclonic	Idiopathic, secondary	<50
Absence	3–10 years	Petit mal	Familial, idiopathic	50
Mixed	>3 years	Petit mal, grand mal	Familial, idiopathic	50
Grand mal	>3 months	Tonic–clonic	Familial, idiopathic	70
Juvenile myoclonic	>12 years	Myoclonic, tonic–clonic, petit mal	Idiopathic, ? familial	90
Secondary				
Grand mal	>3 months	Tonic–clonic	Chronic encephalopathies	50
			Following minor head trauma	>90
			Following breath-holding spells	>90
			Following high fever	>90
Infantile spasms (West syndrome)	0–18 months	Infantile spasms, others	Tuberous sclerosis	<10
			CNS malformation	
			Metabolic disease	
			Asphyxia	
			Infections	
			Others	
Lennox-Gastaut	1–3 years	Myoclonic, others	Same as above	<10
Partial epilepsies				
Rolandic	3–12 years	Focal motor	Idiopathic, familial	>90
Secondary	Any age	Simple, complex, secondarily generalized	Focal or multifocal Brain injuries	Variable

Table 36-3. Relative Frequencies of the Epileptic Syndrome in Children

		Incidence (%)
Generalized epilepsies		31
Primary		
Grand mal	9	
Absence	6	
Myoclonic	1	
Secondary		
Astatic/akinetic	11	
Infantile spasms	4	
Others	<1	
Partial epilepsies		61
Simple	21	
Complex	24	
Secondarily generalized	16	
Unclassifiable		8

(Modified from Alving T: Classification of the epilepsies. An investigation of 402 children, Acta Neurol Scand 60:157, 1977.)

minor head trauma or breath-holding spells. Such seizures probably do not represent an epileptic syndrome.

EVALUATION

The most important step in the evaluation is to determine if the event was a seizure. Children have a variety of "spells" and many movements are not seizures. The differential diagnosis of a seizure is listed in Table 36-5. Because a seizure is a symptom of brain dysfunction, the purpose of the evaluation is to determine an underlying etiology, especially one that is treatable. The history is the most important part of the evaluation, from which one determines both the seizure type and evidence for other neurologic symptoms. The birth history, past medical history, and family history are equally important in determining possible preexisting brain injury which would predispose a patient to seizures. The physical and neurologic exams should corroborate the history. Neurologic signs not explained by the history suggest an acquired illness and indicate the need for a more extensive evaluation. All patients should be examined carefully for neurocutaneous syndromes (tuberous sclerosis and Sturge-Weber syndrome), regardless of the history.

The history and EEG together determine the seizure type. Focal discharges or slowing on the EEG may indicate focal injury to the brain and generalized slowing and disorganization may indicate an encephalopathy. A normal EEG does not exclude the diagnosis of a seizure; the majority of children will have nonparoxysmal recordings. The sooner after the seizure the EEG is obtained, the more likely a paroxysmal abnormality will be found. Certain seizure types, such as absence and minor motor seizures, are more likely to show an abnormal EEG recording. Sleep recordings, hyperventilation, and photic stimulation should be performed to activate seizures and enhance the usefulness of the EEG.

Table 36-4. Etiologies of the West Syndrome

Metabolic abnormalities
  Phenylketonuria
  Maple syrup urine disease
  Hyperornithinemia
  Isovaleric acidemia
  Nonketotic hyperglycinemia
  Pyridoxine dependency
  Leucine-sensitive hypoglycemia
  Tay-Sachs disease
Dyplastic or dysgenetic conditions
  Tuberous sclerosis
  Microgyria
  Ulegyria
  Down syndrome
  Sturge-Weber angiomatosis
  Agenesis of corpus callosum
  Aicardi syndrome
  Schizencephaly
  Lissencephaly
  Porencephaly
  Linear nevus sebaceous syndrome
Prenatal infections
  Cytomegalovirus
  Syphilis
  Toxoplasmosis
Perinatally or postnatally acquired encephalopathies
  Ischemic–hypoxic
  Hypoglycemic
  Traumatic
  Infectious
    Encephalitis
    Complicated meningitis
    Postimmunization (pertussis, influenza)
Intracranial tumors
  Choroid plexus papilloma and others
Unknown

(From Gomez MR, Klass DW: Epilepsies in infancy and childhood. Ann Neurol 13:113–124, 1983.)

The initial history will determine the subsequent evaluation. One should determine if the child has an acute encehalopathy, chronic nonprogressive disease, progressive encephalopathy, or a normal history. The examination and EEG augment the history and determine the extent of the evaluation. Table 36-6 outlines the evaluation. One should always look for a treatable cause whenever possible. If there is no response to therapy or worsening despite therapy, the patient should be restudied. Infants with infantile spasms or unexplained seizures should also be evaluated for possible degenerative diseases.

TREATMENT

The decision for treatment can be difficult. Excluding absence and minor motor seizures, about half of the children presenting with a single seizure will subsequently have further seizures. The prognosis is better for children whose

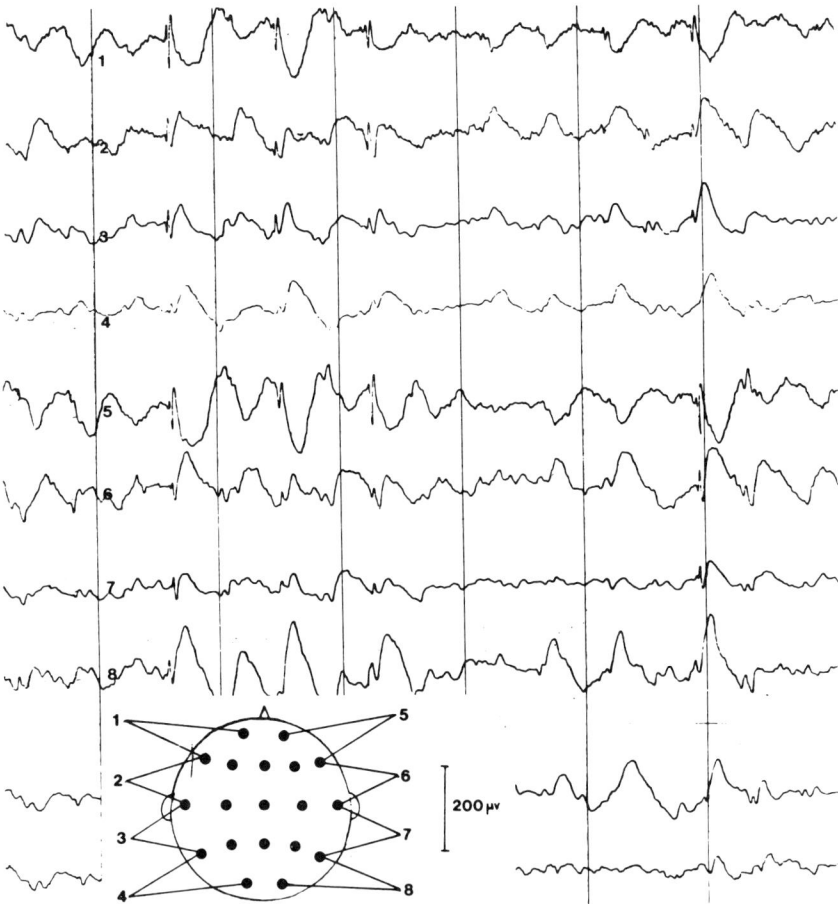

Fig. 36-6. An EEG showing slow spiked wave discharges in a patient with Lennox-Gastaut syndrome.

seizures occurred with an acute encephalopathy (30 to 40 percent remission) than in children with idiopathic seizures (60 to 70 percent remission). It is therefore reasonable to defer long-term therapy for children with a single seizure, especially if associated with an acute illness.

Table 36-7 outlines the use of the major anticonvulsants and complications. Table 36-8 list the less commonly used therapies. Some seizure types respond only to specific anticonvulsants. Absence is the best example of this, in that it rarely responds to drugs other than valproate and ethosuximide. Generalized motor seizures and partial seizures respond to most anticonvulsants with about equal efficiency, except that ethosuximide is not as useful. Minor motor seizures frequently respond poorly to any single drug. Infantile spasms are best treated with intramuscular adrenocorticotropic hormone, 40 to 80 U/day, for 6 to 12 weeks. Approximately 50 percent of cases will have a favorable response but

Table 36-5. Differential Diagnosis of Seizures

Breath-holding spells
Syncope
Hypoglycemia
Hysteria
Pseudoseizures
Fictitious seizures (Munchausen's syndrome)
Complicated migraine
Sleep disturbances
Persistent asymmetric tonic neck reflex
Movement disorders
Decorticate, decerebrate posturing (cerebellar fits)
Apnea
Clonus
"Shudder" attacks

may relapse. Myoclonic, atonic, and other minor motor seizures may respond to valproate or clonazepam and other benzodiazepines (lorazepam, clorazepate). These seizures are often refractory to all therapies. Carbamazepine, phenytoin, and phenobarbital can worsen the seizure control in some patients with minor motor seizures. The ketogenic diet is an alternative to drug therapy. The diet consists of 60 percent medium chain triglyceride oil, 15 percent protein, 10 percent fat, and 15 percent carbohydrate. The child is fasted initially to induce ketosis. The diet is introduced and gradually increased to 150 percent of calculated caloric needs to prevent weight loss.

Table 36-9 list guidelines for the use of anticonvulsants. Simplification

Table 36-6. Guidelines for the Evaluation of Children with Seizures Based upon History

Acute encephalopathy
  Infection: lumbar puncture, complete blood count, culture
  Metabolic: blood chemistries
  Ingestion: toxin screen
  Trauma: CT scan, skull radiographs
  Vascular accident: CT scan, lumbar puncture
Chronic encephalopathy
  Previous brain injury: no further evaluation
  No previous injury:
    Dysmorphism: CT scan, karyotype
    Congenital infection (in infants): lumbar puncture, TORCH titers, CT scan
    Familial: pedigree
    Neurocutaneous diseases: Wood's lamp exam, CT scan
Progressive encephalopathy
  Chronic infection: lumbar puncture
  Mass lesion: CT scan
  Metabolic: blood chemistries, organic acids, NH_4, lactate, amino acids, lumbar puncture biopsy, specific leukocyte or fibroblast enzyme assay
  Chronic intoxication: toxin screen, heavy metals
  Neurocutaneous disease: Wood's lamp exam, CT scan
Normal history
  Normal exam:
    Normal EEG, petit mal, or generalized discharge: no further evaluation
    EEG with focal abnormalities: cautious observation, CT scan
  Abnormal exam: evaluation as for chronic illness

Table 36-7. Anticonvulsant Therapy[a]

Drug	Dose (mg/kg/day)	Schedule (dose/day)	Therapeutic Blood level (μg/ml)	Seizure Type[b]	Complications
Diphenylhydantoin (Dilantin)	5–10	1–2	10–20	GM, PAR, MM	Gingival hypertrophy, hirsutism, rash, mononucleosis-like reaction, bone marrow suppression, megaloblastic anemia
Phenobarbital	3–5	1–2	15–30	GM, PAR, MM	Hyperactivity, impaired learning, depression
Primidone (Mysoline)	10–20	2–3	5–15	GM, PAR	Same as for phenobarbital
Carbamazepine (Tegretol)	20–30	2–3	6–12	GM, PAR, MM	Bone marrow suppression, neutropenia, hepatic injury
Valproic acid (Depakene)	30–60	3–4	50–90	GM, PAR, PM, MM	Hepatic failure (idiosyncratic), hepatic injury (dose related), alopecia, hyperammonemia, tremor, bone marrow suppression, nausea/vomiting, pancreatitis
(Depakote)	20–50	2–3	50–90	GM, PAR, PM, MM	Same as above
Ethosuximide (Zarontin)	20–30	1–2	40–60	PM	Abdominal pain, vomiting, bone marrow suppression, nightmares
Clonazepam (Klonopin)	0.2–0.3	3–4	0.02–0.06	GM, MM	Depression, altered behavior, drooling

[a] The drugs listed are the most commonly used anticonvulsants.
[b] GM = generalized motor, PAR = partial, MM = minor motor; PM = petit mal.

Table 36-8. Less Commonly Used Anticonvulsants

Drug	Trade Name
Mephobarbital	Mebaral
Mephenytoin	Mesantoin
Trimethadione	Tridione
Methsuximide	Celontin
Acetazolamide	Diamox
Phenacemide	Phenurone
Ketogenic diet	

should be the major goal with any therapeutic regimen in order to improve compliance. The use of a single drug is preferrable to multidrug therapy. One should be thoroughly familiar with the indications and complications of any anticonvulsant used. Repeated episodes of drug intoxication should be avoided and one must always weigh the benefit of therapy against its complications. Frequent blood drug levels ensure complicance and reveal unnecessary intoxication. In some instances anticonvulsant therapy may significantly impair learning and behavior, particularly phenobarbital, but others as well, especially multiple drugs used simultaneously. On the other hand, the complications of an untreated seizure disorder are significant. Repeated seizures may cause brain injury and worsening of the seizure disorder ("kindling"), and status epilepticus can cause death or serious injury. Finally, the child with untreated seizures may suffer emotionally, particularly the school-aged child. Each child should be considered individually.

Withdrawing therapy is also an important consideration. There are no absolute guidelines but useful ones are listed in Table 36-10. Meeting these criteria gives about a 75 percent favorable prognosis for remaining seizure free off medication. When medications are being withdrawn, particularly barbiturates and

Table 36-9. Principles of Anticonvulsant Therapy

1. Choose therapy based upon specific diagnosis.
2. Initiate therapy with single drug.
3. Ensure therapeutic drug levels before changing therapy.
4. Change drug if there is a therapeutic failure.
5. Add second drug if first improved control by at least 50%.
6. Monitor levels frequently with multidrug therapy.
7. Use familiar medications.

Table 36-10. Guidelines for Discontinuing Anticonvulsant Medication[a]

1. Two years or more of seizure control
2. Initial ease in establishing control
3. Normal neurologic exam
4. Generalized seizures
5. Normal EEG

[a] Criteria are listed in the order of importance in determining prognosis off medication.

Table 36-11. Febrile Convulsions[a]

Age	Onset, 6 months to 3 years
	Duration, 6 months to 6 years
Fever	Greater than 101°F of a rising fever
Seizures	Generalized, less than 15 minutes
Frequency	Less than two per year
	No more than three ever
Neurologic exam, development	Normal
EEG	Normal

[a] Children who meet these criteria are unlikely to develop epilepsy or have subsequent developmental problems.

benzodiazepines, they must be tapered slowly to ensure against withdrawal seizures.

The role of surgery in the treatment of seizures in children has not been established. The introduction of new anticonvulsants over the past decade has enabled many children with previously poorly controlled seizures or intolerable side effects from other anticonvulsant medications to be satisfactorily controlled. There are still some children who will not have satisfactory control and who can benefit from surgical treatment.

The indications for neurosurgical intervention are (1) failure of medical management at maximal tolerable doses, (2) focal cortical origin of the seizure, and (3) a surgically accessible lesion. Procedures that are of proven efficacy are corticectomy of a seizure focus and temporal lobectomy for seizures arising from the temporal lobe. Hemispherectomy and division of the corpus callosum are questionable procedures except in those instances in which there are preexisting profound neurologic deficits arising from the hemisphere as well as the seizure focus.

If surgery is contemplated, it should be performed at centers experienced with the evaluation, surgical technique, and management of refractory seizures. Much preparation, both preoperatively and intraoperatively, is necessary to ensure maximal benefits and minimal risks from the surgery.

FEBRILE CONVULSIONS

Febrile convulsions are a benign condition of small children. Because fever will often activate a seizure disorder, it can be difficult to determine if a child has simple febrile convulsions or a seizure disorder. Table 36-11 lists criteria for diagnosing simple febrile convulsions. If a child meets these criteria, he is unlikely to develop nonfebrile seizures. The differentiation is more than academic. Simple febrile convulsions imply a benign course with little risk of status epilepticus, learning disabilities, and subsequent epilepsy. For these reasons, prophylactic therapy with anticonvulsants is not indicated.

SELECTED READINGS

Delgado-Escueta AV, Treiman DM, Walsh GO: The treatable epilepsies. N Engl J Med 308:1508–1514, 1983

Dimmer DS, Luders H, Rothner AD, Erenberg G: Complex partial seizures of childhood onset: a clinical and encephalographic study. Cleveland Clin Q 51:287–291, 1984

Dodson WE: Pharmacology and treatment of epilepsy in children. Clin Neuropharmacol 4:1–29, 1979

Gomez MR, Klass DW: Epilepsies of infancy and childhood. Ann Neurol 13:113–124, 1983

Hauser WA, Anderson VE, Loewenson RB McRoberts SM: Seizure recurrence after a first unprovoked seizure. N Engl J Med 307:522–528, 1982

Kurokawa T, Goya N, Fukuyama Y et al: West syndrome and Lennox-Gastaut syndrome: a survey of natural history. Pediatrics 65:81–88, 1980

Kutt H, Penry JK: Usefulness of blood levels of antiepileptic drugs. Arch Neurol 31:283–288, 1974

Lesser RP, Pippenger CE, Lüders H, Dinner DS: High-dose monotherapy in treatment of intractable seizures. Neurology 34:707–711, 1984

Loiseau P, Pestre M, Dartrigues JF et al: Long-term prognosis in two forms of childhood epilepsy: typical absence seizures and epilepsy with rolandic (centro-temporal) EEG foci. Ann Neurol 13:642–648, 1983

Lombroso CT, Fejerman N: Benign myoclonus of early infancy. Ann Neurol 1:138–143, 1977

Markand ON: Slow spike-wave activity in EEG and associated clinical features: often called Lennox or Lennox-Gastaut syndrome. Neurology 27:746–757, 1977

Meadow R: Fictitious epilepsy. Lancet 2:25–28, 1984

Menkes JH: Diagnosis and treatment of minor motor seizures. Pediatr Clin North Am 23:435–442, 1976

Nelson KB, Ellenberg JH: Predictors of epilepsy in children who have experienced febrile seizures. N Engl J Med 295:1029–1033, 1976

Nelson KB, Ellenberg JH: Prognosis in children with febrile seizures. Pediatrics 61:720–727, 1978

Rothner AD: Evaluation of the child with seizures. Cleveland Clin Q 51:267–272, 1984

Sato S, Dreifuss FE, Penry JK et al: Long-term follow up of absence seizures. Neurology 33:1590–1595, 1983

Singer WD, Rabe EF, Haller JS: The effect of ACTH therapy upon infantile spasms. J Pediatr 1980, 96:485–489

Thurston JH, Thurston DL, Hixon BB, Keller AJ: Prognosis in childhood epilepsy. N Engl J Med 306:831–836, 1982

Trauner DA: Medium-chain triglyceride (MCT) diet in intractable seizure disorders. Neurology 35:237–238, 1985

Yang PJ, Berger PE, Cohen ME, Duffner PK: Computed tomography and childhood seizure disorders. Neurology 29:1084–1088, 1979

37

STATUS EPILEPTICUS

Status epilepticus is a pediatric emergency with a 20 percent mortality if untreated. Because a generalized motor seizure lasting longer than 30 minutes probably causes brain injury, prompt and effective treatment is mandatory. The term *status epilepticus* refers to generalized motor seizures lasting longer than 30 minutes. A child who has generalized convulsions repetitively without regaining consciousness between seizures is also considered to have status epilepticus. This is often termed *serial seizures*. Other forms of status epilepticus include partial status.

ETIOLOGY

The causes of status epilepticus are listed in Table 37-1. One of the most common is discontinuance of anticonvulsant medication. This is particularly true with barbiturates, not only because of the loss of anticonvulsive therapy but also because of the effects of barbiturate withdrawal. Metabolic, toxic, infectious, and traumatic etiologies must be considered whether or not the child has a seizure history. A small percentage of children with idiopathic epilepsy will present for the first time in status epilepticus and many "brittle" epileptics will lose control with infections or other stresses despite adequate anticonvulsive therapy.

DIAGNOSIS

There is little confusion about the diagnosis of generalized motor status epilepticus. The characteristics of a generalized motor seizure have been previously described and the difference between a seizure and status epilepticus is the duration of the convulsion. There are a few conditions that should be considered in the differential diagnosis. Patients with increased intracranial pressure and impending herniation and patients with posterior fossa masses often have periods of dystonic posturing. This often takes the form of decerebrate posturing which may look very similar to a tonic contraction of a generalized seizure. These "cerebellar fits" usually accompany an encephalopathy with signs and symptoms of increased intracranial pressure. Certain movement disorders such as chorea and drug-induced dystonias may suggest a seizure disorder; however, the presence of consciousness with the generalized motor activity usually excludes the diagnosis of status epilepticus. Pseudoseizures are another major con-

Table 37-1. Etiologies of Status Epilepticus

Inadequate anticonvulsant therapy
   Poor compliance
   Inadequate dosage
   Gastroenteritis with vomiting of dose
Drug withdrawl
   Prescription lapse
   Change in therapy
   Substance abuse
Matabolic encephalopathy
   Hyponatremia
   Hypocalcemia
   Hypoglycemia
   Hepatic or renal failure
   Others
Infectious encephalopathy
   Meningitis
   Encephalitis
   Abscess
Head trauma
   Open head injury
   Contusion
   Subdural hematoma
Vascular accident
   Intracerebral hemorrhage
   Ruptured arteriovenous malformation
   Venous thrombosis
Mass lesion
   Brain tumor
   Arteriovenous malformation
   Acute hydrocephalus
Intoxication
   Xanthines
   Lead
   Strychnine
   Camphor
   Tricyclics
   Many others
Idiopathic epilepsy

sideration in the differential diagnosis. They may be difficult to distinguish in the patient who has a known seizure disorder, but in the child who is medically naive the pseudoseizure is usually obvious.

TREATMENT

Because of the potentially serious complications of status epilepticus, therapy should be instituted as rapidly as possible. After the patient is stabilized, time can be spent obtaining an adequate history and physical examination. Therapy can be divided into three parts: supportive care, treatment of underlying cause, and pharmacologic treatment of the seizure with anticonvulsive drugs.

Supportive therapy should be instituted to protect the patient from injury, ensure adequate oxygenation, and establish an intravenous access for blood

Table 37-2. Supportive Care for Status Epilepticus

Ensure airway
  Remove foreign bodies
  Aspirate emesis or blood
  Intubate if indicated to ensure adequate oxygenation
Administer oxygen
  4 L/min by mask
Establish intravenous access
  Obtain sample for anticonvulsant levels
  Calcium
  Electrolytes
  Glucose
  Magnesium
  Toxic screen
  Administer dextrose, 10% in 1:4 normal saline, at estimated maintenance rate
Protect patient from injury
  Restrain gently to bed
  Pad bony prominences

sampling and drug administration (Table 37-2). The patient should be placed in a semiprone position to lessen the risk of aspiration if emesis occurs. Because of the high oxygen demands of a patient who is in a generalized motor seizure, oxygen should be administered by face mask. The patient should be gently restrained so that he does not injure himself either by falling or by repetitively striking his extremities or head against hard objects. It is probably unwise to either place an object in the mouth or attempt intubation of an actively seizuring patient. This is apt to cause either aspiration or local trauma. If intubation is acutely necessary, one should first attempt to stop the seizure; if this is unsuccesful, then the patient should be paralyzed. A large-bore intravenous line should be inserted as soon as possible. Samples are drawn immediately for glucose, calcium, magnesium, anticonvulsant levels, electrolytes, and a toxic screen. A Dextrostix test can be performed at the bedside to determine immediately whether or not the patient is hypoglycemic. If so, then intravenous glucose can be administered. This is a rare cause for status epilepticus, however.

After the patient's safety has been ensured, oxygen administered, and an intravenous line established, then specific pharamcologic therapy can be instituted. Table 37-3 outlines the pharmacologic management of status epilepticus. The first drug of choice is diazepam administered intravenously at 0.2 to 0.3 mg/kg. Seizures normally stop within several minutes after its administration, although occasionally this takes longer. The duration of action is approximately 30 to 60 minutes. Lorazepam has similar efficacy but has a duration of action of 4 to 6 hours. The recommended dose is 0.1 mg/kg, but its use in children has been limited. The most serious complication of intravenous diazepam is that of respiratory depression and, less frequently, hypotension. Respiratory depression is more apt to occur in patients who have an underlying encephalopathy or who have been given other respiratory depressant medications, particularly barbiturates. Its rapid action, however, justifies its use despite the risk of respiratory depression. Intubation and assisted ventilation may be required in any patient

Table 37-3. Pharmacologic Management of Status Epilepticus

Initial therapy
1. Diazepam, 0.3 mg/kg iv (0.1 mg/kg/min), or lorazepam, 0.1 mg/kg
2. Phenytoin, 18 mg/kg iv (1.0 mg/kg/min)
3. Phenobarbital, 15–20 mg/kg iv (1.0 mg/kg/min)

Second therapy
4. Paraldehyde, 10% iv infusion to total dose of 0.25 g/kg or 1:1 dilution with mineral oil rectally
5. Valproic acid, 30 mg/kg of suspension rectally

Refractory therapy
6. Lidocaine infusion, 3–10 mg/kg/hr
7. Pentobarbital coma, 5 mg/kg loading dose then 5 mg/kg/hr
8. Diazepam infusion, 0.5 mg/kg/hr constant infusion
9. General anesthesia

with status epilepticus, regardless of treatment. It is much easier to intubate a child who has been given diazepam than one who is actively convulsing.

Because the duration of action of diazepam is brief, a second anticonvulsant of longer duration should be given immediately. Phenytoin is best suited for this purpose. It is given as a slow infusion at 18 mg/kg. The rate of infusion should be approximately 1.0 mg/kg/min. Ideally the patient should be simultaneously monitored for cardiac rhythm and blood pressure. Its major complications are hypotension and cardiac arrhythmias, which are more likely to occur in patients with preexisting heart disease. The onset of action of phenytoin is approximately 15 to 30 minutes. If the patient is still convulsing after administration of phenytoin, then intravenous phenobarbital at 15 to 20 mg/kg should be given. It is unlikely that the respiratory depressant effect of diazepam will still be present at this time. The onset of action of phenobarbital begins 5 to 15 minutes after infusion. With phenytoin or phenobarbital, prolonged seizure control can be obtained because the half-life of these drugs is relatively long and the loading dose will ensure sufficient anticonvulsant levels for the ensuing 12 to 24 hours. If these two drugs are used alone as the initial treatment of status epilepticus, 60 to 70 percent of patients will be controlled. The two-phase approach of giving diazepam to stop the seizure immediately followed by a second drug to maintain seizure control is successful in 80 to 90 percent of patients. If the patient is still convulsing, blood levels of phenobarbital and phenytoin must be obtained to ensure high therapeutic values. Booster doses of 5 to 10 mg/kg can be given or one can repeat diazepam/lorazepam doses while awaiting further data.

If these efforts fail, paraldehyde is probably the next most effective agent and can be given intravenously as a 10 percent solution, but preferably by rectal administration diluted 1:1 with mineral oil at 0.3 mg/kg. The drug is metabolized by the liver, as well as excreted through the lungs. Adequate function of these organs must therefore be ensured. Pulmonary edema and hemorrhage are complications of its use. The drug is also converted to a toxic metabolite with prolonged exposure to light. Valproic acid suspension diluted with water (1:1) and administered rectally at 30 mg/kg has also been shown to be effective in treating status epilepticus.

Ongoing physical assessment and history taking may direct a streamlined approached to the determination of the cause. Results from the laboratory studies obtained at the onset may also determine a specific diagnosis and treatment. If the etiology is still in doubt, then a computed tomographic scan of the head and lumbar puncture will be needed after the patient is stabilized.

Seizures which persist after the previously cited measures usually indicate a severe injury to the brain and refractory status. One can try a continuous lidocaine infusion, and if this fails, it is best to induce coma with pentobarbital, continuous diazepam infusion, or general anesthesia. While the patient is in coma, diagnostic studies such as a computed tomographic scan of the head and lumbar puncture can be performed if the etiology is unknown, and adequate ventilation ensured. Other agents which are not available as a parental injection, such as carbamazepine or valproic acid, can be administered by a nasogastric tube. After these anticonvulsants have reached therapeutic blood concentrations the coma can be withdrawn to determine if the seizures have been controlled.

PARTIAL STATUS

Partial status is a continous partial seizure. It is usually a focal motor seizure with persistent jerking of the hand, face, or other extremity (epilepsia partialis continua). Such seizures may last for hours or months. Frequently children have focal structural or inflammatory abnormalities of the brain and the seizures may be particularly refractory to therapy. Complex partial status can present a very confusing clinical picture. Often the patients have an apparent psychiatric illness because of the fuguelike state in which they present. Since partial seizures rarely interfere with ventilation, the urgency of stopping the seizures is not as great as in generalized motor status, and intravenous diazepam is not indicated.

ABSENCE STATUS AND MINOR MOTOR STATUS

Absence status can appear very similar to complex partial status epilepticus. It consists of continuous attacks of absence seizures without attaining normal consciousness. Some authors consider absence status to be continuous minor motor seizures presenting as clouded consciousness and continuous spike-wave discharges. This is also referred to as electrical status. Intravenous diazepam is effective in stopping these seizures as well.

SELECTED READINGS

Aicardi J, Chevrie JJ: Convulsive status epilepticus in infants and children. A study of 239 cases. Epilepsia 11:187–197, 1970

Aminoff MJ, Simon RP: Status epilepticus. Causes, clinical features and consequences in 98 patients. Am J Med 69:657–666, 1980

Celesia GG: Modern concepts of status epilepticus. JAMA 235:1571–1574, 1976

Delgado-Escueta AV, Waterlain C, Treiman DM, Port RJ: Management of status epilepticus. N Engl J Med 306:1337–1340, 1982

38

HEADACHES

Headache is a relatively common problem in pediatrics and accounts for approximately 10 percent of referrals to a pediatric neurologist. It is estimated that 40 percent of children will have experienced headaches by age 7 and this figure rises to 75 percent by age 15. Headache can be a symptom of serious pathology of the brain in which there are usually other signs and symptoms of encephalopathy. These disorders are discussed elsewhere in this manual. This chapter concentrates on the more common causes of headaches in children, which are usually benign.

PATHOPHYSIOLOGY

The brain itself is anesthetic. The intracranial structures that are sensitive to pain are the intracranial blood vessels, the dural sinuses, and the meninges. These are particularly sensitive to dilatation, stretch, and traction. The soft tissues of the head and neck are also sensitive to pain. The innervation to the head and neck soft tissues and skin is through the trigeminal nerve and the upper cervical spinal nerves (see Fig. 4-4). The supratentorial structures within the cranium are innervated primarily by the trigeminal nerve, and the posterior fossa by the upper cervical roots. Because of common innervation of intracranial and extra-cranial structures, there can be referred pain and poor localization.

EVALUATION AND CLASSIFICATION

The evaluation of a patient with headache rests mainly on the history. Whenever possible, this should be obtained from the child, particularly the location and nature of the pain. Information about the onset, frequency, duration, and associated symptoms or signs can be obtained from the parent (Table 38-1). It is very important to obtain both a family history and a history of previous medical illnesses. The physical examination should include a careful examination of all of the soft tissues of the head and neck, a funduscopic examination, a neurologic exam, and a general physical examination (Table 38-2). A thorough evaluation is necessary in small children because of poor localization and the inability to articulate symptoms. Laboratory test depend upon the suspected etiology.

There are many causes for headaches in children and a classification based

Table 38-1. Historical Aspects of Headache

History	Etiologies
Progression	
Seconds	Neuralgia, hemorrhage, convulsive
Minutes	Migraine
Hours	Muscle contraction, inflammatory
Insidious	Psychogenic, traction
Duration	
Seconds	Neuralgia
Minutes	Convulsive
Hours	Migraine, muscle contraction
Constant	Traction, psychogenic, inflammatory
Intensity	
Mild	Muscle contraction
Moderate	Traction, inflammatory
Severe	Migraine, hemorrhage, neuralgia
Quality	
Throbbing	Migraine
Constant	Muscle contraction, traction, inflammatory
Sharp	Neuralgia
Bizarre	Psychogenic
Frequency	
Paroxysmal	Migraine, convulsive, neuralgia
Constant	Psychogenic, traction, inflammatory, muscle contraction
Occurrence	
Morning	Traction, inflammatory
Afternoon	Muscle contraction
Night	Migraine
Family history	Migraine
Vomiting	Migraine, traction

on etiology is presented in Table 38-3. However, it is more prudent to approach the patient based on the clinical presentation. From the history and physical exam, one can divide the headaches into acute, subacute progressive, chronic nonprogressive, and paroxysmal headaches. Some causes of headache may have more than one mode of presentation.

Acute Headaches

Acute, progressive headaches which precipitate medical intervention may be the first of a paroxysmal disorder or a symptom of an acute, serious neurologic disease. Most of these are associated with an abrupt increase in intracranial pressure or sudden traction on intracranial structures. The headaches in such cases tend to be generalized, severe, constant, and often associated with nausea and vomiting. Alterations in consciousness and other neurologic signs may or may not be present, depending on the etiology. Unless the history is obvious, such as a post-lumbar puncture headache, most patients presenting with a severe, acute onset of headache should have a computed tomographic (CT) scan of the head. A lumbar puncture is generally contraindicated unless the CT scan reveals no mass lesion and one suspects a subarachnoid hemorrhage or meningitis. These disorders are discussed in other chapters of this manual. Treatment

Table 38-2. General Physical Examination for Headaches

Examination	Findings	Significance
Vital signs	Elevated blood pressure	Hypertension
	Fever	Inflammation, infections
	Dyspnea	Hypoxia, hypercarbia
Head, face, scalp		
Auscultation	Bruit	Arteriovenous malformation
Palpation	Swelling, tenderness	Inflammation, trauma, neuritis
Eyes		
Funduscopic	Papilledema	Increased intracranial pressure
	Disk cupping	Glaucoma
	Hemorrhage	Trauma, intracranial hemorrhage
Vision	Decreased	Myopia, neuritis, tumor
Fields	Field loss	Tumor, stroke
Motility	Gaze paralysis	Tumor
	Muscle paralysis	Increased intracranial pressure, tumor
Ears		
Otoscopic	Otitis	Chronic otitis, abscess
Hearing	Decreased	Chronic otitis, tumor
Sinuses		
Percussion	Tenderness	Sinusitis
Mouth		
Teeth	Tenderness	Dental abscess
Throat	Inflammation	Pharyngitis, tonsillitis
Jaw	Crepitus, tenderness	Temporomandibular joint disease
Neck		
Motility	Meningism	Meningitis, posterior fossa tumor
	Limited motility	Arthritis, cervical adenopathy, tonsillitis
	Head tilt	Tumor, arthritis, squint

is aimed at alleviating the underlying cause. Sedating analgesics, particularly narcotics, should be avoided until the etiology has been determined.

Progressive Headaches

Subacute progressive headaches cause greater concern than other types of headache. In most instances the headache progresses over a period of days to weeks and is usually associated with a gradual increase in the intracranial pressure or traction of cerebral structures ("traction" headaches). Patients who have headaches secondary to increased intracranial pressure frequently have a generalized, constant pain, although it can occasionally be described as throbbing. There is a loose association between the location of the headache and its underlying pathology. The headache is often more severe in the morning and may arouse the patient from sleep. Early morning headache and vomiting are classic signs of increased intracranial pressure. The pain often subsides as the child becomes more active throughout the day. Other historical features are a change in personality, deterioration of school performance, and increased somnolence. The physician should look carefully for associated neurologic signs, including papilledema, long-tract signs, and focal neurologic deficits.

A CT scan is necessary in the child with subacute progressive headaches.

Table 38-3. Classification of Headaches in Children

Vascular
  Migraine
  Migraine variants
  Cluster
  Other
    Arteriovenous malformations
    Hypertension
    Venous thrombosis
    Hypoxia, hypercarbia
    Arteritis
Traction
  Intracranial mass
  Hydrocephalus
  Pseudotumor cerebri
  Post lumbar puncture
  Cerebral edema
  Intracranial hemorrhage
Muscle contraction
Seizure
Psychogenic
  Depression
  School phobia
  Conversion
  Malingering
Miscellaneous
  Soft tissue inflammation of head and neck
  Arthritis of temporomandibular joint, cervical spine
  Neuritis, neuralgia
  Meningitis, encephalitis
  Metabolic encephalopathies
  Eye strain
  Fever

If the CT scan is normal, a lumbar puncture is indicated to exclude a chronic infection or raised intracranial pressure secondary to pseudotumor cerebri or other cause. Treatment is directed at the underlying etiology and it is frequently necessary to alleviate the pain with narcotics. In patients with intractable pain one should not be hesitant to use an adequate dose of analgesic. Morphine sulfate at 0.1 mg/kg or meperidine at 1 mg/kg is usually sufficient.

The noncerebral causes of progressive headache are largely secondary to soft tissue disorders of the head and neck (Table 38-4). Sinusitis, dental disorders such as a tooth abscess, and otitis may frequently be misinterpreted as head pain in the younger child. These structures should be investigated closely with skull

Table 38-4. Extracerebral Causes of Headaches in Children

Face, scalp	Abscess, cellulitis, arteritis
Ears	Otitis media, externa
Eyes	Acute glaucoma, orbital cellulitis, neuritis, pseudotumor of the orbit
Sinuses	Acute sinusitis
Mouth	Dental abscess, pharyngitis, abscess, temporomandibular joint disease
Neck	Cervical arthritis, paraspinal mass, cervical subluxation, Arnold-Chiari malformation, torticollis

radiographs, a complete blood count, erythrocyte sedimentation rate, and cultures in patients in whom the etiology is unclear. Severe headache with facial cellulitis is of serious concern because of possible associated dural sinus thrombosis.

Chronic Headache

Chronic nonprogressive headaches are characterized by poor localization and the inability to articulate symptoms. The headaches are often associated with "tension" and occur daily. This probably reflects constant muscle contraction and hence the term *muscle contraction headache*. Muscle contraction headaches can occur in patients who are depressed, have eye strain, or have other disorders of the head and neck. Muscle contraction headaches become more severe as the day progresses and are usually relieved by sleep and minor analgesics such as aspirin. Muscle contraction headaches are unusual in younger children. Rarely, chronic headache is a symptom of an underlying psychiatric or behavioral disorder such as depression, malingering, or school phobia. The etiology of chronic headache is usually apparent after a careful history and physical examination. Further diagnostic studies are not indicated unless specific bony or soft tissue illnesses are suspected or neurologic signs are present on examination. Chronic sinusitis is actually an infrequent cause of headaches in children.

Paroxysmal Headache

Migraine is the most common cause of paraoxysmal headaches in children and it is estimated that 4 percent of children experience migraine. Migraine is caused by a hereditary abnormality of the neurohumoral control of the size of the intra- and extracranial arteries and is often called a "vascular" headache. Abnormal serotonin excretion is thought to be the major cause of migraine headaches, although other neurohumoral compounds have been implicated. Migraine is a biphasic illness caused by initial vasoconstriction followed by vasodilatation of cranial vessels. During the vasoconstrictive phase, ischemia occurs, causing focal neurologic deficits (aura). During the vasodilatative phase head pain occurs. Table 38-5 lists the diagnostic criteria for migraine. There is a high association with motion sickness and many patients suffer their first attacks following head trauma. Certain foods, allergies, exercise, menses, and "stress" will precipitate attacks in other children. Based on the symptoms in the vasoconstrictive phase, migraine can be divided into several types.

Common migraine refers to few or no vascoconstrictive symptoms followed by generalized, constant or throbbing head pain with nausea or vomiting, abdominal pain, and photophobia. The attack may lasts hours and rarely days, with fluctuating pain. A child may have several attacks a year or several a week. Classic migraine differs from common migraine in that the former has an aura consisting of a visual scotoma and the pain is unilateral and throbbing. The scotoma may be black or colored "spots" within the visual fields, or more clas-

Table 38-5. Clinical Diagnosis of Migraine

Major criterion
  Paroxysmal headaches
Minor criteria (minimum of three)
  Aura
  Unilateral headache
  Throbbing pain
  Gastrointestinal symptoms
  Relief with sleep
  Family history of migraine
  Photophobia
Associated features
  Motion sickness
  Somnambulism
  Cyclic vomiting
  Benign paroxysmal vertigo

(From Barabas, G: Management of Headaches in Childhood. Pediatr Ann 12:806–813, 1983. Reprinted with permission Slack Incorporated, Thorofare NJ 08086.)

sically a scintillating scotoma or fortification spectrum. The headache usually follows within minutes of the aura. The headache is severe, lasts several hours, and is associated with vomiting. Sleep almost always terminates the headache.

Complicated migraine is associated with persistent focal neurologic deficits during or after the vasoconstrictive phase. Ischemia of any part of the brain may precipitate these symptoms and signs, which cause quite varied presentations. Some of the more classic syndromes are outlined in Table 38-6. Complicated

Table 38-6. Complicated Migraine and Migraine Variants

Acute hemiplegic migraine	Hemiplegia, hemianopia, asphasia (with right hemiparesis) Resolves within 24–72 hours
Acute confusional migraine	Confusion, combativeness, hyperactivity, restlessness Resolves in 1–24 hours
Basilar artery migraine	Ataxia, vertigo, tinnitis, alternating hemiparesis, vomiting, cortical blindness Resolves in less than 1 hour
"Alice in Wonderland" syndrome	Visual illusions, hallucinations, disorientation, experienced as an aura
Ophthalmoplegic migraine	Cranial nerve III palsy Resolves over days
Benign paroxysmal vertigo	Acute, severe vertigo Resolves in less than 10 minutes
Cyclic vomiting	Periodic vomiting seen in infants and small children
Abdominal migraine	Episodic abdominal pain Resolves in hours
Alternating hemiplegia	Onset in early childhood, repeated episodes of hemiplegia, unilateral or bilateral Other paroxysmal signs Resolves over minutes to hours

migraine can be confused with a number of other acute encephalopathies, especially hemiplegic migraine and acute confusional migraine. In such cases one should usually proceed as if one were evaluating any other acute neurologic disorder. If there is a prior history of similar episodes or a positive family history, then the diagnosis can often be made without further tests.

Migraine variants are "migraine" episodes without head pain. The diagnosis is tenuous in young children. Paroxysmal vertigo of childhood, cyclic vomiting, and abdominal migraine occur in very young children who often develop more specific signs of migraine headaches at a later age. In such cases the diagnosis is made by exclusion of the more common causes of unsteadiness, vomiting, and abdominal pain. Paroxysmal vertigo is the disorder most frequently associated with migraine. This occurs in preschool children and is associated with the sudden onset of severe vertigo to the point where the child is unable to sit or stand. The child usually wedges himself into a corner to try to maintain stability and is terrified of the event. The episode generally subsides over a period of minutes.

Cluster headache is another vascular headache. It is rare before puberty. The cluster headache tends to be retro-orbital in origin and associated with lacrimation, rhinorrhea, and conjunctival injection. The pain is brief and severe but has a shorter duration than most migraine attacks. The headaches usually occur several times throughout the day and frequently will arouse the patient during the night. They occur in clusters between intervals of several symptom-free months. Arteritis is a rare cause of vascular headache in children. Tenderness of an artery and a high erythrocyte sedimentation rate suggest the diagnosis, but biopsy of a cranial artery is necessary to make the diagnosis.

Epilepsy is a rare cause of paroxysmal headache. Occipital discharges on EEG have been recorded in some types of migraine. Some feel that migraine is a form of epilepsy and some children with migraine may respond to anticonvulsants. Most ictal headaches associated with EEG discharges are brief in duration and are associated with other signs of seizure activity. Headaches may also be a postictal phenomenon and can be associated with vomiting.

Paroxysmal headaches associated with metabolic disturbances are exceedingly rare. These include porphyria, amino and organic acidurias, and hypoglycemia. In most instances there are other signs of encephalopathy and these may be confused with basilar artery migraine.

In patients with paroxysmal headaches, one must consider the possibility of an arteriovenous malformation (AVM) or a pheochromocytoma. Headaches associated with AVMs have features similar to those of migraine headaches. Persistent laterality of the headaches and persistent neurologic signs during the headache create suspicion for an underlying AVM. Any child who has paroxysmal headaches and seizures and/or persistent neurologic signs should also be suspected of having an AVM. The evaluation of choice is a contrasted CT scan followed by arteriography. Pheochromocytomas are rare in children but should also be considered in the differential of paroxysmal headaches, particularly those associated with other vascular disturbances.

Also to be remembered in the consideration of paroxysmal headaches are the neuralgias. Trigeminal neuralgia and occipital neuralgia are the two most common. These present as abrupt periods of lancinating pain in the distribution of the affected nerve. Frequently there is a trigger point which will precipitate the pain. In older children, particularly female, trigeminal neuralgia may be a sign of multiple sclerosis. Intermittent ventricular obstruction from a mass lesion can also cause paroxysmal headaches.

TREATMENT OF HEADACHES

The treatment of migraine can be divided in those which are abortive and those which are preventive. Abortive therapy is less successful in young children. Abortive therapy depends upon early recognition of the attack and the administration of medication to abort the subsequent vasodilatative phase. The ergot preparations are the most commonly used; however there is no convincing evidence that this is routinely effective in children. Sublingual tablets are recommended because of their ease of administration and the fact that they will not be lost if emesis ensues. A 4-mg tablet taken sublingually at the first sign of aura and repeated in 15 minutes if there is no abatement of the symptoms may be sufficient to control the headache. A patient should not take more than eight tablets during a week to avoid ergot toxicity.

Prophylactic therapy is usually indicated in the child who has had more than one headache a week or if the headaches are severe enough that they interfere with normal school performance and daily activities. There are many recommended therapies (Table 38-7). None has been shown to be convincingly superior to another, but there have been few controlled trials and there is a significant placebo effect. Propanolol is probably the most widely used. It is contraindicated in those with a history of asthma, heart failure, or depression. Cyproheptadine is more effective in the younger child than in older children or adults. Anticonvulsants have also been recommended for the treatment of migraine, although they are also more effective in younger children. Antidepressants are particularly useful in patients who have tension headaches and an underlying mood disturbance. Calcium-blocking agents have been recently recommended for the treatment of migraine, although there is little information on their use in children. Methylsergide and lithium carbonate are useful in treating cluster headaches, although the former should be used cautiously be-

Table 38-7. Prophylactic Therapy for Migraine

Drug	Dosage	Frequency
Propanolol	1–3 mg/kg/day	tid
Cyproheptadine	0.2–0.4 mg/kg/day	bid
Papaverine	10 mg/kg/day	tid
Phenytoin	5 mg/kg/day	bid
Amitriptyline	1–2 mg/kg/day	hs
Methysergide	0.1 mg/kg/day	tid

cause of the risk of retroperitoneal fibrosis. In general, prophylactic therapy should be continued for 6 months after the headaches are controlled.

Many children respond to nonpharmacologic therapies such as biofeedback. These therapies can be effective but they are expensive and should be reserved for selected patients.

SELECTED READINGS

Barabas G: Management of headaches in childhood. Pediatr Ann 12:806–813, 1983

Belfer ML, Kaban LB: Temporomandibular joint dysfunction with facial pain in children. Pediatrics 69:564–567, 1982

Camfield PR, Metrakos K, Andermann F: Basilar migraine, seizures, and severe epileptiform EEG abnormalities: a benign syndrome in adolescents. Neurology 28:584–588, 1978

Congden PJ, Forsythe WI: Migraine in childhood: a study of 300 children. Dev Med Child Neurol 21:209–216, 1979

Ehyai A, Fenichel GM: The natural history of acute confusional migraine. Arch Neurol 35:368–369, 1978

Golden GS, French JH: Basilar artery migraine in young children. Pediatrics 56:722–726, 1975

Prensky AL: Migraine and migranious variants in pediatric patients. Pediatr Clin North Am 23:461–471, 1976

Rothner AD: Headaches in children: A review. Headache 19:156–162, 1979

39

OTHER PAROXYSMAL DISORDERS

Although seizures and headache are the most common causes of paroxysmal disturbances referred for neurologic consultation, there are many other episodic disorders in children. This chapter discusses some of the other more common paroxysmal disorders. Breath-holding spells are discussed in Chapter 17.

APNEA

Prolonged infant apnea is an arrest of breathing for 20 seconds or longer or for shorter periods of time if associated with cyanosis, pallor, or bradycardia. Lesser periods of asymptomatic respiratory pauses are probably not significant and occur frequently in the preterm infant. Although a major concern, there are insufficient data to determine if there is an association of prolonged infant apnea with sudden infant death syndrome (SIDS). Premature infants with persistent apnea and siblings of SIDS victims are probably at risk for SIDS.

Table 39-1 outlines a classification for the various causes of apnea. If an acute illness or intoxication can be excluded, then the differential is usually among disorders causing respiratory obstruction, seizures, and central apnea. If apnea occurs during wakefulness, then seizures and obstruction associated with gastroesophageal reflux must be considered. If apnea occurs during sleep, then central causes are likely in addition to the others. A careful history will often sort out the most likely presumptive diagnosis.

Table 39-2 outlines the evaluation of the infant with apnea, stressing the treatable causes. Hospitalizing the infant for initial evaluation is recommended in hopes of documenting the characteristics, timing, and severity of the attacks. Prolonged monitoring may yield important clues if interpreted accurately. By simultaneously monitoring the EEG, electrocardiogram, and electromyogram and recording air passage one can determine if the apnea (no air movement) is associated with a respiratory effort (obstructive apnea) or not (central apnea). Electrocardiographic monitoring documents whether cardiac abnormalities are a primary or secondary occurrence, and the EEG determines the presence of convulsive apnea as well as the relationships of apneic episodes to the various stages of sleep.

The treatment of apnea is directed to the underlying cause if it is known.

Table 39-1. Differential Diagnosis of Prolonged Infantile Apnea

Normal respiratory pauses
  Mild apnea associated with choking
  Periodic breathing during sleep
  Occasional 5 to 15-second apneas during sleep
Acute illnesses associated with apnea
  Sepsis
  Acute encephalopathies (any cause)
  Increased intracranial pressure (any cause)
  Infantile botulism
  Respiratory synctial virus infections
  Pertussis
  Hypoglycemia
  Intoxications
Chronic conditions associated with apnea
  Convulsions
  Severe anemia (premature)
  Chronic lung disease
  Gastroesophageal reflux, sensitive laryngeal chemoreceptors
  Cardiac dysrhythmias, "prolonged QT" syndrome
  Abnormalities of respiratory control
    Immature respiratory center
      Apnea of prematurity
      Excessive periodic breathing
    Respiratory center dysfunction
      Obstruction sleep apnea
      Idiopathic sleep apnea
      Ondine's curse
      Drug-induced or post-traumatic hypoventilation/apnea
      Arnold-Chiari-associated apnea
      Posterior fossa tumor
      Dandy-Walker malformation
      Leigh's syndrome
    Idiopathic apnea at infancy

Patients with Ondine's curse and severe obstructive apnea may require assisted ventilation during sleep. Apnea of prematurity often responds to theophylline. There are insufficient data to determine whether home monitoring prevents SIDS in these children. However, a home monitoring system is often recommended for children with prolonged infant apnea or others who are at risk for SIDS.

Table 39-2. Clinical Evaluation of Prolonged Infant Apnea

Complete blood count
Serum electrolytes, glucose, calcium, magnesium, urea nitrogen
Urinalysis
Chest radiograph
Electrocardiogram
Barium swallow, scintiscan, esophageal pH monitoring
EEG, awake and asleep
Monitoring of simultaneous electrocardiogram, EEG, electromyogram, and thermistor
Computed tomographic scan of the head

Table 39-3. Causes of Vertigo in Children

Middle ear disease
  Acute serous otitis media
  Acute bacterial otitis media
  Chronic otitis media
    Cholesteatoma
    Abscess
Inner ear disease
  Meniere's disease
  Otosclerosis
Vestibular nerve disease
  Vestibular neuronitis
  Acoustic neuroma
  Mononeuropathy
    Vasculitis
    Meningitis
Brain stem
  Cervical neck disease
  Malformation of the cranium and brain stem
  Tumors of the posterior fossa
  Vascular insufficiency
    Cerebrovascular accident
    Migraine
      Paroxysmal vertigo of childhood
      Basilar migraine
Cerebral cortex
  Seizures
Other
  Intoxications
  Hypoglycemia
  Head trauma

VERTIGO

Vertigo is the illusion of movement. The symptoms include a sensation of spinning and tumbling, light-headedness, or environmental motion. The mechanism of balance is very complex and involves integration of sensory input from the vestibular nerves, cerebellum, vision, and muscle proprioception by the vestibular system. This information is consciously sensed by the cortex of the temporal lobe. The major cause of vertigo is an imbalance of input to the vestibular system or, more rarely, hallucinatory activity of the temporal lobes caused by spontaneous electrical discharges, as seen in the aura of many complex partial seizures. Of the nonconvulsive causes for vertigo, there are usually eye signs, with the slow component nystagmus or deviation of the eyes toward the side of greater input to the vestibular system. By convention, the direction of nystagmus is the direction of the rapid phase.

Although vertigo is not a particularly common complaint in children, the causes are many (Table 39-3). Middle ear disease, either purulent or serous, is common in childhood but rarely causes a complaint of vertigo. Chronic middle ear disease with cholesteatoma formation or abscess is frequently associated with vertigo. Inner ear disease, particularly Meniere's disease, is rare before puberty and is associated with fluctuating hearing loss, a sense of fullness in the ear, and often a positive family history. Benign positional vertigo occurs in adults and the vertigo is associated with changing head position. Vestibular neuronitis may be a postinfectious disease. It can cause severe unsteadiness and vertigo but generally resolves over 6 to 8 weeks. There is no associated hearing loss.

Disease of the eighth cranial nerve includes compression from bony entrapment or tumor and as a consequence of bacterial or other meningitis. Eighth cranial nerve tumors and meningiomas are associated with neurofibromatosis but rarely occur before adolescence. In diseases which affect the eighth cranial nerve, hearing is often impaired and brain stem evoked responses usually demonstrate delayed conduction of the eighth cranial nerve.

Central causes of vertigo include many intoxications and occasionally metabolic disturbances. Cervical neck disease and malformation of the cranium and brain stem may cause mechanical distortion of the vestibular system or vascular supply and a sensation of unsteadiness. Vascular disease in childhood is uncommon and has an etiology different from that of adults (see Ch. 34). Strokes occurring in the brain stem are frequently associated with vertigo. Benign paroxysmal vertigo and other migraine syndromes can cause episodic vertigo in children (see Ch. 38). Diseases of the brain stem causing vertigo include tumors, particularly pontine gliomas, and multiple sclerosis. Vertigo may be associated with seizures, particularly with the aura of a partial complex seizure arising from the temporal lobe. Certain medications and drugs, including alcohol, affect the brain diffusely and frequently vertigo is a major symptom.

If the vertigo is brief in duration or infrequently paroxysmal and a careful history and physical exam reveal no other signs or symptoms, then further evaluation can be deferred and the patient observed. If a hearing deficit or other neurologic signs are detected on examination, then a structural lesion should be excluded by performing a CT scan. The brain stem auditory evoked response and audiogram can localize eighth cranial nerve disease. An EEG is indicated for those patients with suspected seizures.

SYNCOPE

Syncope, or fainting, is a frustrating entity in which the etiology is usually not determined. It is rare in younger children but becomes more common in adolescence. Syncope is brief loss of consciousness in which the patient often has symptoms of light-headedness or dizziness and a blurring or dimming of vision prior to loss of consciousness. The patient can usually describe the preceding symptoms.

The most common causes and the differential diagnosis are listed in Table 39-4. In the simple faint, decreased perfusion of the brain stem is the most common cause and usually results from hypotension. A vagal response to pain, seeing blood, or other unpleasant experience is a common syndrome and is similar to the pallid breath-holding spells of infants. Orthostatic hypotension, vestibular basilar insufficiency, and the subclavian steel syndrome are similar

Table 39-4. Differential Diagnosis of Syncope in Childhood

Hypotension
    Hyperresponsive vagal reflex
    Vertebrobasilar insufficiency
    Cardiac dysrhythmia
    Hypovolemia
    Subclavian steal syndrome
Atonic seizures
Hypoglycemia
Hysteria

causes. Cardiac dysrhythmias are rare causes for simple syncope; however, exertional syncope suggest an underlying cardiac disorder, particularly aortic stenosis. Atonic seizures usually coexist with other seizure types but can manifest themselves by a sudden loss of posture or tone. Hypoglycemia is rare and, when present, is associated with other symptoms, which include sweating, tachycardia, and anxiety. Fainting is often a hysterical symptom.

The evaluation is usually limited to a careful history and physical examination, including measurement of the supine and upright blood pressure and trying to reproduce the symptoms if the patient is able. Electrocardiographic monitoring and EEG may be necessary in some cases. The treatment is directed toward the underlying cause if determined.

SLEEP DISTURBANCES

Sleep disorders can be divided into those which occur only during sleep and those which cause excessive sleep (Table 39-5). Sleep myoclonus and nightmares are normal phenomena, occurring at all ages. Myoclonus begins shortly after going to sleep and consists of recurrent or isolated jerks of muscles or groups of muscles. Myoclonus on arousal from sleep is often associated with a seizure disorder. Nightmares are frightening dreams and are usually remembered by the child. The subject is often related to an event that occurred prior to going to

Table 39-5. Sleep Disorders

Sleep-related disorders
    Sleep myoclonus
    Nightmares
    Pavor nocturnus (night terrors)
    Somnambulence (sleep walking)
    Seizures
Hypersomnolence syndrome
    Narcolepsy
    Obstructive apnea
    Substance abuse, intoxications
    Depression
    Carbon dioxide retention
    Kleine-Levin syndrome

bed. Excessive nightmares can signify an emotional problem. Night terrors (pavor nocturnus) occur at the end of stage IV sleep; pavor nocturnus is common in adolescence but can occur in younger children. It is characterized by the child appearing alert, confused, disoriented, and terrified. It lasts for variable periods of time and afterward the child returns to sleep without memory for the event the following morning. Sleepwalking has similar features. Night terrors can be treated with low-dose diazepam before bedtime.

Some seizures occur more frequently at night than at any other time. This is particularly true of rolandic seizures, which may have partial features or become generalized. Return of enuresis in a previously continent child and blood stains on the pillow are clues of nocturnal seizures.

Of the hypersomnolent syndromes, sleep apnea is the most common. A history of snoring or other respiratory noises during sleep is evidence of airway obstruction. Hypertrophy of the adenoids or tonsils are the usual causes, although retrognathia and other causes for an obstructed airway can occur. Daytime sleepiness occurs because of the interruption of nocturnal sleep. Obstruction of the airway repeatedly awakens the child, causing sleep deprivation.

Narcolepsy is a rare disorder in childhood. Excessive nocturnal and daytime sleeping are the usual symptoms. Associated symptoms are rare in children but become more frequent as the child matures. Cataplexy is a sudden loss of postural tone with brief unresponsiveness following sudden excitement. Hypnagogic hallucinations and sleep paralysis occur just prior to or more frequently just after arousal from sleep in which there is vivid dreamlike awareness with the inability to move. Narcolepsy can be diagnosed by showing a shortened rapid eye movement latency on EEG. The patient is asked to try and go to sleep and if rapid eye movement sleep develops in less than 5 minutes, then narcolepsy is likely. The patient can be treated with stimulant medications in the daylight hours, such as dextroamphetamine and methylphenidate.

There are many other causes for excessive sleep. Most of these are psychiatric or emotional in origin. Depression, substance abuse, and an altered sleep–wake cycle should be considered in every child. The pickwickian syndrome is caused by CO_2 retention and is usually found in children with morbid obesity.

OTHER PAROXYSMAL DISORDERS

There are a number of familial episodic disorders, including familial intermittent ataxia, familial intermittent chorea, episodic dystonia, and a few inborn errors of metabolism that have intermittent encephalopathy. The etiologies for these disorders are unknown except for the metabolic diseases. Intermittent maple syrup urine disease, pyruvate dysmetabolisms, Refsum's disease, porphyria, hyperammonemias, organic acidemias, and a few others can cause acute encephalopathy often associated with ataxia or seizures. Those disorders are discussed in Section 5.

Disturbances of the hypothalamus can cause a number of vegetative symptoms. Tumors in this area cause abnormal growth and maturation, personality changes, and unusual behaviors. The diencephalic syndrome causes marked failure to thrive with normal caloric intake. The Kleine-Levin syndrome causes episodic hypersomnolence and hyperphasia.

Finally, some children experience episodic senseless combativeness and anger (rage attacks). The etiology is unclear. Some also have epilepsy but many do not. Carbamazepine has been used to treat this and other episodic behavioral disorders.

SELECTED READINGS

Anders T, Weinstein P: Sleep and its disorders in infants and children. Pediatrics 50:312–324, 1972

Eviatar L, Eviatar A: Vertigo in children. Pediatrics 59:833–838, 1977.

Kattwinkle J: Neonatal Apnea: pathogenesis and therapy. J Pediatr 90:342–347, 1977

Rein AJJT, Simcha A, Ludomirsky A et al: Symptomatic sinus bradycardia in infants with structurally normal hearts. J Pediatr 107:724–727, 1985

Rigatto H: Apnea. Pediatr Clin North Am 29:1105–1116, 1982

Yoss RE, Daly DD: Narcolepsy in children. Pediatrics 25:1025–1033, 1960

INDEX

Note: Page numbers followed by f denote figures; those followed by t denote tables.

Creeping, development of, 13f
Crying, asymmetric, 34
Cutaneous abnormalities, 28t
Cutaneous sensory innervation, 41f
Cytomegalovirus, 99, 99f–100f

Dandy-Walker malformation, 138, 138f
Death, brain, 308, 308t
Debrancher deficiency, 211
Deep tendon reflexes, 43t
Deliquency, 183
Dementia, 229
Denver Developmental Screening Test, 16f–17f
Depression, childhood, 180–182, 181t
Dermal sinus, 132f, 134–135
Dermatomyositis, 296–299, 297f–298f
Development
  assessment of, 16–18, 16f–17f
  environmental influences on, 10–11
  nervous system, 9–10, 10f–11f
  normal, 12, 13f–14f, 15t
  of recruitment and plasticity, 11–12
Developmental disorders, pervasive, 182–183, 183t
Developmental screening tests, 83–84, 84t
Devic's disease, 228–229
Digital subtraction angiography, 62
Drug-induced neurologic disorders, in newborn, 102t
Duchenne muscular dystrophy, 287–289, 289f
Dysautonomia, familial, 116–117, 274
Dysmorphic syndromes, in mental retardation, 150, 153t
Dysostosis multiplex, 221f
Dystonia musculorum deformans, 239

Eaton-Lambert syndrome, 281
Electroencephalography, 49–50, 50f–53f. See also individual procedures.
  abnormal, 50, 54f
  electrode placement in, 49, 51f
  general principles of, 49, 50f
  in neonatal seizures, 106–107
  posterior dominant rhythm in, 49, 53f
  sleep, 49, 52f
Electromyography, 57–58, 57f
Electrophysiologic procedures, 49–58. See also individual procedures.
Electroretinography, 56
Elimination, disorders of, 186
Embryology, 129–133

Emery-Dreifuss dystrophy, 290, 290f
Encephalitis
  herpes simplex, 347
  herpes simplex type II, 99–100
  mumps, 347
Encephalitis periaxialis concentrica, 229
Encephalocele, 132f, 134
Encephalomyelitis
  disseminated, 351–352
  subacute necrotizing, 236
Encephalomyelopathy, postinfectious, 351–352
Encephalomyopathy, mitochondrial, 231, 231t, 232f
Encephalopathy
  with acquired metabolic disturbances, 101–102, 101t
  bilirubin, 102
  hypoxic-ischemic, 91–92, 93t
  metabolic, 195–209, 306t. See also individual types.
  myoclonic, 354
  neonatal, 91–103, 92t
Enuresis, nocturnal, 186
Environment, development and, 10–11
Ependymoma, 375f
Epidural cranial abscess, 336, 337f
Epidural spinal abscess, 336–338, 337t–338t
Epilepsy, 391–395, 394t. See also Status epilepticus.
  clinical features and classification of, 394t
  relative frequency of, 395t
Epileptic encephalopathy, 232
Epiloia, 244–245, 246f–247f
Episodic illnesses, 3–4
Erb's palsy, 128
Evoked response, 50–54
  brain stem auditory, 51–53, 55f
  somatosensory, 53–54
Excitation contraction coupling, 277
Extremities
  abnormalities of, 28t
  lower, muscle innervation of, 40t
  upper, 39t
Eye
  abnormalities of, 25t
  involuntary movements of, 36t

Facial nerve injury, in forceps delivery, 127–128
Facioscapulohumoral dystrophy, 292f, 293